CONSUMING PASSIONS

16 20
32
74

CONSUMING PASSIONS

FEMINIST APPROACHES TO WEIGHT PREOCCUPATION AND EATING DISORDERS

Edited By

CATRINA BROWN

A N D

KARIN JASPER

SECOND STORY Press

CANADIAN CATALOGUING IN PUBLICATION DATA

Main Entry under title:
Consuming passions: feminist approaches to
weight preoccupation and eating disorders

ISBN   0-929005-42-2

1. Eating disorders.   I. Brown, Catrina
II. Jasper, Karin

RC552.E18C66 1993   616.85'26   C93-093732-5

Edited by Beverley Beetham Endersby

Printed and bound in Canada

*Second Story Press gratefully acknowledges the assistance of the
Ontario Arts Council and the Canada Council*

Published by
SECOND STORY PRESS
760 Bathurst Street
Toronto, Ontario
M5S 2R6

CONTENTS

III COMMUNITY EDUCATION AND POLITICAL ACTION

ACKNOWLEDGEMENTS

Many people have shared in the production of this book. We thank, first of all, the contributing authors for making their knowledge and experience available here and for putting aside the many demands on their time to work on these essays. The partnership of the women at Second Story Feminist Press not only made this project possible, but made working on it a pleasure. In particular Lois Pike's considerable organizational talents and sense of humor helped keep the project on track, in more ways than one. To Beverley Endersby, the editor, we extend our appreciation especially for her thoroughness with the first draft and for her willingness to adjust to our timelines. We also want to acknowledge the partnership we have built with one another through the mutual support and mutual challenge this project has required. Finally, we are deeply appreciative of our clients for what they have taught us and what they have given to us.

Special thanks from Karin: I thank Allison for putting up with my "bear-in-the-cave" routine during this project and for expressing the fact that she didn't like it. For handling more than half of our shared responsibilities while I worked on this book as well as for his conversation and editorial comments, I thank Sandy. Most of all I appreciate the quality of attention he brings to what he does. I also thank my colleagues at the College Street Women's Centre for the encouragement and enthusiasm they expressed for this book, as well as their cheerful acceptance of a lesser contribution from me while I have been working on it.

Special thanks from Catrina: I am indebted to Don Forgay for his invaluable and ongoing care, support, encouragement, and intellectual challenge which have nourished me through this book and over the past ten years. I have relied upon and benefitted from his generosity and ideas, and my work has been enriched and deepened.

We are grateful to Don for suggesting the name we chose for the book.

PREFACE

Over the past ten years significant challenges have been made to the coercive and tyrannical ideal of thinness and the pressure it puts on women to diet. While most women continue to police and control their bodies in an effort to attain this ideal, increasing numbers have discovered that dieting does not work and have begun to realize that it is possible to live free from weight preoccupation and chronic dieting. These women are learning to accept their bodies as they are, in their various shapes and sizes. Instead of enduring constant hunger, self-denial, deprivation, and preoccupation with food and eating, these women have empowered themselves to eat without guilt, to enjoy their bodies, and to live in peace with themselves. We hope the writings of women in Canada who have contributed to these changes can help others to establish a sense of freedom from weight preoccupation and eating disorders.

This book encourages women to liberate the pleasures of their bodies, to accept their desires and appetites, and to enjoy the power of a full, embodied existence. It affirms the belief that women are participants in their own "making." Thus, while we recognize that eating "disorders" and weight preoccupation have a social context, we do not subscribe to the view that women are simple puppets of a patriarchal society. We especially want to avoid the commonly accepted conclusion that society's obsession with weight is predominantly a product of pernicious media influence. Such a perspective degrades women by falsely assuming their passivity and inevitable victimization.

In order to understand complex behaviours, attitudes, and experiences, we must get beyond simplistic explanations for them. If we want to foster the "empowerment" of women, we cannot focus on the narrow issue of women's conformity to the "tyranny of slenderness." Despite the asymmetrical power relations and inequalities of social conditions between men and women that characterize most aspects of life in modern society, we can act individually and collectively to empower ourselves and create social change.

We believe this collection of essays benefits not only individual women who are trying to understand their own weight preoccupation, but therapists and other helpers who want to provide caring, knowledgeable, and effective support to women who seek their help. While critiques of the social pressure to be thin have become quite common among feminists and within the women's health movement, very little has been written to guide us in practice. This book aims to go beyond the debunking of the "beauty myth" by opening a discussion among therapists, community workers, and activists of some of the ways to adopt in practice a fat-positive, nondiscriminatory, and pro-woman approach, and by encouraging individual women who want to be free of the endless cycles of dieting and weight preoccupation to use this book to help themselves.

We have tried to be as comprehensive as possible within the scope of a single volume, choosing to emphasize issues not previously widely discussed from a woman-centred perspective. This book explores childhood trauma, alcoholism, sexual abuse, and sexual violence in relationship to the development of eating disorders and weight preoccupation. It also challenges the effectiveness of dieting, some commonly held notions about healthy eating and exercise, and the oppression of fat people in our society. It examines feminist ways of working as clinicians and activists, challenging the traditional medical model in which the individual is separated from her social and cultural influences. In broad terms, the essays collected here place weight preoccupation, eating "disorders," and our experiences of our bodies within the context of Western patriarchal society. By intentionally avoiding the construction of a monolithic set of arguments or ideas for practice in this book, we encourage the reader to enter into dialogue with the diverse points of view represented by the contributing authors.

The women's movement today is very concerned with diversity and complexity in understanding women's experiences in society. While white middle-class feminists have had a long history of universalizing their experiences as all women's, today a concerted effort is being made in feminist theory and practice to recognize difference as well as similarity in women's experiences. This means that the women's movement has become increasingly committed to examining a wide range of views and experiences in exploring issues in women's lives. Thus, whereas women of colour, Jewish women, Native women, women with disabilities, lesbian women, and economically disadvantaged women have frequently been excluded when feminism has talked about women's experiences, in this book we have tried to include as many voices as possible in an effort to bring forward a perspective that encompasses the complexity of women's experiences.

As feminists we want to avoid medicalizing or disease-oriented language. Some readers will be uncomfortable with our use of the terms "eating disorders," "anorexia," and "bulimia." Because these terms originated in psychiatric literature, they are associated with a medical or disease model, the very model we criticize here. We have chosen to use these terms because they are easily understood, having become part of everyday language. We do not accept, however, the medicalization or psychiatrization of eating disorders. Women who develop anorexia or bulimia should not be singled out as pathological. Their behaviour and thinking need to be understood within the context of a culture which produces weight preoccupation among women.

This book presents alternatives to traditional frameworks that dichotomize what is "normal" or "abnormal," or that adhere to rigid formulas for what a person should weigh or eat. We wish to cultivate a climate which accepts diversity in body size, shape, and eating behaviour, and a social context that encourages women to meet their physical requirement for food and their needs for emotional nurturance.

Words like *obese* and *overweight* perpetuate the "normal"/"abnormal" dichotomy in that they have a pejorative connotation and imply a deviation from some objective standard, something "wrong" and in need of correction. Authors who have used these words have put them in quotation marks. However, in general we recommend reclaiming the word *fat*. While it has connotations of disparagement for many people, it has the advantage of simply describing, as does "thin," a body type. Often we speak here in broader terms, such as "weight preoccupation" or "weight and shape issues," which include anorexia and bulimia.

Mainstream approaches to women's preoccupation with weight often view women as mentally ill. Women's experiences are pathologized and their behaviours and feelings are removed from the context of their actual lives. Removing behaviour from its context makes it seem "irrational" or "crazy." This book argues that women are not crazy or mentally ill when they are weight preoccupied or develop eating "disorders." Rather, in controlling food and weight, women exercise some degree of control over their lives. Within the context of a weight-preoccupied and fat-prejudiced society, women "speak" with their bodies. This book argues that eating disorders are not separate from most women's experiences of their bodies and eating, but instead are understood to exist on a continuum of weight preoccupation. The essays collected here will allow the reader to see some of the ways in which behaviours and emotions associated with weight preoccupation and eating disorders have meaning: how they make sense and how understanding that they do can be helpful in the resolution of weight, shape, and eating issues.

— *Catrina Brown and Karin Jasper*
Toronto, 1993

·I·
CONTEXT

INTRODUCTION

WHY WEIGHT? WHY WOMEN? WHY NOW?

Catrina Brown and Karin Jasper

The idea that thinness is attractive, desirable, and healthy is so pervasive in Western societies that it often goes unchallenged, despite the fact that it has not always been, nor is it everywhere the case. Widespread preoccupation with weight, dieting, and exercise has escalated to such a degree that it is an accepted, encouraged, and rewarded aspect of social life, and in North America has launched a multibillion-dollar industry. Alongside the social obsession with thinness and dieting is an alarming incidence of anorexia and bulimia among women. Women are seduced by the promises of happiness, success, and love that thinness is presumed to fulfil and risk their health in desperate attempts to achieve its rewards.

Why has weight preoccupation among women proliferated over the past twenty years? Why has the thin body come to be so valued, particularly in Western societies? What aspects of women's lives today does thinness symbolize? Why weight? Why women? Why now? The thin beauty ideal is not simply an aesthetic style, it is a metaphor for the effects of social and economic changes on women's lives. We argue that the idealized thin body, which is increasingly lean, muscular, and "surgically enhanced," reflects the fragmented and contradictory expectations women experience in Western societies at a time when they have achieved greater equality, yet continue to be oppressed in fundamental ways. Thus, much can be understood about the world women live in through examining the pervasiveness of weight preoccupation.

By exerting control over their bodies, women hope to gain self-esteem and an increased sense of power and control over their lives. Powerlessness and dissatisfaction can be replaced by the self-satisfaction, social approval, and sense of accomplishment won through weight and shape control. Women's bodies become the arena for their expressions of discontent and protest. Focusing on "improving" their bodies in order to feel better *about themselves* distracts them from the actual sources of their discontent. As the expressions of protest become obscured, a socially and politically generated problem becomes personalized. When women say they feel better when they are thinner, they really mean it. They actually feel better about themselves. Complex dissatisfactions are transformed by being shifted onto the body. Unhappiness fades and an uneasy well-being emerges as the body changes shape.

Generally through this essay we refer simply to "women" in Western societies, without specifying race/ethnicity, class, sexual orientation, or age. Although some epidemiological research has been published, especially in the last six years, the studies are yet too few and too small to allow firm conclusions to be drawn. It was originally thought that eating disorders affected primarily young, upper-class women; however, it now seems that more women of lower economic classes and more women who are older have difficulties related to food, weight, and shape (Rand and Kuldau 1992). Lesbian women seem to have higher ideal weights than heterosexual women or gay men, but are more dissatisfied with their bodies, more concerned with weight, and more often dieting than are gay and heterosexual men (Brand, Rothblum, and Solomon 1992). One study of Native American women reports that weight control is very important, and purging behaviours are common, especially among those who are heavier than average and including those who are older (Rosen et al. 1988). We found no studies reporting on the incidence of eating disorders among disabled women; however, it is possible that their lack of social power might lead them to seek greater control over their lives through their bodies. Western women still seem to be at greater risk for eating disorders than Black, Asian, Arab, Greek, Japanese, or African women, but the degree of westernization women of all backgrounds are exposed to seems to increase their risk (Dolan 1991). Dolan states that current reports must be read with caution — biased results may be occurring because research projects and clinical sampling operate within the dominant culture's framework. Researchers and clinicians may not be aware of the extent of eating problems among non-whites because they do not ask the right questions or recognize the symptoms of those who are outside their framework. Nevertheless, all studies we know of confirm that women are at greater risk than men. Therefore, we refer to women in Western society in general, knowing that many non-white women are affected and that the numbers may be greater, but are not likely smaller than studies already show.

WOMEN AND THEIR BODIES

Historically, women's social value has been inseparable from their bodies. Their social role has been identifed with and expressed through their bodies: in bearing children, in satisfying men's sexual needs, and in the labour of caring for men's and children's emotional and physical needs. Interestingly, "ideal" body images for women tend to shift in tandem with changes in women's social roles. The most notable among such transformations has been that from the ideal of being rounded and fertile-looking that predominates when women's role as childbearer has been most important (Beller 1977; Bruch 1973), to the thin and muscular look of today. A declining emphasis on women's fertility followed industrialization in Western societies, and as women experienced advances in economic, political, and social life, thinness came to symbolize wealth, independence, and freedom. Instead of the fertile rounded look being glorified, a thinner body ideal that emphasized non-reproductive sexuality became valued.

Where body size and shape are crucial to their social value, women learn to focus on appearance. As a result, policing and controlling appearance becomes an imperative for achieving both inner satisfaction and social success. Women internalize the fashionable body image, recognizing that how they appear affects how they are valued and treated. How women feel when they compare themselves with other women, including women depicted in the media, in advertising, and in the fashion industry, shapes their experience of their own bodies and selves. Self-esteem becomes deeply connected to body size and shape. In continuously scrutinizing and altering themselves, women anticipate being scrutinized and evaluated, and attempt to have some control over the results (Berger 1972).

Because the way women's bodies look bears greatly on how other people relate to them and is directly connected with women's economic value in society, women learn that looking good is a form of currency in the world. Even now that more (predominantly white, middle-class) women are gaining social power, appearance figures in women's social value far more than it ever has for men. While women are now encouraged to be successful in the public world, they are still "given approval for continuing and even increasing their investments in their bodies" (Polhemus 1978, p. 120). It is no wonder, then, that women learn to believe they can change their lives by changing their bodies.

The female body has the power to create and nurture life. Yet, too often, women learn that their own appetites are to be controlled or denied rather than being indulged and enjoyed as sources of pleasure. Eating has become a major area of conflict for women as they are expected to provide physical sustenance and nurturance to others but must deny themselves food, or police their own eating in order to maintain the right body shape. Passionate, unrestrained eating is itself seen as unfeminine or unattractive, while dieting and asceticism are acceptable and encouraged. Mira Dana and Marilyn Lawrence (1988, p. 35) suggest that, "given the conflict and contradictory meaning which women's bodies hold for us, it is hardly surprising that the body is often the arena within which women unconsciously choose to express conflict which they feel in their lives."

The body is an instrument of communication which mediates social life. Examination of variations in body ideals through history shows that they are closely related to cultural values and social relations and highlights the shifting meaning associated with body ideals in relation to women's social position. In both modern and traditional patriarchal society women's reproductive and sexual roles have had direct expression in body ideals (Brown and Forgay 1987). Today's body ideal emerged through the effects of industrialization, women's entry into the labour force and the public sphere, and feminism and increased social equality for women. As is shown below, the contemporary thin ideal expresses the current circumstances in which women's oppression co-exists with women's emancipation.

THE BODY SPEAKS: EMERGING BODY FASHIONS AND THE SOCIAL POSITION OF WOMEN

One of the earliest known representations of human form is the "Venus of Willendorf," a statuette dating from about 25,000 B.C. It depicts a female body of magnificently large proportions, that, in today's medical terms, would be considered "morbidly obese." During the Stone Age, the making and using of the statuette likely would have been part of ritual and ceremony designed to bring scarce resources forth from nature (Paglia 1991). People had little control over food supply or fertility, and this statuette represented the desire for sufficient food and fertility to sustain human life. At times when food is scarce and mortality rates are high, a rounder, fatter, body type tends to be valued.

In Europe, towards the end of the Middle Ages and the beginning of the Renaissance, a rounded, fertile look for women continued to be emphasized. However, artwork from this period suggests that several beauty ideals existed (Seid 1989), including a slim female body with rather short legs and a full, rounded, pregnant-looking belly. Both the bride in Jan van Eyck's 1434 painting *Giovanni Arnolfini and His Bride* and Eve in Jan and Hubert van Eyck's 1432 painting *The Ghent Altarpiece* illustrate this ideal. The emphasis on the belly in these works reflects the conditions of a Europe plagued by disease and pestilence; it is probable that a fertile or pregnant look was reassuring against the ubiquitous fear of death.

In the sixteenth and seventeenth centuries the art of Raphael, da Vinci, Titian, and Rubens depicted even ampler bodies, while Bronzino and Cellini painted nudes representing a more slender, though not at all thin, ideal. Consistently, until the eighteenth century, we see evidence of more than one beauty ideal; we see men's bodies, as well as women's, idealized in nudes; and we know that, outside court society, few people would have had access to artworks or the economic means to dress fashionably, and that, therefore, the vast majority of people would not have expected to.

From the eighteenth century onwards, a number of significant changes occurred (Seid 1989). The food supply, which had previously been unreliable, began to stabilize, giving rise to restraint as an expression of refinement. In emerging industrial society, where the transfer of property through inheritance was relatively less important, arranged marriages declined. Women began having to "attract" male partners; thus, appearance played a greater role than it had previously for women seeking mates. Corresponding with this need to attract a partner, a new seductiveness combined with innocence became evident in women's fashions. Men's fashions, by contrast, changed less radically, and whereas female nudes became explicitly erotic, male nudes gradually ceased to be a genre in art.

In the Victorian era in North America, restrictive women's fashions were emblematic of a conservative social code that enforced the strict separation of spheres for men and women. Because the arrival of German and Irish immigrants to America had ended an era of scarce labour, the social position of middle-class women changed from one of greater equality of work opportunities to one in which staying at home was encouraged. During this time, the "cult of the lady" emerged.

The beauty ideal for women, as epitomized in the American "Steel Engraving Lady" of the 1830s (images for magazines were produced from engravings in steel), was an expression of this society's values and perhaps a reaction against the undesirable consequences of industrialization. This look emphasized qualities of delicacy, gentility, slenderness, and etherealness, though by current standards, only the waist was thin (Banner 1983; Seid 1989). A hearty appetite was considered unladylike, and doctors reinforced this view by arguing that women's digestive systems were too delicate for "heavy meats" (Seid 1989). The thin, delicate appearance for women was a mark of gentility and implied that a husband or father had wealth (Seid 1989). The ideal also emphasized youth and purity, reflecting nineteenth-century romanticization of childhood and the simultaneous infantilization of women. The youthful aspect of the ideal offered a new optimism and rejuvenation for this period consistent with the promise of upward mobility carried by growing industrialization (Banner 1983).

Still, very few women would have expected their own bodies to match perfectly the ideal represented by "ladies" in the steel engravings. Because clothing was not mass produced, women would either have made their own clothing or had it made, accommodating their own unique proportions. Styles varied by age — mature women were expected to be large and, although a very fat person was considered unhealthy, a somewhat fat person was not (Seid 1989). In addition, a competing "antifashion ideal" that was "rosier, healthier, plumper and stronger" (Seid 1989, p. 67) was promoted by early feminists and others concerned with the ill effects of the steel-engraving look. By the 1850s, the pale, frail look was unpopular.

After the American Civil War, a more "voluptuous" beauty ideal represented the postwar increase in the importance of fertility (Banner 1983). Lillian Russell, a popular American beauty of the time, was by today's standards a very large woman. Towards the turn of the century, as fashions once again changed, she, became one of the first public figures we know of who dieted. At two hundred pounds, she felt pressure to lose weight reflecting a new emphasis for women on having the right body shape and size and, more generally, a rising concern for eating the proper amount of "healthy" food (Seid 1989). The promise of industrialization to increase control over nature likely contributed to the development of this new emphasis.

Towards the end of the Victorian era, Lillian Russell was replaced by the tall and athletic "Gibson Girl." Middle-class women of the late nineteenth century were expected to adopt the fashion of the day while simultaneously expressing a "unique personality" necessary for romantic love — fashionable beauty became a greater avenue for upward mobility through marriage. According to Wilson (1985, p. 123), appearance became increasingly intertwined with identity in this period. It was, she states, "the beginning of Self as a Work of Art, the 'personality' as something that extended to dress, scent, and surroundings, all of which made an essential contribution to the formation of 'self' — at least for women" (1985, p. 123).

The early twentieth century saw the introduction in North America of several new body ideals. At the turn of the century, a very narrow-waisted hourglass figure was popular and required the use of tightly laced corsets (only women of the urban upper and middle class would have worn these). Women could eat very little and had difficulty breathing with ease while wearing them. Fainting, headaches, and uterine problems were common complaints (Banner 1983).

By 1910, Mary Pickford and Clara Bow embodied the new, small, boyish ideal. The flapper era, with its flat-chested, straight-bodied, and shorter-hemline look, celebrated women's emerging social mobility and independence (Lurie 1981). Certainly, the feminist "dress reformers" played a role in influencing the popularity of this fashion, their intention being to free women from the restrictiveness of the previous long, heavy, and crinolined fashions. Increased physical mobility mirrored advances in the social mobility and independence of women. The suppression of curves suggested a freer sexuality for women with less emphasis on reproduction, but implied that women's sexuality was still limited and controlled (Seid 1989).

Women's reproductive role was affected by the changing social and material conditions of industrialization. The shift from an agrarian to an industrial society created a new occupational environment away from the home. Improved standards of living also resulted in a decrease in infant and child mortality. It was no longer necessary for urban middle-class women to be pregnant throughout their lives. These factors contributed to freeing women from the confines of the reproductive role and represented a further stage in the emancipation of women. The look associated with thinness was symbolic of this change (Brown 1987a). As sex became eroticized in popular culture, its associations shifted to pleasure and away from reproduction (Epstein 1983, p. 88). With that shift, roundness, which had always been an image of fertility and reproduction, gave way to thinness, which came to be associated with the pleasure of sexuality.

While rural societies traditionally viewed plumpness as a sign of prosperity and thinness as a reminder of famine, urban society during the early 1900s saw thinness for women as a symbol of freedom from hard physical labour and, therefore, as a sign of success for their husbands and fathers. During this period of increased automation and gains in social wealth, the pursuit of fashion again suggested leisure, pleasure, and self-indulgence, all status symbols of the wives (and property) of rich men (Banner 1983). For complex reasons then, including the increased liberation of women during the first wave of the women's movement, our society adopted a clear preference for thinness in women (Bennett and Gurin 1982).

In the first thirty years of the twentieth century, a growing medical bias against fat developed, body size became connected with health, the science of nutrition began to use of the concept of the calorie, and growing prosperity made fashion and health messages available to larger numbers of people (Seid 1989). At the same time, inexpensive mass-produced clothes in standard sizes came on the market, democratizing fashion by making fashionable clothing accessible to most women for the first time. However, increasing standardization also meant that, in practical terms, women encountered the idea that their bodies were wrong when the standard size didn't fit them (Seid 1989). Thus, a serious, multi-determined social investment in slimness took hold, evidenced in 1917 by the first best-selling book on weight control, Dr. Lulu Hunt Peters's *Diet and Health, with Key to Calories* (Seid 1989).

In the 1930s, the social climate changed in response to threatened food shortages as a result of two world wars and the Depression. Attitudes towards the body at this time were ambivalent, as seen in the March 1933 issue of Butterick's *Delineator* magazine, which carried an ad for a weight-loss product, and one for a yeast-fortified beer with the caption: "Dangerous to be skinny. New discovery adds solid, healthy flesh quicker than beer."

After the Second World War, women were required to leave their jobs and return to the home in order to reopen jobs for men returning from war. Emphasis on reproduction generally follows war, but the baby boom generation born out of the postwar era also signified the success of a postwar public campaign aimed at women to reclaim the role of "homemakers," short-circuiting any inclination they may have felt to remain in the public sphere as equals to men. Having fewer children on average than previous generations helped the new suburban families of this period to maintain a higher standard of living. The slim yet curvaceous body ideal of the time allowed for emphasis on women's return to their roles in reproduction, as mothers and housewives, but also on the increased freedom and mobility provided by suburban living, higher levels of education for women, and the economic success of their husbands. It was perhaps the first time in history that women in large numbers had a personal experience of what emancipation could bring, through having worked in the public sphere in responsible positions during the war and through access to higher education. Just as they could taste emancipation, women were once again restricted by the limitations of the private sphere.

Body weight was well on its way to being seen as an indication of character as well as of health. Fatness was connected with poor moral character because it was mistakenly identified with gluttony. The distinctions between "overweight," "obese," "plump," "chubby," and so on slowly died, eventually leaving only two categories — fat and thin (Seid 1989). Just the same, the era differed from our own in that it still differentiated styles suitable for adolescents from those suitable for adult women, and though the emphasis was on thinness, what counted as thin was far closer to "average" than our current standard.

In the late 1960s, the radical politics of the civil rights movement, the revived women's movement, and the hippie subculture influenced a rebellious, natural or unadorned look, which emphasized youth. For the first time, standards of beauty were challenged by a variety of racial and ethnic looks that were seen as attractive (Banner 1983). But while "Black is beautiful" made an appearance, the fashion icon of the time was a white English schoolgirl called Twiggy, who, at 5' 7 1/2", weighed 91 pounds. Her emaciated shape perfectly expressed the values placed upon youth and thinness and gave new meaning to the fashionable image of etherealness. The recommended route to perfecting the female body seemed to be getting rid of it altogether. The emphasis on sexual freedom and youth culture of the hippie era was offset by this prepubescent body shape. It managed simultaneously to de-emphasize differences between men and women and to communicate a very sexualized yet innocent image. For young women who had grown up with frustrated mothers struggling to reconcile their heightened awareness with their lack of real power, the childlike body was also insurance against being defined through reproductive capacity, against being burdened by the real responsibilities of having children. Its immateriality promised the freedom to ascend to heights never before reached by women.

In the 1960s, television eclipsed film as a primary influence on what was considered beauty in North America (Banner 1983). Mass communication through television, the growing sophistication of advertising, and vivid images in full-colour magazines ensured the promotion and consumption of new ideals throughout Canada, the United States, and Europe. The result was a greater emphasis than ever before on outer image, both instead of and as a measure of inner worth. In addition to the changing role of women, television, advertising, fashion magazines, celebrity fashion models, and the mass marketing of clothing comprised a very powerful coalition of influences shaping our ideals of beauty.

The widespread communication of a very thin beauty ideal corresponded with an increased incidence of anorexia and the advent of bulimia in the 1970s. Not a new phenomenon, anorexia had first been diagnosed as a medical illness in 1874 by Lasegue in France and in Britain by Gull in 1873. The first Canadian case reported was by P. R. Inches in the *Maritime Medical News* in 1895. Anorexia had remained a rather obscure "illness" until the 1970s when it, and bulimia, became practically epidemic among women and an explanation that went beyond the language of "medical illness" was required. Eating disorders seemed to reflect the shifts and uncertainties in women's lives as they entered the labour force in soaring numbers and the second wave of the women's movement took hold.

In the 1980s, ever new rigours were recommended for those wanting to avoid the scourge of fat. Increased exercise was required to meet the new more muscular, but still thin, ideal, and "healthy eating" became synonymous with various forms of food fetishism designed to ward off fat as well as a number of vaguely defined illnesses (Seid 1989). Cosmetic surgery became touted as a way of perfecting the body. With the fashionable reappearance of large breasts came a corresponding rush for breast-augmentation surgery, but the newest surgery to emerge was liposuction. An article in the *Toronto Star* in the late 1980s described liposuction as useful for correcting the "violin deformity," an indentation between hips and thighs on most women's bodies. It is one thing to distinguish between actual and ideal body shapes. It is another to describ a typical female body shape as a deformity. Increasingly, "eating right," losing weight, and perfecting the body with all means available came to be seen as the road to perfecting the self and achieving happiness. Women's fashion magazines now exhorted women to "take charge" through controlling body shape, and to "control yourself" through eating calorie-reduced foods. By the end of the 1980s, most North American women regularly dieted to lose weight and said that they disliked their bodies.

Today's continuation of the thin body ideal for women is more substantial than its Twiggy predecessor and includes a limited range of shapes that can all be characterized as thin and muscular and are glamourized as "being fit." It ranges from the delicate but toned look commonly seen in fashion magazines, to the more obviously muscular look of Jane Fonda. Unlike the ideals of most other periods, today's ideal female body is very low in body fat and muscular, and tends to have tight abdominal muscles, thighs toned by many hours in the gym exhibited in Spandex outfits cut high on the hip, discernible biceps, and large yet perky breasts. This image expresses both the strength and the sexiness consistent with the "superwoman" ideal of today. This perfect all-round woman is expected to perform the contradictory roles of the nurturing and caring mother; the soft, sexy, and giving wife; and the sexually independent, competitive, and ambitious, career woman. The current body ideal embodies all of these qualities, conveying through the body the contradictions women face in their lives today.

While feminist analyses of the current body ideal have tended to focus on the shift in women's social power, emphasizing either women's continued oppression in a male-dominant world or women's increased social equality, most fail to consider the contradictory nature both of women's lives and of the body ideal. Susan Wooley (1987) argues that women are expected to make their bodies more masculine in an effort to fit into the masculinist labour force. Kim Chernin (1981) views the thin body ideal as an expression of society's resistance to women's increased social power. She argues that, at a time when women have achieved greater equality, the thin body ideal portrays women as small, vulnerable, weak, and powerless. She points out a correspondence in the development of the "women's reduction movement" of the 1960s with its emphasis on losing weight, and the feminist movement as it re-emerged in the 1960s. Chernin notes that, while the women's reduction movement promised increased happiness and self-esteem through weight loss, the feminist movement increased its efforts to improve the possibilities for women's happiness through social change. However, Chernin does not address the feminist movement's own ambivalence about the new body ideal, despite its potential to be damaging to women. The thin ideal was too perfect a symbol of women's freedom from "anatomy is destiny," or the limitations of women's reproductive role in society.

Other feminist writers suggest that the emergence of the thin body ideal parallels women's increased social power. Janice Cauwells, for instance, believes that the thin body represents women's increased equality, and communicates the superwoman image of the competent, sexy, and successful woman (1983). Similarly, Ann Hollander maintains that the thin body ideal that emerged in the 1920s, and continues today, symbolized increased equality in the image of women as mobile, independent, and active (1980).

Susie Orbach (1986), however, has observed that the thin ideal of today represents increasingly contradictory messages about what it means to be a woman; the thin body expresses the ambivalence of society towards increased social power for women. According to Orbach "today's role confusion is negotiated by transforming the body" (1986, p. 24). Similarly, we argue that the current body ideal is a complex metaphor for the contradictory aspects of women's lives today. It portrays both women's continued oppression and their growing emancipation, alongside women's conformity and resistance to these conditions.

From the 1960s to today, thinness appears to be an antipatriarchal rebellion. The thin body image expresses liberation through its connotations of mobility, independence, sexuality, and freedom;

however, it can also be said to express women's continued oppression in that, despite its current muscular manifestation, it also connotes diminutiveness, dependence, and vulnerability, through its delicacy and smallness. A recent resurgence of Twiggy-like images reflects our era's continued ambivalence towards women's power. The liberation of women attempts to define woman as more than her body; however, the same body type that symbolizes patriarchal influence also symbolizes liberation. The thin body image, then, incorporates both the patriarchal conditions of women's lives and women's opposition to patriarchy. Although many feminist analyses suggest that the pressure for women to be thin, and thinness itself, reflect women's oppression in patriarchal society, we suggest that a more layered and complex analysis allows us to understand the contradictory elements related to women's oppression and emancipation.

Recently, Catherine Steiner-Adair (1990), a psychologist who is a research associate with the Project on the Psychology of Women and the Development of Girls, at Harvard University, has described in developmental terms the effect of these contradictions on girls who are becoming young women. She suggests that girls face two developmental double binds, the first of which is related to body development. At puberty, both boys and girls face the challenge of coming to terms with a body that is biologically different from the one they've been living with, but for boys there is consistency between the characteristics they are supposed to demonstrate as they become young men and the changes in their bodies. The development of muscle, the increase in height, the lowering of the voice are associated in our culture with power, effectiveness, and authority. For girls, in contrast, there is an inconsistency between what their bodies are going through and the characteristics they are supposed to demonstrate as the "New Woman," such as assertiveness, independence, and self-control. They are betrayed by an increase in body fat required for menstruation, as fat is a cultural sign of powerlessness, ineffectiveness, and lack of control. This bind has the following result: a female who is effective and in control in her life, but who has a fat body, or has fat on her body, will probably feel this fat belies her effectiveness and control. A female who starts out not feeling or being effective and assertive will probably feel that the fat on her body makes her failure immediately evident to everyone. In both cases, the learned dissatisfaction with their bodies' normal fat levels will probably drive these girls and women to lose weight.

The second double bind is related to self development. Steiner-Adair describes girls as spending a lot of time during the first eleven years of their lives learning the ins and outs of relationships. During this time they use a wide range of emotions in talking about themselves and about relationships, and they are very realistic, saying that it's not always possible to be both nice to someone else and true to oneself at the same time. Their tendency is to try to resolve conflict, which they accept as a part of relationship, through the use of empathy in order to deepen friendship. Beginning around age twelve or thirteen, and certainly by the age of fifteen or sixteen, some major adjustments are required of girls. As they begin to relate more and more to boys, they come up against barriers to practising relationships in the way they are used to. Boys learn to relate differently: their play with one another is more rule-based and more competitive, often culminating in finding out who is the winner and who is the loser. (The adjustments boys have to make to tolerate this kind of relating have their own problems). However, girls learn, according to a superficial and idealized model of caregiving that seems to come into play as heterosexual relationships begin, that it is their role to be the primary caregiver and maintainer of these relationships. Clearly the role of the ideal nurturer as one who experiences no conflict between what is good for herself and what is good for the other is inconsistent with what girls know about relationships from their own experience during the first eleven years of their lives. They have to "forget" what they know in order to approximate this ideal. Typically girls lose confidence at this time in their lives.

In terms of the self-development double bind, girls are encouraged to show both the traditional characteristics of the abundant caregiver and the characteristics of the "New Woman," who looks after herself before anyone else. Girls, then, are getting contradictory messages about their role in relationships and what is expected of them as individuals growing up in a society that values independence, individuality, and competitivenes. These contradictions raise conflicts for girls that make them doubt themselves. Feeling self-doubt in the context of our current body ideal, girls often try to generate self-esteem by losing weight, a strategy that is reinforced by the body-development double bind.

THINNESS AS METAPHOR:
WOMEN'S FRAGMENTED IDENTITY

Weight preoccupation can be understood as the product of the coincidence of the prevailing body ideal and the fragmented identity women experience in their ambiguous and contradictory social role. Uncertain how to proceed with their lives through a maze of conflicting expectations, possibilities, and desires, many women have attempted to gain control of their lives by controlling their bodies. Weight is something that can be controlled, and exercising such control can, at the same time, satisfy a major social expectation: being sexually attractive. Indeed, it requires a strong sense of self and high self-esteem to resist the social pressure to be thin (Lawrence 1984).

Anorexia nervosa can be described as a "psychological bridging mechanism" for women as they enter the public sphere (Orbach 1986, p.103). Entry into a masculinist culture requires that women retain qualities traditionally associated with femininity, but which the society devalues, and also adopt and value what have traditionally been male workforce characteristics. Tremendous conflict also exists between social expectations and women's subjective experience of their capacities. While feminist pressure has resulted in gains in opportunity for many women, there have not been corresponding changes in the culture that would fully support women in taking advantage of those opportunities, including expansion of the role that men take in domestic labour and in caring for relationships and children. Feminists have expressed concern about the "double day" required of women as they continue to perform most of the domestic labour in addition to their work in the labour force. The burden of this double day is compounded by the lack of adequate childcare services provided by society. Such changes, even if they are forthcoming, will be slow. In the meantime, anorexia, bulimia, and weight preoccupation today may be the most common ways women have to cope with the desperation and uncertainty they feel.

In the face of such conflicting, unrealistic, and indeed oppressive social expectations, it is no wonder that women experience tremendous conflict about having their own emotional needs met. In fact, the way a woman deals with food and eating may reflect how she deals with both her own and others' needs (Dana and Lawrence 1988). Eating behaviour, can be seen as a metaphor for the receiving and giving of nurturance.

Metaphorically, then, a woman who eats emotionally is aware that she needs something but is not aware of what it is; is usually able to nurture others, but receives little nurturance back. Conversely, the anorexic woman tends to deny or minimize her needs and has difficulty taking anything in. Because relationships are often experienced as intrusive, she focuses on self-sufficiency and absolute self-control. The bulimic woman, in contrast, may experience elements of both, as she can take things in but has difficulty sustaining or absorbing the good or nurturance in them. She acknowledges she has needs, although she is not comfortable with them. Indeed, she may have a pervasive sense of guilt about her needs and feeding herself. While this metaphor seems to have general applicability, the issues for individual women are bound to be complex and, in some cases, may be quite different.

It is clear that the issues women face with meeting their own needs is a reflection of women's psychology, their life situations, and the social roles they play. Women have too often learned to take care of others' needs at their own expense. The particular intersection of this issue with the demands made on women in the workplace for more individualistic, less other-orientated behaviour creates internal conflict. Because food and the body are themselves conflictual issues in women's lives, it is logical that they become the arena in which women react to the conflict and distress they experience in other areas of life.

The physical and sexual violence that many women and children are subjected to contributes significantly to a lack of control and a fragile sense of self. Attempting to attain self-esteem and a sense of being in control through controlling the body is a significant issue for many women who have experienced such abuse. Many develop serious weight-preoccupation issues. Other childhood traumas including various forms of deprivation, violation, or neglect teach girls that their worlds are not emotionally or physically safe. While most women learn that their needs are insignificant and unworthy, this lesson is compounded for those who have experienced such trauma, increasing the chances that they will develop eating disorders.

We argue that women may express conflicts in their lives through their bodies and food at this time in history for two important reasons: the propagation and internalization of the thin body ideal, and the conflictual relationship women in our society tend to have towards food and the body. The violence and childhood traumas women experience in their lives add an additional layer, and seem to increase the likelihood that women will develop weight preoccupation or eating disorders as a consequence of looking for a greater sense of control and self-esteem by regulating food intake or body shape. These factors together make "eating disorders" a viable response during this contradictory and uncertain period of women's history.

In this section of the book, a number of these themes are elaborated. Kim Buchanan discusses the prevalence and significance of weight preoccupation in the lives of Black women in Western society.

In the context of racism, the meaning of weight preoccupation shifts.

Catrina Brown describes a continuum approach to understanding weight preoccupation and eating disorders. In laying out the criteria for diagnosing eating disorders, medical practitioners create the impression that there is a clear and qualitative distinction between women who are anorexic or bulimic and those who are not. This impression obscures the significant similarities among all women who are preoccupied with weight and shape in our culture, pathologizing some as "ill" and rewarding and normalizing others who "just diet."

In her essay on fat oppression, Beth MacInnis discusses the pervasiveness of weight prejudice and fat intolerance in our current beliefs about health and fitness, and in the related practices of health professionals. She explores the idea that fat oppression acts as a form of patriarchal social control.

Research on the effects of weight-control practices, the health risks of being over or under average weight, and the role of genetic factors in determining weight is often complex and inaccessible. In reviewing this information, Donna Ciliska disputes the assumption that fat is unhealthy and presents a compelling case against dieting.

Some of the most compelling arguments being offered in promoting weight-loss efforts among women link fitness and health with thinness. This link, argues Helen Lenskyj, has been exploited in the sports and fitness industries at the expense of many female athletes, both competitive and recreational. Rooted in the heterosexist and male-dominated sports culture, it serves to enhance the power and authority of male coaches while disempowering women. Some women-centred alternatives are suggested.

Once free of obsession with body size and shape new avenues are opened to appreciate our bodies as sources of pleasure and passion. Farah Shroff describes some ways in which pleasure and passion related to eating and sexuality are socially mediated and how women might be able to enjoy their bodies more.

◆

CREATING BEAUTY IN BLACKNESS

Kim Shayo Buchanan

As a Black feminist, I was quite hesitant to write about beauty and body image. Although I have discussed the issue with a number of my Black women friends, my concern over such an individualistic matter seemed somehow self-indulgent, given the numerous more urgent issues — poverty, police violence, miseducation of ourselves and our children, racist immigration policies, sexual and physical assault, inadequate child care, and employment discrimination, to name just a few — that currently face Black women and Black communities. Discomfort with appearance pales in comparison.

But the material inequalities that result from white supremacy can have a debilitating effect on the health and self-esteem of individual Black women. As Opal Palmer Adisa (1990, pp. 13–14) puts it: "Did you ever wonder why so many sisters look so angry?... Stress from the deferred dreams, the dreams not voiced; stress from the broken promises, the blatant lies; stress from always being at the bottom, from never being thought beautiful, from always being taken for granted, taken advantage of; stress from being a black woman in white America. How long do you think you can hold your breath without asphyxiating? Yes, black women do commit suicide!"

The stress of being a Black female in a misogynist, anti-Black culture that denies our humanity, and often denies Black women our basic physical needs, has damaging effects on our psyches and helps to place Black women at higher risk for some health crises, such as stroke, heart disease, and hypertension (White 1991, p. 28).

Black feminists, then, have rightly prioritized addressing the structural inequalities of racism and sexism. African American feminists such as Angela Davis (1983) and bell hooks (1981, 1992), for example, have placed more emphasis on representations of African women in the dominant culture than they have on the ways Black women see ourselves. Meanwhile, white feminists who write about body image, such as Naomi Wolf (1990), often fail to acknowledge the particular concerns that Black women face because of the combination of racism and the "beauty myth." Because relatively little has been published on the subject of Black women and body image, I turned to my own experience and that of other Black women to identify appearance issues that particularly concern us. African women are subject to the same pressures to attain an ideal of beauty as are white women in North American society, but efforts to approach the blonde, thin, young, white ideal are made at even greater cost for Black women. Weight preoccupation is not a central concern for many Black women, but weight is one among many factors that preclude Black women from attaining "beauty" according to the cultural archetype. Three issues came up again and again when I talked with other Black women: skin colour, hair texture, and body size.

Black women in Canada live in a culture of white supremacy that not only constructs white privilege and Black subordination, but also produces a racist ideology that makes that inequality seem natural and inevitable. The white-supremacist aesthetic negates or denigrates ("darkens") all that is associated with Africa and Blackness. Julia A. Boyd (1990), an African American feminist therapist, points out that this anti-Black ideology erodes the self-image and self-esteem of Black women. Blackness is a symbol of the inferiority of Black women and men: "Most folks in this society do not want to openly admit that 'blackness' as sign primarily evokes in the public imagination of whites (and all the other groups who learn that one of the quickest ways to demonstrate one's kin-ship within a white supremacist social order is by sharing racist assumptions) hatred and fear" (hooks 1992, p. 10).

In her essay "Revolutionary Attitude," bell hooks argues that "loving blackness" is a political stance that can subvert the ideology of white supremacy (hooks 1992, p. 1–7). While I am not con-vinced that individual self-love and self-esteem in themselves threaten entrenched white domination, they do provide an essential grounding for Black women and men to mount an effective chal-lenge to it.

Most Black women are very concerned with physical appear-ance because, like all other women, our "beauty" or lack of it deter-mines our value in Western society (Collins 1990, p. 80). But the Western tradition of dichotomous thinking has created a concept of beauty that has always been two-edged: "Blue-eyed, blond, thin white women could not be considered beautiful without the Other — Black women with classical African features of dark skin, broad noses, full lips, and kinky hair" (Collins 1990, p. 79). So, when beauty emerged as a dimension of female value in the nineteenth century, the construction of economically privileged white "ladies" as beautiful and virtuous was made possible by contrasting them with degraded, ugly Black womanhood (hooks 1981, p. 32).

Western Black women learn at an early age that our Blackness is abnormal and ugly. As Audre Lorde (1984, p. 151) says, "We are Black women born into a society of entrenched loathing and con-tempt for whatever is Black and female. We are strong and endur-ing. We are also deeply scarred." Black women and men who emi-grate to the West from African countries experience a shocking transition. In African countries, despite Western influence, Blackness is normal. It is taken for granted, much as white Canadians do not often notice their whiteness. Suddenly, on arrival on Canadian soil, African looks signify to others inferiority, ugli-ness, and shame. Several continental Africans living in Canada have told me, "I wasn't Black until I came here."

Bizarre and irrational as the pathologization of Blackness is, the negativity which defines Western images of Africa and Blackness has a profound effect on the self-image and self-esteem of Black children, male and female: "My six-year-old niece has an ulcer. Where does that come from? This kid used to put chalk on his face and hide beneath the desk. My son's name is Osaze which means 'One whom God loves', it's a name from Malawi. He came home and wanted his name changed to Tom" (Brand and Sri Bhaggiyadatta 1986, p. 54).

Both boys and girls learn that whiter is better. But the anti-Black aesthetic is even more damaging to Black girls and women because this culture ties women's self-esteem so closely to our appearance. In her essay "Eye to Eye," Audre Lorde (1984, p. 149) describes her childhood as the darkest of three sisters:

> They were goodlooking, I was dark. Bad, mischievous, a born troublemaker if there ever was one. Did *bad* mean *Black*? The endless scrubbing with lemon juice in the cracks and crevices of my ripening, darkening, body. And oh, the sins of my dark elbows and knees, my gums and nipples, the folds of my neck and the cave of my armpits!

COLOUR

Although feminist theorists such as Susan Faludi (1991) and Naomi Wolf (1990) point out that white women are forced to struggle for an unattainable ideal of femininity, never feeling beautiful enough, they choose to write about beauty as though Black women did not exist. All women are objectified when they are judged by their physical appearance and heterosexual appeal. However, as Patricia Hill Collins (1990, pp. 79–80) points out:

> [White women's] white skin and straight hair privilege them in a system in which part of the basic definition of whiteness is its superiority to blackness. Black men's blackness penalizes them. But because they are men, their self-definitions are not as heavily dependent on their physical attractiveness as those of all women.

But African-American women experience the pain of never being able to live up to externally defined standards of beauty — standards applied to us by white men, white women, Black men, and, most painfully, one another.

The beauty ideal is even more unattainable for Black women than it is for White women because Blackness is considered — in itself — ugly.

"From childhood on, if you read books, watch television, see movies, beauty is always a white girl with blonde hair and blue eyes. It is something that works its way deep into you," a Dutch Asian woman observes (quoted in Chapkis 1986, p. 60). This Nordic ideal is a cultural self-image that doesn't even reflect the way white North Americans really look. Natural blonde hair is actually extremely rare on Canadian adults. One Black woman put it succinctly: "Albinism is considered the most attractive." So the light-skinned Black woman with straight hair who most closely resembles the blonde ideal has traditionally been deemed the most attractive by whites and by Westernized Black men and women (Boyd 1990, p. 227; hooks 1992, p. 73).

European characteristics are considered beautiful in themselves. In Toni Morrison's *Jazz*, (1992, p. 201), Felice, a young, dark-skinned Black woman, describes her murdered friend: "Dorcas should have been prettier than she was. She just missed. She had all the ingredients of pretty too. Long hair, wavy, half good, half bad. Light skinned. Never used skin bleach. Nice shape .... If you looked at each thing, you would admire that thing — the hair, the color, the shape. All together it didn't fit."

Similarly, while traveling in the Caribbean and Latin America, Black nationalist Ann Cook noted that "no matter whether the language of the countries I visited was English, French, Spanish, Dutch or Portugese, there were phrases for 'good hair' and 'marrying light to improve the race' " (1970, p. 152). This colour prejudice persists today. For example, a dark-skinned Black woman I know was in a relationship with a mixed-race man who looks white. White strangers would approach them in the street and tell them, "Your children will be so beautiful!"

The white people who "complimented" my friends this way probably thought they were being anti-racist in supporting a "mixed" relationship. But my friends were deeply offended. Their children would be deemed Black in North American culture, but because they would look more European, they would be considered beautiful, for Black people. Clearly, Black and white people who think that "mixed" children are all good-looking have accepted that "marrying light" does improve the Black "race."

Because light skin is more valued in a white-supremacist culture, it does confer some privileges: in Toronto, young Black women and men find that racist whites treat light-skinned Black people more favourably than they do their darker peers because they see them as "less Black" (James 1990, p. 16). No wonder, then, that a Black South African woman recalls that, as a child, she longed for blonde hair and blue eyes: "It wasn't just that these things were supposedly beautiful, but they seemed to represent a special kind of life, the life I imagined white people had" (quoted in Chapkis 1986, p. 69).

No wonder, either, that a few Black people have turned to chemical skin lighteners. A 1980 advertisement in *Pace*, a Black women's magazine, equated paleness with a prosperous lifestyle: "Clere for your own special beauty. We are a successful people and have to look successful. We use Clere for a lighter, smoother skin. Now, Clere will work its magic for you, and make you more beautiful and successful" (quoted in Chapkis 1986, p. 89).

Today, skin bleaches are euphemistically called "fade creams" and advertise their ability to "even out skin tone." Little, however, has changed — the August 1992 issue of *Essence*, for example, carried this advertisement: "Nothing succeeds like Palmer's Skin Success Fade Cream."

Historically, though, Black women who were "pretty" — i.e., European-looking — did not necessarily benefit from this distinction. "Harriet Jacobs, an enslaved light-skinned woman, was sexually harassed because she was 'beautiful,' for a Black woman"

(Collins 1990, p. 81). The light-skinned Black woman is defined by white society as more "beautiful" because she looks like a tanned white woman. But her attractiveness has an added frisson of the sexually exotic, since white men define her, and all Black women, as available for sex (Collins 1990, p. 81; hooks 1992, p. 74).

Dark-skinned women fare even worse: "Nowadays, black women are included in magazines in a manner that tends to reinscribe prevailing stereotypes. Dark-skinned models are most likely to appear in photographs where their features are distorted. Biracial women tend to appear in sexualized images" (hooks 1992, p. 72).

Most contemporary Black people recognize the preference for European features as a manifestation of internalized racism. Nonetheless, most Black North American women continue to process their hair.

HAIR TEXTURE

bell hooks (1992, p. 73) observes that when dark-skinned models with African features are featured in white fashion magazines such as *Vogue*, they are often posed nearly nude against a background that evokes the stereotypical image of the Black woman as "sexual primitive." Currently, darker-skinned models with non-European features tend to be photographed wearing ridiculous long, straight wigs (hooks 1992, p. 71). This reflects an "aesthetic that suggests black women, while appealingly 'different,' must resemble white women to be beautiful" (hooks 1992, p. 73).

Orlando Patterson (quoted in Collins 1990, p. 90) argues that hair texture is much more important in assigning status than is skin colour, since the differences between African and European are much more pronounced in hair than in skin, and those differences persist longer with intermixing.

Good hair is straight hair. Bad hair is natural — kinky, nappy, African hair. *Essence*, a popular Black women's magazine, occasionally challenges this anti-Black aesthetic by running articles that celebrate Black women's natural hair texture, or by creating space for

Black women and men to discuss the social meaning of straightening African hair. However, this magazine also relies heavily on advertising for chemical "relaxers" and the many expensive conditioners and moisturizers that this damaging process necessitates. There were thirteen ads for such products in the September 1992 edition alone, as well as those for wigs, hair extensions, and, most disturbing and harmful of all, chemical skin bleaches. Perhaps to reassure the dubious consumer, some hair products carry ironic names such as "Affirm" and "African Pride."

Some Black women have internalized the idea that processed hair is superior to their natural hair texture. On an Oprah Winfrey show in 1991, Winfrey asked three Black singers who process their hair whether they felt that relaxing their hair had anything to do with their feelings about being Black. Gladys Knight's answer was revealing: "Whatever you feel like you can do to improve upon yourself, do it, because you've got to feel good about yourself" (quoted in Gregory 1992, p. 91).

Tania, a Black South African woman, observes the colonial impact of imposed white beauty norms: "By taking away a people's culture and pride in their appearance, you literally change the way they see themselves" (quoted in Chapkis, 1986, p. 69).

Nonetheless, most Black women who "relax" their hair are comfortable with their Blackness and express no desire to look more white. My Black friends who straighten their hair tell me that they do it because processed hair is "easier to take care of" or because they "prefer" the look. I find that my own natural hair is much healthier and easier to take care of now than it was when it was "relaxed." But, as Patricia Hill Collins (1990, p. 81) points out, "Institutions controlled by whites clearly show a preference for lighter-skinned Blacks, discriminating against darker ones or against any African-Americans who appear to reject white images of beauty. Sonia Sanchez reports, 'sisters tell me today that if they go in with their hair natural or braided, they probably won't get the job.' "

Black women's concern that employers prefer straightened hair is well founded. In 1987, Cheryl Tatum, a hotel cashier, and Renee Randall, a cafeteria food server, were fired from their jobs for refusing to unbraid their cornrows. Sydney Boone, a hotel telephone operator, was ordered by her employers to wear a wig over her braids if she was to keep her job. All three women pursued their cases with the U.S. Equal Employment Opportunity Commission (Wheeler 1988; Sanchez 1988; *The Washington Post,* 1988). Pamela Mitchell, a Mariott Hotel receptionist in Washington, D.C., had to pursue a complaint with the D.C. Office of Human Rights to defend her right to wear a hairstyle that represented "part of her African heritage" on the job (Duke 1988).

While Mitchell won her case (Sanchez 1988), few Black women have the time, the money, or the will to take their employers to court over their hair. Several Black university students who braid their hair have told me that they will relax their hair when they start looking for full-time work. And they are realistic: Black people who are seen as rejecting white beauty standards will be penalized. As bell hooks (1992, p. 17) says:

> On our jobs, when we express ourselves from a decolonized standpoint, we risk being seen as unfriendly or dangerous.
>
> Those black folks who are more willing to pretend that "difference" does not exist even as they self-consciously labor to be as much like their white peers as possible, will receive greater rewards in white supremacist society.

In an *Essence* article discussing Black women's intense relationship with our hair, Brenda Wade, a clinical psychologist, frankly acknowledged that "I know that to get asked back on shows like *The Today Show,* I would be more acceptable to most of the audience if I had straight hair. As Black women, we straighten our hair to look more acceptable to white society" (quoted in Gregory 1992, p. 91). Straightening our hair, then, is not so much a rejection of ourselves as an adaptation to the reality of white supremacy: "For black women, learning to comply publicly with white standards has been not as much a choice as a dictate necessary for survival" (Boyd 1990, p. 231).

One of my friends, a Black feminist law student who has considered the racial implications, but continues to relax her hair, argues that relaxed hair does not emulate white hair because the styles that Black women create are completely different from those of white women. In fact, a look around downtown Toronto shows that white women copy Black women's hairstyles, from cornrows to combing their hair tightly off the face into a high bun.

So while Black hair is defined by mainstream white society as inferior and unappealing, at the same time, the styles that Black women (and men) evolve are considered the cutting edge of "cool" fashion. As long as styles such as natural hair, braids, and dreadlocks are seen as apolitical fashion statements, they are admired, and even copied by whites. This trend reflects a consumer attitude towards cultural and racial differences in the social mainstream. "Within commodity culture, ethnicity becomes spice, seasoning that can liven up the dull dish that is mainstream white culture" (hooks 1992, p. 21).

Thus, while Blackness is considered ugly, Benetton has mounted a successful advertising campaign that features very dark Black people with natural hair; "exotic"-looking Asians; and very pale, Nordic-looking whites. Racial difference is unthreatening as long as it is confined to colour and style in the context of cultural consumerism. But the distinctive styles Western Black people wear evolved within Black communities created by displaced Africans as havens from white supremacy and as sites of resistance to it. Multicultural tourism fails to acknowledge that Blackness in North America means "more than just skin color and hairstyle, but a generational lifestyle that is rich in culture and value" (Boyd 1990, p. 229).

BODY SIZE

Evelyn White, editor of *The Black Women's Health Book*, observes that almost 35 percent of African-American women between the ages of 20 and 44 exceed the "ideal" weight for their height and age by more than 20 percent (1991, p.28). Some 50 percent of African-American women between 45 and 55 years old are also defined as obese. As Rosemary L. Bray (1992, p.54) points out: "When you consider how many Black women are raising children alone and how gleefully social commentators lay every problem Black children have at the feet of their drained and exhausted mothers; then you think about the disproportionate number of us who are poor and have no idea what having enough means, you begin to get a sense of the emotional weight we carry."

Rosemary Bray goes on to say that Black women bear heavier responsibilities than Black men and other women: "We are forever working, loving, volunteering, scolding, nurturing and organizing — but nearly always for others" (1992, p.54). Often, Black women's support systems — families, churches, and each other — revolve around preparing and sharing food.

But the fat Black woman finds herself even more despised than the fat white woman. In the eyes of racist whites, her body evokes the racist-sexist stereotype of the Black mammy, the opposite of the thin, blonde ideal (Bray 1992, p.90). bell hooks (1981, p.84) observes that, historically, slave nursemaids were typically young Black women with few family attachments. Southern white men and women created the Black mammy image as old, fat, and somewhat unclean — in order to reassure themselves that white men would never be attracted to them. This insidious stereotype can further undermine a fat Black woman's self-esteem. "We are just *too* much to be tolerated, so excessive that we should be hidden, kept from view, trotted out only to be laughed at. And that is a contagious attitude, an attitude that makes every woman who hates her body a little more filled with self-hatred, a little more disgusted, a little more intolerant of herself" (Bray 1992, p.90).

Fat Black women have to deal with a thin, white ideal that they can never achieve. The more a Black woman identifies with white beauty standards, the more she will value thinness (Gray et al. 1987, p.739). For example, only five British women of colour had been diagnosed with eating disorders by 1989; "problems of racial identity were prominent in these patients, four of whom had been cared for by white women" (Dolan 1989, p. 73).[1] Fortunately, Black communities accept fat on women far more than the white beauty standard allows (Rand and Kuldau 1992, p. 43; Gray et al. 1987). Traditionally, African American communities had a feminine ideal that was realistic and sexy: "Women's bodies were substantial. They had breasts and hips and curves and softness" (Bray 1992, p. 54). This ideal is refreshingly tolerant of real women's bodies. It persists today in a "cultural standard from our African heritage that allows for more voluptuousness and padding on Black women" (White 1991, p. 28). African cultures present an alternate vision of feminine beauty that allows more Black women to be comfortable with their size, and to enjoy it.

All of the Black women and men that I have talked to agreed that, although white men seem to find thinness an important criterion of attractiveness, Black men are much more appreciative of female curves. Black men often openly admire Black women who would be considered overweight by white beauty standards. Part of the reason for this is that a large, round butt is considered a sign of heightened sexuality in the "black pornographic imagination" (hooks 1992, p. 63). It is hardly surprising, then, that social researchers find that "almost twice the percentage of white as black girls wished for smaller hips and thighs" (Hsu 1987, p. 120). Skinny women are not considered as attractive as women who are "built."

Many Black women — especially, it seems, women from Africa and the Caribbean — carry their weight with pride and style. In many poor countries, excessive thinness is a sign of poor health (Chapkis 1986, p. 166). In Tanzania, where my extended family lives, men expect their wives to gain weight after they get married: "If she doesn't get fat, people will think I'm not taking good care of her!" men often say.

Senegalese filmmaker Osman Sembene observes the same fat-positive thinking in West Africa. In his film *Camp Thiaroye*, a

Senegalese war veteran asks a tailor to make his girlfriend two dresses — one tight, one loose. "Why?" the tailor asks. "Is she fat or thin?" The veteran replies: "She used to be fat, but she writes me that she's gotten thin because she misses me so much. But when she sees me at home, she'll be happy, and she'll get fat again!" Thus, it appears that, despite increasing Western influence, many African cultures continue to celebrate real women's bodies.

CREATING BEAUTY IN BLACKNESS

African American feminist bell hooks (1984) argues that Black women's location at the bottom of the hierarchies of race and gender provides us a "privileged perspective" from which to analyse those systems of domination. The dominant white culture has deemed Black women ugly (or, at best, as exotic imitations of "beautiful" white women). African women and men have always had to challenge the unlikely European image of beauty that white culture presents as ideal, and we have: "The oppositional black culture that emerged in the context of apartheid and segregation has been one of the few locations that has provided a space for the kind of decolonization that makes loving blackness possible" (hooks 1992, p. 10).

To keep our self-respect and to restore our pride, politicized Black women and men — artists, writers, nationalists, and feminists — are engaged in creating a cultural space that validates and celebrates Africa and our Black bodies. "We are laying claim to our selfhood, making bold to assert ourselves as women .... We write in order to create new models for our young, and a new fortitude" (Ngcobo 1987, p. 1)

This responsibility extends to popular Black North American culture. *Essence*, the largest Black women's magazine in North America, for example, is in many ways typical of mainstream women's magazines. It features articles on beauty and health, although its (relatively few) articles on dieting, unlike those in white women's magazines such as *Cosmopolitan* and *Glamour*, explicitly relate weight loss to health, and not to slimming. But unlike white women's magazines, *Essence* consistently features light, dark-skinned, and brown models with various hair lengths and types. Unlike any mainstream white women's magazine, Essence often uses fat models as well as typical thin women in its fashion editorials.

The pro–Black woman content of the articles in *Essence* is undermined, however, by the numerous advertisements it carries, for hair relaxers and for products such as makeup, cars, and cigarettes that continue to feature thin, light-skinned, European-looking models almost exclusively. But there is an evident effort in this popular magazine to resist the dominant white aesthetic and reconstruct real Black women, in all our sizes and shapes, as beautiful.

Outside the commercial pressures of mainstream publication, Black women are freer to construct alternative images of Black beauty. For example, Marlene Nourbese Philip, a Toronto poet and writer, deliberately works to appropriate the English language to create empowering Black images. She challenges the white construction of Blackness as unbeautiful in her book of poetry, *She Tries her Tongue: her silence softly breaks* (1989, p. 20): "when we hear certain words and phrases, such as 'thick lips' or 'kinky hair', the accompanying images are predominantly negative .... From whose perspective are the lips of the African thick or her hair kinky? Certainly not from the African's perspective. How then does the writer describe the Caribbean descendants of West Africans so as not to connote the negativity implied in descriptions such as 'thick lips'?"

Works such as Philip's poem "Meditations on the Declension of Beauty by the Girl with the Flying Cheek-bones" and African American filmmmaker Julie Dash's *Daughters of the Dust*, reflect the beauty of African women in all our diversity. Dash says that, through her work, she wants to "continue to challenge ... the conventional images of black women on screen" (Rule 1992, p. C15). Black women in contemporary film are typically portrayed as either mammy or slut (hooks 1992, p. 74).

The characters in *Daughters of the Dust* do not conform to these traditional representations; yet Dash resists the facile white aesthetic that says Black women can be "beautiful," as long as we look like Whitney Houston or Rae Dawn Chong. The little-known actresses in this film are stunning — and they look like real Black women. They represent a range of sizes and ages. Their natural hair is styled in beautiful and unusual ways. All but one of them are dark-skinned. And all of them are beautiful. "I wanted it to be healing, cleansing and empowering, so when they leave the theater people feel good about themselves," Dash explained in an interview (Rule 1992, p. C15). A viewer could never emerge from Dash's film believing that Black women must look alike — and white — to be beautiful.

The tall, hungry, blonde, blue-eyed ideal of the "beauty myth" is unattainable for most women of any race. It rests, then, on the fundamental premise that real women are not beautiful. Artists and writers such as Dash and Philip are restoring a vision of female beauty that challenges this belief. The images that they create powerfully show that Black women are beautiful in our real bodies. Works such as theirs are steps towards creating what Patricia Hill Collins (1990, p. 88) calls an "alternative feminist aesthetic" that "involves deconstructing and rejecting existing standards of ornamental beauty that objectify women and judge us by our physical appearance. Such an aesthetic would also reject standards of beauty that commodify women by measuring various qualities of beauty that women broker in the marital marketplace."

Currently, the struggles of liberal white feminists such as Naomi Wolf to resist what she calls the "tyranny of beauty" are receiving unusual attention in the popular media. But Wolf bases her argument on what she believes to be the experience of Western women: "As the economy, law, religion, sexual mores, education, and culture were forcibly opened up to include women more fairly, a private reality [the beauty myth] colonized women's consciousness" (Wolf 1990, p. 16).

As Black women, we do not have individual access to powerful positions within these institutions, nor is inclusion the kind of "liberation" that Black feminists seek. "Only those who find Jeane Kirkpatrick and Margaret Thatcher shining examples of feminism will believe that this sort of individual success is the same thing as women's liberation" (Chapkis 1986, p. 84). Black feminist theory has focused, instead, on the ways in which racism, sexism, and economic inequality are integral components of existing political and social institutions; it is relations of power, not women's bodies, which need to be radically transformed.

The creation of a feminist aesthetic is not an end in itself. Rather, it is a small part of a wider struggle against systemic patriarchy and white supremacy, and the lethal conditions that they create. bell hooks (1992, p. 50) warns against "the narcissistic-based individual pursuit of self and identity [that] subsumes the possibility of sustained commitment to radical politics." A healthy individual identity is meaningless in the absence of commitment to collective effort for fundamental social change.

As Black women, we need and deserve to love ourselves; but this self-love must be grounded in a wider commitment to working with and for our communities if we are to challenge the white supremacy that creates the conditions that force us to struggle for our identity and for our very survival.

◆

NOTE

1. This is not to suggest that problems with racial identity are the sole explanation for the incidence of eating disorders among Black women; obviously, women of colour share many of the beauty imperatives that white women respond to in this society. Rather, the issue here is that the less restrictive weight standards in African and disasporic cultures have to some extent as Hsu (1987, p. 120) points out, "protected [Black] females from developing the eating disorders."

THE CONTINUUM:
ANOREXIA, BULIMIA, AND WEIGHT PREOCCUPATION

Catrina Brown

Preoccupation with weight among women is not restricted to a few women, nor does it include only women who are bulimic or anorexic. Dieting and weight control have become an accepted and rewarded way of life. Today, women who are not concerned about their weight are the social anomaly. Anorexia (self-starvation) and bulimia (bingeing and purging) are the extremes on a continuum of weight preoccupation among women in affluent Western societies.

The statistics are alarming: almost 95 percent of anorexics and bulimics are women (Bemis 1987; Striegel-Moore, Silberstein, and Rodin 1986); up to 20 percent of female college students are bulimic (Garfinkel and Garner 1982) and 79 percent experience bulimic episodes (Halmi, Falk, and Schwartz 1980). The statistics for dieting and weight preoccupation in our society are no less alarming: by age 18, 80 percent of women have dieted to lose weight (Sternhell 1985), and by age 13, 60 percent have already begun to diet (Friedman and Maranda 1984).

The weight-preoccupation continuum often includes fear of fatness, denial of appetite, exaggeration of body size, depression, emotional eating, and rigid dieting. Only a matter of degree separates those women who diet, work out, and obsess about their body shape and calorie intake from the more extreme behaviours of anorexia and bulimia. We cannot stigmatize anorexia and bulimia as individual pathologies or diseases, at the same time that we approve, even praise, the behaviour of those women who exercise and diet to attain the culturally prescribed body ideal. The tendency to separate the social obsession with thinness from anorexia and bulimia allows the latter to be treated as individual problems and isolated diseases, disconnected from popular culture in patriarchal society.

Many women diet throughout their lives, repeatedly gaining and losing weight (Orbach 1978). While most women report feeling better about themselves when they lose weight, this sense of well-being is precarious: dieting has a very high "failure" rate, and 90 to 95 percent gain back even more weight than they lost, which likely contributes to the continuous dieting among women (Chernin 1981; Dyrenforth, Wooley, and Wooley 1980; Robinson 1985). Many women come to believe that losing weight is the key to solving the major problems in their lives (Millman 1980; Orbach 1978). Through weight loss they expect to feel more confident, to like themselves better, to be more outgoing, and to be happier.

When the body doesn't measure up, most women feel they themselves don't either. For many women, having the wrong body overshadows their talents, positive attributes, and accomplishments. Several years ago talk-show host Oprah Winfrey had a very public weight loss of 67 pounds, and proudly pronounced that nothing she had ever accomplished had meant as much to her, nothing had made her feel more in control of herself, nothing had made her feel better about herself. Nothing else, it seems, counted.

One survey of 33,000 women found that 75 percent felt they were too fat (Sternhell 1985), and, of these, 45 percent were actually "underweight" according to height/weight charts. If the more liberal revised 1983 height/weight charts advocating higher acceptable body weights had been used instead of the 1959 Metropolitan Life Insurance figures, even more of those women would have been considered "underweight." Clearly, not only anorexic women overestimate body size and think they are fat when they are thin. Most women have difficulty accepting their bodies, and the problems of anorexic and bulimic women are just more extreme forms of a common experience. Women tend to appraise their bodies in relation to an "ideal," and against this measure they find that their bodies are never good enough. Thus, the "distorted" perception of body image typically associated with anorexia is not unlike that of the average woman (Lawrence and Lowenstein 1979, p. 42).

A feminist approach to eating disorders and weight preoccupation recognizes how the conditions of women's lives shape their experience with weight and eating. Although Western women today have made inroads in attaining gender equality, the sense of control women feel they have over their lives and themselves is very precarious. Weight preoccupation among women is not simply a manifestation of widespread acceptance of an ideal presented by the media. The ambiguous halfway point between the demands of liberation and of traditional femininity in which women find themselves, is such that controlling the body and eating behaviour is one of a few meaningful and promising ways to establish an acceptable sense of self. By focusing dissatisfaction on the body, women often displace the real sources of their unhappiness. Women's collective preoccupation with weight is testimony that we have a long way to go, yet it is evidence that we are struggling, both conforming to and resisting the conditions of our lives.

Those who have adopted the continuum concept of women's eating and body-image problems tend to stress the differences rather than similarities between women who are labeled anorexic or bulimic, and women who are weight preoccupied (Garner, Olmstead, and Garfinkel 1983; Garner, Olmstead, Polivy, and Garfinkel 1984). The starting-point for understanding eating problems, then, is one that focuses on the differences in women's experiences. Such a framework obscures the fact that anorexia and bulimia are widespread problems among women, and that these problems must be situated in relation to the weight preoccupation typical of most women in Western society. A framework which emphasizes the similarities between women on a continuum of troubled eating and weight preoccupation allows for a feminist understanding and approach to working with women.

A continuum framework which recognizes that there are more similarities than differences among anorexic and bulimic women and those who diet and exercise to control their weight allows us to question traditional understandings of eating disorders. The continuum approach challenges the idea that anorexic women are substantially more disturbed, or that their behaviour provides a form of psychological organization which is radically different from that of women preoccupied with weight. Indeed, it is both characteristic and acceptable within contemporary Western society for women to displace feelings, needs, and dissatisfactions onto their relationship with their eating and their bodies.

The relationship women have with their bodies and eating is shaped and given meaning within the larger context of women's lives in patriarchal society. How women deal with their bodies and their psychological distress is mediated by socially acceptable strategies. It is therefore objectionable to label those who adopt more extreme measures as psychopathological, disordered, or diseased while simultaneously encouraging and rewarding dieting and weight preoccupation as healthy and normal when much of this more common behaviour is, itself, very extreme.

We can distinguish differences in degree of behaviour and the subsequent results of this behaviour without adopting a framework or starting-point that emphasizes difference and separates anorexic and bulimic women's experience from that of those who are less preoccupied with or have less invested in controlling their bodies. It is possible to be committed to a feminist approach which opposes the disease- or medical-model view of "eating disorders," and yet recognize that phenomena that can be described as "anorexia," "bulimia," or "weight preoccupation" exist.

Imagine the following situation:

Cathy has decided that today she will not eat because she "pigged out" yesterday. She rides her bike to work determined that if she makes herself exercise she will lose weight. All day she feels hungry, but is pleased that she hasn't eaten anything. She feels very in control; however, as evening progresses she can't stop thinking about the food she is craving to eat. If she can make herself not eat for a few more days then maybe she can eat whatever she wants. After pumping out 60 sit ups she goes to bed hungry feeling a little thinner. (Brown and Forgay 1987, p. 12)

Is Cathy anorexic or bulimic, or is she just like many women who are desperate to be thin? It is impossible to tell, but what is clear is these experiences differ only in degree. If we examine the American Psychiatric Association's criteria for anorexia and bulimia, we find that, at least in part, these descriptions fit behaviours exhibited by most women. How is it possible that such behaviours are routinely framed as psychiatric disorders when most women share them?

Many women who would not be considered anorexic or bulimic by the medical and psychiatric establishment adopt lifestyles that revolve around weight control and cycles of starving and bingeing. Dieting often precedes bulimia, as food deprivation is frequently followed by binge eating if food is available. The desire to eat is a natural response to starvation whether it is self-induced or the result of famine. This inability to stop eating when food is available is a common reaction among all people who are denied essential food intake (Bruch 1973; Keys et al. 1950). People who are starved have been found to become preoccupied with eating and to talk incessantly about food, and among some anorexic women the need to eat when starving themselves of food precipitates binge eating.

Many women who become weight preoccupied find themselves at different places on the continuum over their lives. Some women exchange anorexia and emaciation for bulimic bingeing and purging. Bulimic women may, at some points, vomit to purge, and at others use laxatives, diuretics, or exercise. Bulimic women may stop purging but continue to binge and find themselves gaining weight. These shifts, in themselves, are not uncommon and suggest that the psychological underpinnings remain quite similar, regardless of what form the weight preoccupation takes.

According to the American Psychiatric Association's *Diagnostic and Statistical Manual of Mental Disorders* (*DSM-III-R*), the diagnostic criteria for anorexia include an intense fear of becoming fat, a disturbed body image that involves feeling fat even when thin, loss of at least 15 percent of one's original body weight, refusal to maintain a normal body weight for one's age and height, and no known physical cause for the weight loss (American Psychiatric Association 1987). Yet most women are afraid of becoming fat, and most overestimate their body size. Many women try to keep their weights at levels lower than those considered "normal" for them. The psychiatric criteria provoke a number of questions. What happens when a fat woman loses 15 percent of her body weight, refuses to eat, becomes preoccupied with losing weight, and ceases to menstruate? Is she anorexic, even though she is fat? At what point does she become "anorexic"; that is, is she "normal" one day and "anorexic" the next? Although her feelings about her self, her life, and her behaviours may have remained consistent over time, not until she has actually become emaciated do people consider her to have a problem. Prior to the emaciation, her behaviours and psychological stance are likely to be encouraged and rewarded.

Presumably, anorexia develops over time, as emaciation and amenorrhea do not occur spontaneously. The psychiatric criteria reflect a poor understanding of the degree of desperation and anxiety the average woman in our society experiences around eating and her body shape and size. Not only are the psychiatric descriptions of anorexia nervosa and bulimia removed from the overall social context that precipitates weight obsession, they are static and fixed rather than fluid and temporal. Within such mainstream approaches, one simply is anorexic or has "recovered." This either/or evaluation perpetuates the understanding and treatment of these problems as diseases. Conversely, when anorexia and bulimia are framed as part of a continuum of weight preoccupation among women an alternative evaluation is possible, one that reflects a different understanding of women's psychological distress in society.

The psychiatric criteria themselves change over time, suggesting that the characteristics associated with anorexia and bulimia are not immutable, but socially defined. For instance, in 1980 the *DSM-III*, required women to have lost 25 percent of their body weight, revised down from 15 percent in 1987. As the criteria for anorexia have become less stringent, more women are able to fit the diagnostic label. Since the 1980 delineation of eating disorders in the *DSM-III*, a new code called "Eating Disorder Not Otherwise Specified" has been added to the *DSM-111-R*. While the 1980 criteria for eating disorders could already be criticized for being so broad as to describe most women, the 1987 addition now includes: "a person of average weight who does not have binge eating episodes, but frequently engages in self-induced vomiting for fear of gaining weight"; "all of the features of Anorexia Nervosa in a female except absence of menses"; and "all of the features of Bulimia Nervosa except the frequency of binge eating episodes" (1987, p.65).

These labels and criteria are not sacrosanct; rather, they reflect the powerful and dominant medical paradigm. This paradigm represents a particular way of understanding the social world and human problems. For example, "drapetomia" was a label once used to describe Black Americans who had attempted to escape slavery and human bondage. Homosexuality was, until recently, considered a psychiatric problem, and its psychiatric criteria were outlined in the *DSM-III*. The proposed diagnostic category "Masochistic Personality Disorder" was critiqued by feminists, but replaced by another sexist diagnostic label, "Self-defeating Personality Disorder" in the *DSM-111-R*. Another proposed diagnostic category is "Late Luteal Phase Dysphoric Disorder," which defines Premenstrual Syndrome as a psychiatric disorder. These labels and diagnoses reflect a particular understanding of social relations.

They define and often reinforce socially hegemonic ideologies concerning race, sexual orientation, and gender. While women's suffering has often been born out of the confinement, limitations, and expectations of patriarchal society, individual women have been institutionalized, drugged, and labeled as disordered. This approach to women's pain and suffering depoliticizes the social origins of the problems; invalidates and delegitimizes women's experiences; and negates women's expression of pain, dissatisfaction, and resistance.

By splitting women's fear of being or of becoming fat away from the context of their feelings and experiences, the medical model is unable to understand the meaning of these fears. When contexualized, women's fear of fat makes perfect sense. However, we must take a closer look at what this experience is really like for women. Anorexic women's lives, like those of most women preoccupied with weight, are dominated by fixations on food, thinness, and weight control, and by a personal sense of inadequacy and lack of control. A lifestyle evolves out of these feelings of inadequacy and ineffectiveness that centres on attempts to reduce these feelings through control of the body. Hyperactivity and exercise are further ways anorexic women and many weight-obsessed women seek to control the body. An anorexic woman's physical activities are often rigidly and ritualistically structured, like her other behaviours, in an attempt to gain a feeling of personal control, and with it a sense of personal adequacy. She will deny her skeletal appearance and impending death, desperately holding on to the only control she feels she has over her life: control over her body. While anorexic women usually know they are not fat, they feel fat, and like most women preoccupied with weight, they experience this feeling as untenable.

When an anorexic woman describes herself as "feeling out of control," she is often expressing that inner feelings of inadequacy make her feel very helpless. If she is already feeling inadequate, the conflicting needs to eat and to be thin exacerbate that inadequacy. She feels overwhelmed in the face of the demands she places on herself to achieve and do well. Anorexic women have often been described pejoratively as "perfectionistic," yet this tendency is, in part, often an expression of the need to please and receive approval from others. This need to please others is not uncommon among women socialized in a male-dominant culture where women learn to take care of others' needs at their own emotional expense. Despite anorexic women's achievements and successes in life, they usually feel they are failing, regardless of how they appear to others. For most women, the need to receive approval from others and to achieve in the world is a way to feel better about oneself.

Anorexia is something women do for themselves — it is an uncertain attempt to achieve self-empowerment and well-being. The result is what Marilyn Lawrence calls a "control paradox": the more anorexic women feel the need to exert control over their bodies, the more out of control they often are (Lawrence 1979; Brown 1990a, 1990b). An anorexic woman is communicating to others, and herself, that something is gravely wrong — that she is very unhappy. Her behaviours and her body serve as a statement of her frustrations, and she may perceive them as the only way she can express feelings so they do not impinge upon or upset others. She has learned in her life that she cannot risk the direct communication of her feelings. She is frustrated with her inability to develop a sense of self she can accept and that she feels others will accept as well. Some have suggested that anorexic women are struggling to develop a self (Chernin 1985; Friedman 1985; Orbach 1986).

Initial success with weight loss often brings praise from others and encouragement to continue to lose weight. The control established over the basic human urge to eat, especially when starving, is compelling as it makes the anorexic woman feel stronger. The anorexic woman feels she should be able to control her urge to eat. She experiences a personal sense of failure if she succumbs and eats, a reaction that is also common among bulimic women and most dieters. Conversely, women often feel a sense of power and personal satisfaction when they can contain and curb their appetites, even when they are emaciated and near death. The accomplishment of self-control, not weight or food intake in themselves, becomes the central issue. For anorexic and bulimic women as well as dieters, controlling the body becomes one viable way to feel more in control of one's self and one's life. It is a control such women are usually unwilling to let go of unless an alternative means of gaining control over their lives is established.

Anorexic women struggle to meet their own emotional needs. Their bodies communicate their deep emotional fragility and the need for emotional nourishment. Most dieters exert significant control over themselves and their eating, often denying and depriving themselves of food and the comfort it offers. But this pales in comparison with the degree of denial and deprivation anorexic women achieve, which parallels the degree of emotional deprivation many of them have experienced in their lives. Paradoxically, the sense of achievement or accomplishment this denial and deprivation produces makes anorexic women feel powerful.

Bulimia is perhaps more widespread among women than is anorexia. Bulimic women may be of any weight, from very thin to fat by social standards, depending on their "set-point" or physiologically programmed body weight, and the extent and nature of the bingeing and purging. Both anorexic and bulimic women live lives dichotomized around feeling in control and feeling out of control, and both states they associate with eating and not eating. Bulimic women often feel they have found the perfect private solution to the pressure to be thin since they can eat as they like, control their weight, and please others simultaneously. In this sense, bulimia conforms more to social expectations of women, as bulimic women's behaviour remains hidden and secret, and their emotional turmoil is obscured from others' vision. Such is not the case with anorexic women whose unwillingness to eat is often displeasing to others, and whose emaciation is mute testimony to their emotional suffering.

The *DSM-III-R* criteria for bulimia include recurrent episodes of binge eating of high-calorie food over a short period of time when one is alone (American Psychiatric Association 1987). Binge eating stops because of fullness, sleep, or vomiting, and is followed by depression and a self-deprecating mood. Bulimia is characterized by repeated attempts to lose weight by following very prescriptive diets, by self-induced vomiting, or by overuse of laxatives or diuretics, and by frequent weight fluctuations of at least ten pounds. Diagnostic criteria also include an awareness there is a problem with the eating behaviour, and that, like anorexia, it is not caused by a physical disorder.

Bulimic women's binge/purge cycles often convey the ambivalence they feel towards feeding and nourishing themselves. While eating is always connected to how we feel and what we need, for some it becomes the central way of fulfilling emotional needs. Many "compulsive" or "emotional" eaters use food in an attempt to fill up the "emptiness" they feel inside, or as a distraction from dissatisfaction or unhappiness.

Many similarities exist between dieters who binge and bulimic women who binge and purge. While binge eating is frequently a response to dieting, many women report emotional reasons for bingeing. Dieting is often especially difficult for those who depend on food to meet their emotional needs. It will not provide weight loss for these women for, as soon as the diet is over, eating will be resumed as the way to meet emotional needs. For many, binge eating is a way to give comfort and nurturance to oneself. Dieting is then experienced as both physiological and emotional deprivation. Bingeing can be called "comfort eating" as it often provides a distraction from uncomfortable feelings and produces the desired effect of numbing emotional pain. Conversely, some women feel they punish themselves by eating until they are in physical pain. Purging is equally as important as bingeing; most women purge through vomiting or laxative use, and even exercise, as a way to provide a release of emotional tension, especially anger. The bingeing and purging of bulimic women plays out an internal emotional drama involving uncertainty, vulnerability, emotional neediness, and rage. Bingeing and purging behaviour is not unlike the "slashing" or "cutting" some women do to express and release their pain.

We live in a culture which encourages women to nurture others but to expect emotional denial and deprivation for themselves. It is, then, not surprising that women have difficulty getting their needs met, or that they often feel some ambivalence about having their own emotional needs nurtured. These experiences are reflected in anorexic and bulimic women's treatment of their bodies, eating, and selves.

Histories of sexual abuse or physical battery are common among women with anorexia and bulimia.[1] Such women often have difficulty expressing anger at the abuser and blame themselves, taking out their anger on their own bodies (Wooley and Wooley 1986). Abuse of the body also sets women up to have difficulty with their own physical and emotional boundaries. Abusive histories often produce a poor sense of self, a lack of control or safety in life, and difficulty establishing positive relationships. Many of these issues are reflected in women's struggle with weight and eating.

The "psychiatrization" of relatively normative behaviour in the *DSM-III-R* criteria for anorexia and bulimia suggests that the psychiatric profession tends to be very distanced from women's experiences in our society. Most women acknowledge they binge eat, or eat for emotional reasons. When they "binge" eat they tend to eat high-calorie sweet food, or "junk" food, and this bingeing is almost always done when they are alone. Women admonish themselves for this behaviour and promise themselves they will diet or exercise in compensation. They tend to feel guilty, ashamed, and out of control. Paradoxically, women tend to feel very bad about themselves after comfort eating. The fact that this phenomena has become a subject in popular culture, such as the "Cathy" comicstrip, illustrates the normativity of this experience.

In 1987 compulsive exercise was added to the use of laxatives, diuretics, and vomiting in the *DSM-III-R* criteria for bulimia.[2] Many women who exercise compulsively share the same attitude as women who purge, that is: "I can have my cake and eat it too." Bulimic exercisers attain a tremendous sense of control over their lives through the control they achieve over their bodies. Compulsive exercising, like dieting, is often admired and encouraged, although it is as much a part of the problem as self-starvation, vomiting, and laxative use among many women. While these behaviours are all part of the continuum of weight preoccupation, and may express women's psychological distress, they need not be considered psychiatric disorders.

Adopting a continuum model of weight preoccupation encourages a greater sense of identification with the experiences of women who become anorexic or bulimic. Too often a we/they dichotomy is perpetuated even among those feminists who are knowledgeable about weight and shape issues. When we place the entire continuum of obsession with weight within a social framework, we can see the similarities between the dynamics propelling the development of eating disorders and those of most women's obsession with weight and shape in our society.

The degree of psychological conflict women experience about weight, shape, and eating is an important indicator of position along the continuum of weight preoccupation. Clearly, most women in Western societies would like to be thin. Feeling thin or achieving thinness is an accomplishment, and often produces a corresponding increase in self-esteem and a feeling of having control over one's life. For anorexic and bulimic women, the self-esteem enacted through controlling their bodies is pivotal. The "extremeness" of the anorexic woman's starvation or the bulimic woman's bingeing and purging is often an indication of there being more at stake.

Yet anorexia and bulimia are not centrally about weight or eating. Rather, those behaviours represent an attempt to deal with psychological distress in women's lives. Viewing these behaviours as "dieting gone crazy" frames these problems in terms of weight and eating and can obscure larger and often more substantial issues. To address the real issues or problems in women's lives, helpers must assist women in discovering why they focus on weight and eating.

A feminist approach to eating disorders differs from the medical model analysis and treatment of these problems. Where the medical model tends to offer an asocial, decontextualized, and highly individualized explanation of eating disorders, a feminist model seeks to understand the connection between women's relationship to our bodies and the conditions of our lives. Traditional approaches to working with eating disorders tend to focus on weight and eating, the chief objective being behavioural change. The emotional rollercoaster women often ride in relation to how they are feeling about their bodies and eating is much larger than simple concern about weight and shape, although arguably there is no such thing as simple concern about weight and shape for women. For each woman who diets, who thinks about the size of her thighs, who starves herself during the week so she can "pig out" or "binge" on the weekend, thinness offers many rewards.

For many women, thinness represents feelings of being in control, successful, attractive, valued, worthy, lovable, sexually attractive, and powerful. However, some women feel too vulnerable and powerless when they feel thin and are more comfortable at a higher body weight. Fatness for most women, though, means feeling out of control, powerless, unattractive, unworthy, devalued, ashamed, and like a failure. Women's investment in attaining thinness is a completely rational phenomenon, given the degree of fat prejudice and hatred that exists in our society. We believe we will be better off if we are thin and we know with a certainty we will be punished for being fat.

It is not just anorexic or bulimic women who refer to "feeling fat" or "feeling thin." What does it mean to feel thin or to feel fat? The feeling has very little to do with actual body size. Most women who say "I feel fat" mean "I feel bad"; when they feel thin, they feel good. Ultimately, by focusing our dissatisfaction on the body rather than on the condition of our lives, nothing significant changes.

Traditional psychiatric accounts describe anorexic and bulimic behaviour in such a way that such behaviour appears bizarre and irrational. These accounts do not address the way women's behaviours are connected to how they feel. Women's own stories of their experiences are almost never included in the institutionalized

accounts. By presenting a disembodied, detached, and pathologizing view of women's experiences, traditional frameworks silence
women.

How can we pathologize women's fear of being fat, or their
investment in controlling their bodies when these are among the
few legitimate mechanisms women have for developing a sense of
control over their lives? We need to hear the voices of individual
women as they struggle through their relationships with weight and
eating. The body and eating are embedded with meaning in all cultures. Both eating behaviour and how the body is presented and
adorned express meaning about individuals and society. The
woman who starves herself to sixty pounds is making a meaningful
statement; she is not crazy. Indeed, she desperately needs to be
heard and will not be ready emotionally to relinquish self-starvation until she is. Bulimic women who spend the better part of their
waking day bingeing and purging are desperately communicating
and expressing the chaos they feel about their lives. Other women
who exercise for hours every day often do so not only for the sake
of fitness, but to feel a greater sense of self control. Hence, weight-
obsessed women will continue their behaviour until they no longer
need it as a way to be heard.

Western culture continues to invest a woman's appearance with
extraordinary significance in judging her overall value. In Western
societies, appearance is inseparable from identity, social value, and
hence self-esteem. Women learn they should not feel good about
themselves unless they look a particular way. We are told by family,
friends, lovers, doctors, journalists, and the media that we cannot
feel good about ourselves if we are fat. What women value about
themselves commonly reflects the values of society. Some, however,
have begun to question the validity of these beliefs, as is evident
from the numbers of women who have been active in challenging
the social values of thinness and hatred of fatness.

Each time we diet, each time we judge our personal value on
the basis of appearance, each time we criticize others or feel better
than them based on how they look, each time we positively reinforce

weight loss, or even each time we sit around in groups and complain in a comradely way about our bodies, we contribute to the perpetuation of the pressure to be thin. As women, we are not simply victimized by social values and pressure, but take an active role in keeping the phenomenon of weight preoccupation alive. Overcoming weight preoccupation, giving up dieting, or accepting one's body as it is, is by no means easy, but the only way off the treadmill is for women themselves to reject the value of thinness and rebel against its tyranny. We need to recognize the strength and courage it takes to rebel against predominant social values. Most importantly, we must recognize the necessity of our doing so.

◆

NOTES

1. Research on and documentation of the relationship between sexual abuse and eating disorders have become more widespread. The following writers have observed a connection between sexual abuse and eating disorders through either clinical work or research: Abraham and Beaumont 1982; Bass and Davis 1988; Beckman and Burns 1990; Brown 1990a, 1990b; Beaumont, Abraham, and Simpson 1981; Brown and Forgay 1987; Buchok 1990; Calam and Slade 1989; Goldfarb 1987; Hall et al. 1989; Hambridge 1988; Kearney-Cooke 1988; Miller 1990; Oppenheimer et al. 1985; Palmer et al. 1990; Root 1988; Root and Fallon 1988, 1989; Runtz and Briere 1986; Schecter, Scharwtz, and Greenfield 1987; Sloan and Leichner 1985; Smolak, Levine, and Sullins 1990; Waller 1991; Wooley and Wooley 1986.

2. Some women avoid sleep in an effort to burn calories, and others chew food but do not swallow it. Diet pills can be used by women to compensate for periods of unrestrained eating. Strong prescription diet pills used to curb appetite are often stimulants and thus interrupt sleeping and eating patterns. The behaviour of women using these pills can resemble that of anorexia.

FAT OPPRESSION

Beth MacInnis

Many qualities and characteristics define a person, but when I reflect upon me the first characteristic that comes to mind is fat. My memories of childhood are a blur of physicians and nutritionists, each pushing a different diet at me. Success or failure was measured by the results of weekly weigh-ins. When the scales showed weight loss, I would be filled with pride, and could anticipate verbal praise as well as tangible rewards from family members. When the scales showed a weight gain, I would be lectured about "cheating" and would endure the silent yet resounding disappointment of family members. The shame I felt would be amplified by well-intentioned family members who felt it their duty to comment on every morsel of my food intake.

My family harboured a great hope that I would grow out of my fatness, but by early adolescence it became apparent that this was not to be. At age thirteen I was hospitalized by a psychiatrist, in an attempt to monitor my eating habits. This experience of being hospitalized with other children who were battling life-threatening illnesses did not result in the desired weight loss, but did leave me feeling demoralized.

During my teenage years the pressure to "do something" about my weight increased. The offer of tangible rewards was replaced with the threat of an unhappy, unmeaningfull life (i.e., you'll never have a boyfriend, you'll be miserable all of your life, you'll never be able to have nice clothes). Despite these threats I steadfastly refused to discuss my weight or diet — a stance I maintained for many years. I did not recognize the political implications of my experiences as a fat woman until I began exploring weight and shape issues from a feminist perspective. While this essay is not a personal narration, its writing is rooted in my own personal experiences.

Women's preoccupation with weight and the current ideal of thinness have to be examined within the context of fat oppression if we are to understand the sociopolitical factors that perpetuate weight preoccupation and weight prejudice. Fat oppression, the fear and hatred of fat that result in discriminatory practices, is so commonplace in Western cultures that it is rendered invisible. However, evidence exists in abundance to suggest that society hates fat, particularly on women, and persecutes women who do not meet or are not actively striving towards the ideal of thinness. In effect, "fat" has become a prejudicial term, synonymous with "stupid, lazy, and ugly." It is my belief that the medical community has played a significant role in perpetuating, if not shaping, pervasive fat-oppressive attitudes. It is also my belief that a feminist analysis can provide insight into the roots and purpose of fat oppression.

LEGITIMIZING THE MYTHS

Science consists of observations and opinions held together by a set of beliefs known as a paradigm. Paradigms are useful organizational tools in that they provide a frame of reference from which research questions are generated and their results interpreted. However, paradigms are not objective in so far as they reflect a particular world view. Given that science as a community of endeavour has been dominated by men, it has been suggested that its world view is characterized by patriarchal norms and values (Benston 1989). In fact, it could be argued that science, cloaked in the myth of objectivity, functions to perpetuate patriarchal ideology.

"Obesity" researchers operate under a paradigm which posits that an ideal weight exists, that weight is governed by conscious control, and that fat people are overfed (Mayer 1983a). Arising from this view comes a theory which states that fatness is a physical abnormality somehow linked to the consumption of too much food. Efforts to maintain this paradigm have led to a circular definition of overeating as eating enough so that one gains weight. Simplistically, "overweight" people are those who eat too much food. By extension of this definition, chronic dieters who gain weight on 800 calories a day would be defined as overeaters (Bovey 1989). Medical ideology related to body size that posits a distinct relationship between food, eating, and weight is presented as a collection of uncontestable truths. These "truths" have come to reflect more than a physiological understanding of the relationship between food and weight; they represent a moral code by which health-care professionals judge clients. That is, fat people are perceived to be gluttons who are the authors of their own misfortune. Evidence to challenge the assumptions under which obesity researchers operate is available, but not widely accessible.

In a review of medical studies of "obesity," Susan Wooley and Wayne Wooley (1979) found that well-controlled research studies do not support a causal relationship between food and fat; that is, valid medical studies suggest that the food intake of "obese" individuals does not differ from that of those considered to be of "normal weight." Furthermore, Wooley and Wooley cite a study of the physiology of dieting which revealed that fat has little to do with food intake and lack of willpower, and much to do with an internal control system, known as a set-point, which dictates how much fat a body should carry (Bennett and Gurin 1982). Losing weight requires that a person eat less than the body needs to function. When a thin person engages in such eating habits, it is called self-starvation; when a fat person consumes less than the body needs to function, it is called dieting (Kelly 1983). Even when food intake is decreased, the body fights to maintain fat reserves by using protein from the heart and muscle and by slowing the basal metabolism rate. Attempts to control food intake and reduce weight to a level below a body's natural set-point are rarely successful because the body intervenes to increase appetite and weight until the set-point is achieved. If the body is continually starved, it will work to store fat to protect itself against the next famine, and the set-point will be raised. Raising the set-point allows the body to maintain its weight at fewer calories than before dieting (Tenzer 1989). This important aspect of the physiology of dieting explains why 95 percent of all diets not only fail, but often result in postdieting weight gain. In fact, it has been hypothesized that dieting, long thought to be the primary treatment for obesity, may be the primary cause of it (Wooley and Wooley 1979).

The notion of treatment typically presupposes some form of pathology, and fat people are encouraged to diet for health reasons. "Obesity" was once thought to be directly related to heart disease, high blood pressure, and diabetes; however, Susan Wooley and Wayne Wooley's review (1979) suggests there is little medical evidence to support such a claim. In fact, some health-care professionals now recognize that the health risks associated with chronic dieting are more substantial (Nopper and Harley 1986).

Nonetheless, the medical community continues to construe fat as an unhealthy, abnormal, and abhorrent state, despite the lack of empirical evidence to validate such claims. Given that dieting is generally ineffective, medical professionals have searched for alternative means to combat fatness. For instance, physicians prescribe medications such as Furosemide to assist in weight reduction. The possible side-effects of such medications include insomnia, dry mouth, facial swelling, vomiting, disturbances to blood chemistry, low blood pressure, and "mental illness" (Greaves 1990). Should medication not result in the desired weight loss, several surgical procedures now exist to "treat" fat women. The intestinal bypass involves removing most of the small intestine so that the stomach is linked almost directly to the anus. Food passes through the system so quickly that it is hardly digested. It is estimated that one to fifteen of every hundred women who have this procedure die as a result of it (Mayer 1983b). Those who survive can anticipate such side-effects such as malnutrition and permanent diarrhoea. Gastric stapling, another form of surgery, involves implanting surgical staples in the stomach to radically reduce its capacity to hold food, setting an upper limit of 3 to 10 ounces. Eating more than this maximum causes severe pain and vomiting. It is estimated that 4 percent of women who opt for this surgery die during the operation (Wolfe 1983).

In view of the mortality rate for these procedures one would assume that a woman's condition would have to be life-threatening before a surgeon would perform either of them. However, the evidence suggests the contrary, that the majority of these operations are performed for cosmetic reasons. Surgeons justify performing these procedures by claiming that the patient suffers a psychosocial handicap. Attaining a more socially acceptable body appears to result in psychosocial rehabilitation.

One must examine why the medical community continues to perpetuate the myths that fat people are abnormal and unhealthy, despite medical evidence to the contrary. Susan Wooley and Wayne Wooley (1979) suggest that our beliefs about fat are so ingrained that health-care professionals will be slow to change attitudes about fat. Until attitudes change, the medical community will continue to be active agents of fat oppression, as evidenced in their "treatment" of fat women. Recognizing that the medical community is part of a patriarchal system is fundamental to understanding why practitioners by and large continue to validate a cultural stereotype of attractiveness at women's expense. That fat women are willing to risk their lives and endure tremendous pain to attain the ideal of a thin body attests not only to the oppression that fat women face, but also to the value placed on this ideal. A feminist analysis is necessary to an understanding of why women engage in the relentless pursuit of thinness.

DISPELLING THE MYTHS

The ideal body is a sexist construct that serves to control women. To be a women is to be a body: to be looked at, appreciated, and ultimately owned. In patriarchal societies women are often ranked according to their approximation to the body ideal; those who most closely approximate it are given status, and those who fall outside of the prescribed beauty/body boundaries are devalued. The notion of a beauty/body ideal not only separates women from one another, but serves to separate a woman from herself by dividing the body into a series of parts to be judged. Study after study reveals that women harbour a deep dissatisfaction with, even hatred, of their bodies. The message that the only legitimate means of accessing power is through the body places women in competition with one another. We measure our success, worth, and power against another women's body size and appearance. We are encouraged to compete for the ultimate reward: the attention and admiration of males.

The rewards of approximating the beauty/body ideal are tangible. Studies show that good looks are socially rewarding. Women who approximate the cultural body ideal date more often, have access to a wider selection of mates, marry earlier, and have greater access to jobs. However, body ideals may change several times in one woman's lifetime, keeping women ever vigilant. Fluctuations in the body ideal tell us about women's place in society and about the economics of the time. When life is precarious and resources scarce, fat connotes wealth and survival, and is thus highly desirable. In times of prosperity, and when women have banded together to effect social change, body ideals become restrictive, and the ideal women is small, childlike, and passive. It is not coincidental, then, that during the second wave of feminism, when women were demanding mass social reform, the body ideal dropped to 23 percent below the average woman's weight (Wolf 1991). As women began to enter the workforce in greater numbers, domesticity as a form of mass social control lost ground, and was replaced by increased pressure to conform to a narrowly defined beauty/body ideal. Restrictive body ideals leave women with the clear message that, regardless of the gains we have made, we still don't own our bodies.

Chernin (1988) suggested that hatred of fat stems from misogyny. In women-oriented societies, God is a female and she is usually fat (Kelly 1983). In a misogynistic society, women are not to take up space, use up resources, or nurture themselves. Fat women are perceived to violate all of the rules, including those that govern what it means to be a woman, and are deemed to be deserving of society's contempt.

Hatred of fat tends to be internalized by women, regardless of body size. By age 18, 80 percent of all women have dieted to lose weight. Women are encouraged to look at their large bodies as the source of failure in their lives. Women expend a great deal of time, energy, and money attempting to reduce body size. Subsequently, attention is focused inward and diverted away from the culture that despises women's natural bodies. Chernin (1981, p. 106) observed that a woman in such a culture "will not seek to change her culture so that it will accept her body; instead she will spend the rest of her life in anguished failure at the effort to change her body so that it will be acceptable to her culture."

Until recently, understanding fat oppression as a form of social control has not been a subject for feminist analysis; in fact, early feminist analysis perpetuated that oppression. In virtually all forms of feminist analysis, feminists assert that society and not individual women need to change. As a result of hegemonic fat-oppressive attitudes, different standards were applied to fat women. Fat women who turned to feminism to understand the political nature of their oppression would find little comfort in the writing of feminists, such as Susie Orbach, author of *Fat Is a Feminist Issue*, who brought fat into the realm of feminist thought and analysis. Orbach's early work (1978) suggests that, through nondieting and self-acceptance, women will lose weight and attain their true selves.

Underlying such an analysis are the assumptions that fat is abnormal, that women choose their body sizes, and that the choice to be fat represents some unresolved psychological conflict. Similarly, in *A New Approach to Women and Therapy*, Miriam Greenspan presents a case-study entitled "Bonnie's Story: Fat as the Great Refusal." In this case-study, Greenspan states: "as a patient, the chances of her shedding her fat were quite slim" and concludes that "Bonnie's fat was the outward and direct manifestation of a suppressed wish to defy the cultural conventions by which women are groomed to be beautiful" (p. 269). Both Greenspan (1983) and Orbach (1978) reinforce cultural standards of attractiveness, construe fatness as pathology, and fail to recognize that what makes fat a problem is society's hatred of it.

Laura Brown (1987) draws a parallel between fat oppression and homophobia. Both serve to keep women from deviating from male-defined normative behaviour. Lesbophobia is a form of social control that keeps women from loving each other; fat oppression is a form of social control that keeps women from loving ourselves. Neither fat women nor lesbian women are seen as actively trying to please men, and are subjected to ridicule, scorn, and contempt. Fat women, like lesbian women, are marginalized, stigmatized, and devalued. It is of interest to note that Brown has observed less evidence of "eating disorders" among lesbian women, and suggests that, "once having successfully challenged the rules against loving a women, a woman may be less likely to impose other patriarchal norms, such as conventions of attractiveness and size, on herself" (p. 299).

Unlike Greenspan, who asserts that fat women choose not to adhere to conventions of beauty, Brown suggests that lesbian women are more likely to challenge conventions of attractiveness; that is, Brown recognizes that body acceptance is an act of resistance, whereas Greenspan appears to see it as an indices of pathology.

Overcoming our socialization and learning to accept our natural body size is just one, albeit a significant, step towards liberation.

A fat women who accepts her body must still live in a society that hates it. While the relationship between race, class, and fat oppression have not been well examined, the consequences of not approximating the cultural body ideal are real. For many women, poverty is one such reality. "Obesity," as defined by the medical community, is seven times more common among working-class women than among women of other socioeconomic status; in fact, the American socioeconomic group with the highest percentage of fat members is that of Black women below the poverty level (Mayer 1983b). It cannot be stated that fat determines socioeconomic status. It is, however, noteworthy that trends between weight and class, evident for women, are not as well defined for men. Nancy Worchester and M. Whatley (1985) posed the question of whether, in our Western society, a woman's body build is a factor in determining her economic status. Given that nonobese women are more likely to be accepted into college than obese women (Canning and Muir 1966), combined with the reality that fat women face the reduced likelihood of being hired for jobs, a woman's body build may impact on her economic status. Within the framework of a feminist analysis, this finding should not be particularly startling, given that in a patriarchal society a woman's primary value is derived from the extent to which she approximates male-defined beauty/body ideals. Consequently, men of higher economic status are less likely to "settle" for a woman who does not reflect the cultural beauty ideal.

The relationship between body size and economic status is evident in such expressions as "a woman can never be too thin or too rich." Somehow thinness is seen to conform to the North American values of hard work and self-denial: being thin is virtuous and a sign of economic success, but being fat is shamefully lower class (Mayer 1983a). Thus fat represents low social status and lack of self-control (Greaves 1990). That women have to be thin to get and keep jobs, and to attract male attention, makes the pursuit of thinness not only a matter of aesthetics, but a means of economic survival (Székely 1988).

Understanding the consequences of not approximating the ideal of thinness helps illuminate why weight preoccupation constitutes the norm. In the book *Shadow on a Tightrope* (Schofielder and Mayer, eds. 1983), fat women recount numerous forms of abuse they experience, ranging from verbal harassment to job discrimination, to physical assaults. The stories of fat women are remarkably similar. Everyday oppressive experiences include taunting from strangers; encountering bus, theatre, and airline seats which are too small; not being able to purchase clothing in the same stores as their "normal-sized" sisters; being constantly assailed with the message, for example, weight-loss ads, that they are not okay; and being subjected to the conversations of "normal sized" friends and co-workers who complain of being "too fat." These are not isolated experiences of oppression; rather they make up the fibre of a day, a week, and a lifetime, for the fat woman in Western society.

That women support a multibillion-dollar-a-year weight-loss industry attests to the normative nature of dieting. Part of the revenues generated are used to bombard women through advertisements in the mass media, making it virtually impossible to escape the message that "thin is in." Ads promoting weight loss are generally vague about its supposed health benefits; however, the use of health-care professionals to endorse weight-loss products implies that fat is unhealthy. These ads exist in a society where fat women are actively discriminated against because of their fatness. For example, a woman in the United States was expelled from a nurses' training program because she was deemed to be too fat. Thus, what weight-loss ads offer women is the hope of social rewards, economic security, and a sense of self-control, albeit fleeting.

A feminist analysis provides a useful framework in which to explore how we experience our bodies. Our preoccupation with weight and body size is not neurotic; rather, it is a reflection of our innate understanding of how we are valued. Regardless of the gains women have made, our bodies continue to be the battlefield where our oppressors wage their war.

In a society where 80 percent of women have dieted before age eighteen and 76 percent of women consider themselves too fat, it is safe to conclude that fat oppression exploits all women. Feminists have revealed the body ideal to be a sexist, heterosexist, racist, ageist, and classist construct. Consequently, the mechanisms that exist to oppress fat women are complex and interwoven, and freeing ourselves from them will be difficult. Shattering the myths about fat and naming fat oppression are the first steps in the process.

◆

WHY DIETS FAIL

Donna Ciliska

DESIRE FOR THINNESS

The culturally prescribed "ideal" body size for women in the Western world is very thin. Professional models, the standard against which we most commonly measure beauty, are now 23 percent lighter than the average North American woman (Sheinin 1990). The 1985 Health Promotion Survey (Health and Welfare Canada 1988a) disclosed that 70 percent of all Canadian adult women (including heavy, average-sized, and thin women) wanted to reduce their weight. Thirty-six percent of women who were of normal weight believed that they were overweight (Millar 1991). Consequently, it is estimated that, at any given time, 40 percent of all women and 61 percent of adolescents and young adult women are dieting (Berg 1992), and for socially dictated, cosmetic reasons rather than health reasons. Girls as young as five years have reported restricting their food intake because they were afraid of getting fat (Feldman, Feldman, and Goodman 1986). This fat phobia has led to billions of dollars being spent annually for weight-loss products, programs, and paraphernalia, and has contributed to some women suffering from poor nutrition; an increase in the incidence of eating disorders; wider prevalence of body dissatisfaction, resulting in diminished self-esteem and its attendant symptoms of depression; weight gain, escalation of discrimination against "over-weight" people; and diminished bank accounts. All diet programs result in some weight loss for most people. However, very few result in weight-loss maintenance. In addition to lack of long-term benefit, there are also attendant hazards. This essay focuses on the lack of effectiveness and the hazards of dieting, and some of the myths that perpetuate the pursuit of weight loss.

DEFINITION OF "OVERWEIGHT"

There is no one definition of what constitutes being "overweight" or "obese." Different researchers and clinicians use different measures, ranging from a few pounds above some ideal (as in the Metropolitan Life tables of ideal weight) to 100 percent above a population average based on sex, age, and height. Because definitions vary, so do estimates of prevalence. Body Mass Index (BMI) is gaining international acceptance as a measure of body size. Your BMI is calculated as your weight in kilograms divided by your height in metres squared. Thus someone who weighs 75 kilograms (165 pounds), and is 1.65 metres (5 feet 5 inches) tall has a BMI of 27.5 ($75/1.65^2$). However, no international agreement has been reached on what BMI is too large or too small. An expert consensus panel (Health and Welfare Canada 1988a) recommends the adoption of BMI for adults, ages 20 to 65. They have stated that a BMI of 20 to 25 is considered "a good weight for most people"; 25 to 27 "may lead to health problems in some people"; over 27 indicates an "increasing risk of developing health problems"; less than 20 also "may be associated with health problems for some people" (Health and Welfare Canada 1988b). BMI does not consider body build as a factor. Thus a very muscular person could have a BMI indicative of health risk, but have very little body fat. The literature from Health and Welfare Canada has made an important advance by identifying that people at a low weight are at risk, and advises against further weight loss, although it stops short of recommending weight gain. The focus on weight loss perpetuates discrimination against people who are at the higher weight ranges. Also, it ignores conflicting evidence supporting the myth that being "overweight" is synonymous with having health problems. However, use of the BMI standard is gaining acceptance among health professionals for deciding when weight loss will be recommended.

On the basis of the BMI calculation, 50 percent of Canadians aged 20 to 65 are at the recommended BMI range of 20 to 25; 27 percent (20 percent of women, 32 percent of men) have a BMI over 25; 23 percent (15 percent of women, 5 percent of men) have a BMI under 20. Thus, in terms of the argument that weight impacts on health, men are at greater risk because of being "overweight" and women are at greater risk because of being "underweight" (Health and Welfare Canada 1991). However, substantially fewer men than women seek weight-loss programs. Clearly, women's desire for thinness is esthetically, not health, based.

As is true of most physical measures, the weight of a group of women of a particular height is normally distributed. That means, a few women are very thin, a few are very heavy, and most are in the mid-range. Yet, society tells women to reject the normal distribution and to aspire to a position at the lower end of the scale. Medicine categorizes the upper end of the weight range as a chronic disorder. We need to work towards acknowledgement that there is no magic number defining "overweight." The term itself should be avoided. We do not use "overheight"; however, we have no descriptive term, the equivalent of "tall," that is free of the baggage of negative connotation. For many people, particularly women, being "overweight" is no more a disorder than being "normal" weight; that is, many women have no health problems at all, even though they are at the high end of the weight distribution.

Weight, like height, seems to be strongly genetically influenced. There is not much action that can be taken to change the expression of height or weight. Various studies have investigated the heritability of weight. Studies of families and fraternal and identical twins have supported that fact that genetics are more important than environment in determining the weight of adults (Bouchard,

Perusse, and Leblanc 1988; Stunkard, Foch, and Hrubec 1986; Stunkard et al. 1986).

HEALTH RISKS AND "OVERWEIGHT"

How strong is the evidence that there are health risks associated with being "overweight"? Are there health reasons to diet? The findings of many large-scale population studies conflict. A group of experts convened by Health and Welfare Canada to develop guidelines for healthy weights reported that there generally is a U-shaped curve relating weight to mortality and morbidity. Very low weights and very high weights are associated with increasing risk: "excess weight is associated with hypertension, diabetes, elevated serum cholesterol, endometrial and colon cancer. Furthermore, obesity is a heterogeneous condition: that is, not all obese individuals are unhealthy. There are also many individuals within commonly accepted weight standards who have elevated serum cholesterol, hypertension or diabetes" (Health and Welfare Canada 1991, p. 93). This statement from Health and Welfare Canada is emblematic of the ambiguity that surrounds associations of weight with health risk. That is, high and low weights are associated with disease and death, but the linkage is far from conclusive. People can be very heavy and very light without being unhealthy. Also, "associated with" does not mean "causes"; in other words, high or low weight may have no causal relationship with disease or death, but merely coincides with it at increasing levels of frequency in cases where weight is at the extreme ends of the high-low scale.

Contrary to the idea that any degree of "overweight" is dangerous, documented evidence exists that there are health benefits associated with "moderate overweight." These benefits include lower risk of developing osteoporosis, and increased survival associated with lower cardiovascular risk and lower rates of suicide (Ernsberger and Haskew 1987). Osteoporosis is decalcification, or softening of the bones, such that the bone is susceptible to breaking. The fractures often occur in the legs or the spine. Any activity that puts stress on the leg bones, such as walking or carrying more weight, helps the bones to keep their calcium, and, thus, stay stronger. Several large studies have found that being above the recommended weight for height actually decreases your chance of dying from heart disease, although the mechanisms that allow this to happen are unknown. Similarly, the mechanism that leads to the reduced rate of suicide is also unknown, even very surprising, given the social stigma attached to being "overweight." Also, while one might expect the incidence of depression or other emotional problems to be higher, they are the same for "overweight" as for average-weight people.

Genetic factors, the location of fat on the body, "yo-yo" dieting (with resultant fluctuation in body weight), and intake of fats in food contribute to risk and may be more powerful predictors of mortality and morbidity than is the degree of "overweight." Genetically, predisposition to disease in general is more directly linked to gender (being male) and family history than to weight. In relation to fat distribution on the body, the apple shape (abdominal fat) is associated with greater risk for cardiovascular disease and diabetes mellitus than the pear shape (femoral-gluteal fat) (Bjorntorp 1987). A waist measurement that exceeds the hip measurement increases the likelihood of diabetes and cardiovascular disease to a greater degree than does being "overweight" (Kissebah, Freedman, and Peris 1989).

The high prevalence of dieting in our society has led to the common finding that body weight in adults fluctuates over time, rather than remaining stable. Several investigators have begun to link the "yo-yo" pattern of weight loss and regain to health risks. Six studies have found positive significant correlations between weight fluctuation and death from all causes, and most found the same relationship with heart disease (Lissner and Brownell 1992). The strongest evidence was collected in the Framingham study, a large-scale population study that started with healthy adults, and has been collecting data now for thirty-two years on the same people to identify cardiovascular risks. Lissner and colleagues (1991) found that, in that population, the variability in weight was associated with greater risk of heart disease and death but unrelated to cancer, for men and women. Thus, the risks associated with being "overweight" may be partially, or mostly, those associated with weight fluctuations as a result of repeated dieting. While risk factors for heart disease, diabetes, and some cancers are improved at the initiation of a weight-loss program, the extreme difficulty of maintaining weight and the subsequent regain and rebound may actually increase risk for these illnesses and death, beyond levels associated with a stable high weight. Also, since the period of weight loss is brief, it is impossible to evaluate whether health is actually improved through weight loss for women who have any of those illnesses.

Nutritional intake is a predictor of heart disease and various cancers; however, the measure is not just calories consumed, but amount and type of dietary fat. A high intake of saturated and total fats is associated with increasing risk of coronary disease, and bowel and breast cancer (Health and Welfare Canada 1989).

Ironically, another factor associated with increased health risks for larger women is the fact that they avoid regular preventive medical check-ups and delay seeking medical treatment for problems out of fear of recrimination from health practitioners for "allowing" their weight to be so high. Many have encountered health-care workers who have attributed all existing conditions — from colds to persistent headaches — to weight. Certainly health practitioners are becoming more aware of the ineffectiveness of weight-loss programs and the dangers of dieting, but they retain their misconceptions about health risks associated with being "overweight," and many retain their weight prejudice. We need to move to the point where "helpers" ask women if they are willing to *risk* their health, through dieting, to be thin, rather than suggest that they will *improve* their health through dieting.

In addition to increased risk of cardiovascular disease and death from all causes associated with weight fluctuations, dieting has been implicated in the development of many other problems.

Studies have shown that dieters, during the weight-loss phase, may improve self-esteem and reduce depression. They feel they are doing something positive for themselves, that they are being effective. However, this short-term benefit is offset by the effects of long-term nutritional deprivation, depression, anxiety, anger, mood swings, and binge eating and chronic eating disorders. Moreover, after a period of weight regain, self-esteem, self-confidence, and happiness drop lower than the levels before the weight-loss program was started (Garner and Wooley 1991); the dieter feels that she has failed again, and generalizes this feeling, and repeated cycles lower self-esteem even more.

Each diet changes the body composition as well. Muscle mass is lost and, when weight is regained, it returns as fat. Keys and associates' classic study (1950) of men in semi-starvation showed that, over six months, 25 percent of weight was lost, body fat fell by almost 70 percent and muscle by 40 percent. After the subjects started eating ad lib, weight rebounded to 110 percent, and body fat to 140 percent, of original levels. Thus each diet replaces some muscle mass with fat, making the next weight-loss attempt more difficult.

Clearly, dieting is not risk free. Are the benefits worth the risks? There is little controversy about the ineffectiveness of dieting. Virtually all programs lead to weight loss, but very few people are able to maintain their lower weight. In a review of studies of weight-loss programs with follow-up beyond one year, Kramer and colleagues (1989) found an average weight loss of 7.3 kilograms at the end of the treatment, 5.8 at one year, 5.0 at two years, 3.6 at three years, and 2.4 at four years. Weight loss at the end of these programs was unremarkable and not maintained. While commercial weight-loss clinics sometimes report initial successes, rarely do they report how many people are able to maintain their weight loss over a period of time. Similarly, clinical programs seldom report even a one-year follow-up, but those that do show that about 90 percent of people who enter weight-loss programs have regained the weight they lost by the end of one year. Of those who have gained weight, most gain more than they lost. Only recently have studies appeared that report more favourable results, but the programs in such studies have been extensive (one- to four-year) maintenance programs (Bjorvell and Rossner 1990; Brownell and Jeffery 1987). People who stay in a program for maintenance have been more successful in maintaining some weight loss. However, large drop-out rates are common. Clearly, as well as contributing to health risks, dieting offers virtually no long-term benefits for most people.

WHY DO DIETS FAIL?

Diets fail, but is that failure simply attibutable to lack of willpower? First, diet programs are based on the assumption that "overweight" people overeat, and that weight loss will follow when calorie intake is reduced below bodily needs. However, several studies have shown that there is no difference in quantities of food, speed of eating, bite size, or total caloric intake between "large" people and the general population (Stunkard et al. 1980). Second, because body weight is affected by a variety of factors, including genetic and physiological ones, giving all overweight people the same program is bound to lead to failure.

Evidence exists that supports the theory that body weight is "defended" around a certain predetermined level known as an individual's "set-point." Whether this internal control is genetically determined is still being debated. However, there is agreement that, when an individual tries to go below set-point, metabolic rate (the rate at which one uses up calories) decreases to match the reduction in calorie intake, conserving energy and weight. Similarly, when a person tries to exceed set-point, metabolism speeds up to use calories, and keep weight from increasing. The farther one tries to get from set-point, the more difficult it becomes to lose or gain weight. For those trying to lose weight, metabolism can drop as much as 25 percent; that is, the body uses 25 percent fewer calories during daily activities. This adaptation to lower calorie intake has great survival value during periods of famine; however, it is a source of great frustration to women pursuing the ideal of thinness.

One argument against the set-point theory is based on the fact that some people experience wide fluctuations in weight, as much as 50 kilograms or more, during their adult lives. Such variations may be the result of conscious control, as in extreme overeating, or as in a severe reducing diet, followed by the inevitable weight gain. Or, it may also indicate a failure of the set-point mechanism in stabilizing weight.

Another argument against set-point is that it cannot be directly measured. The closest one can come to identifying an individual's set-point is to base the estimate on an individual's weight during one year of adulthood characterized by moderate physical activity and normal food intake. (One year is considered sufficient time to readjust metabolism following a reducing diet.)

OTHER "TREATMENTS" OF "OVERWEIGHT"

Exercise programs, pharmaceutical interventions, stomach or intestinal surgery, and liposuction are some of the many "treatments" developed for "overweight." Exercise has long been considered an essential component of weight-reduction efforts. It is now evident that, even though the actual calories expended during exercise are minimal, it may help to maintain metabolic rate and muscle mass during low-calorie diet programs. However, exercise will not prevent the fall in metabolic rate that accompanies severe calorie reduction, and is not effective as a sole means for reducing weight. Exercise is a positive addition to weight-loss programs as it has a beneficial effect on fats in the bloodstream, and thus cardiovascular health, as well as on the body's processing of carbohydrates (Calles-Escandon and Horton 1992). However, the same could be said about exercise alone, without the goal of weight loss; not only does it have positive physical effects, but it enhances body appreciation, mood, and self-esteem (Folkins and Sime 1981).

Considerable research is being undertaken on drugs intended to reduce weight primarily through suppressing appetite or increasing metabolism. Although the researchers claim effectiveness, they also point out that drugs currently available are effective only in the short term (one to three months) and that weight regain follows discontinuation of treatment (Bray and Inoue 1992).

Stomach stapling and gastric bypass surgery have been recommended only for the "severely obese" (usually defined as those with a BMI greater than 40). The U.S. National Institutes of Health Consensus Development Conference on Gastrointestinal Surgery for Severe Obesity (1991) indicated that only short- and intermediate-term effects of such surgery have been observed, and long-term effects are unknown. Yet, they concluded that such surgery resulted in substantial weight loss, with lowest weights reached at eighteen to twenty-four months, and some regain within five years. Secondary findings included improvement in many related conditions such as irregular breathing during sleep (sleep apnea), diabetes mellitus, and hypertension. Surgery subjects reported feeling satisfied, content, happier, and more sociable, although the duration of such improvements is unknown. However, not all reported effects were positive: 10 percent or more of surgery patients suffered complications immediately following surgery, such as infection, ulcers and blood clots; others developed later complications, such as nutritional deficiencies, persistent vomiting or abdominal pain, significant late post-operative depression, and failure to lose weight. The Consensus Conference statement concluded that, if there are no coexisting medical problems, a variety of nonsurgical treatments or *no further treatment* (emphasis mine) should be explored before surgery is considered.

Liposuction is not recommended for generalized fat, but rather for "sculpting," for cosmetic treatment of people of average weight who want fat removed from one specific area, such as the neck or thighs (Ersek et al. 1986).

Weight-loss attempts of any kind — dietary, exercise, drugs, or surgery — have proved to have short-term success and intermediate- to long-term failure, with the added insult of a weight rebound above the original starting-point. Weight is predominantly biologically determined, and fat-conserving mechanisms are activated when attempts are made to reduce weight. Weight is distributed on a continuum like height, but we are socially conditioned to find only the lower weight range for weight desirable. But where does that leave women who are not built like models? It is easy to advise about fat acceptance, and even cognitively to agree with it. It is very difficult, however, to accept emotionally and to resist the allure of diet-industry advertising, and to deal with the level of discrimination and self-disparagement that exists. Certainly the anti-dieting movement is growing among both the general public and therapists and health professionals. Where women seeking help would once have found only advice, it should now be possible for them to find support.

◆

RUNNING RISKS:
COMPULSIVE EXERCISE AND EATING DISORDERS

Helen Jefferson Lenskyj

The relationship between women and physical activity is both complex and contradictory. It has taken many decades of women's resistance to put to rest traditional myths of female frailty that medical professionals, clergymen, physical educators, and the popular press began promoting in the late nineteenth century. By the 1970s, two related trends were evident in Canada: more women in the general population were exercising for recreational purposes, and more female athletes were participating in national and international sporting competition.

In the 1980s, with growing awareness of eating disorders among women, debates began to appear in the medical literature over the relationship between "compulsive" or "obligatory" exercise and eating disorders. Concerns were raised about the women with eating disorders who were using recreational physical activity solely for weight-control reasons, as well as the women active in competitive sport who were developing eating disorders. In relation to the sportswomen, several possibilities were raised: that women with a so-called predisposition towards eating disorders were attracted to competitive sport, or that participation in competitive sport triggered or even caused eating disorders, or that both explanations had some validity.

This essay addresses both the problem of eating disorders among competitive female athletes, and the relationship between compulsive exercise and eating disorders among women in the general population who are recreational athletes/exercisers. In discussing the social-cultural context, the two related issues of societal pressure on women towards ultrathinness and abusive and harassing behaviour by male coaches are also examined.

FITNESS, FEMININITY, AND FEMINISM

From the 1970s on, there was growing feminist resistance and activism in two areas that have important implications for an analysis of compulsive exercise and eating disorders: social constructions of femininity and male violence against women.

First, feminists challenged the socially constructed formula of fitness = ultrathinness = heterosexual attractiveness, a formula reinforced by televised exercise programs, media advertising, and fitness fashion. Thinness and (some) muscularity through exercise constituted simply one more "man-made" hoop through which women were expected to jump in order to meet societal standards of what it meant to be attractive to men. For women of all sexual orientations, standards of feminine attractiveness were constructed in a way that favoured thin, white, middle-class women; it was primarily women from this class and race background who had the necessary money and time to devote to exercise for self-improvement purposes.

Second, feminists in the 1970s continued their campaigns against male sexual violence, and there was growing public awareness about the problem of sexual harassment and sexual abuse of girls and women by men in positions of power over them: fathers, teachers, employers, professors, etc. Only in the last few years have male coaches been added to the list of men who may abuse their power and authority over girls and women. Of particular relevance to the issue of eating disorders is sexual harassment on the part of male physical educators, coaches, and instructors, often taking the form of public humiliation and ridicule of girls and women who have not kept within some arbitrarily specified weight range.

Developments in North American women's movements since the 1960s, together with growing general public interest in the benefits of regular physical activity, have contributed to women's increased participation. Within women's self-help health movements, traditional disease models of women's health were challenged, and many women were discovering the empowering effects of sport and physical activity on both the mind and the body. National campaigns promoting regular exercise, such as Participaction, were also responsible for some of the changing attitudes and practices, including women's heightened awareness of the health benefits of regular physical activity.

Despite the impact of the feminist movement(s), many women remained susceptible to the powerful media messages concerning thinness and heterosexual attractiveness. Women who began jogging and taking aerobic exercise classes were often motivated by the promise of quick weight loss in the fitness industry's advertising campaigns. Self-destructive behaviour on the part of physically active women, notably exercise obsession in combination with dangerous eating behaviours, was one outcome of societal pressure on women to achieve thinness through physical activity.

FEMINIST ACTIVISM AND WOMEN'S SPORT ISSUES

In competitive sport, increases in female participation occurred throughout the 1970s and 1980s, aided by the affirmative action programs of provincial and national sports organizations. Lobbying by liberal feminists was a central factor in pushing governments to develop affirmative action programs in sport. Outside of mainstream sport, however, some radical feminists successfully established woman-centred alternatives, such as soccer and softball leagues that were organized on feminist principles and valued recreation, fun, and friendship above winning. Many of these initiatives involved women who were openly lesbian and were attempting to create a lesbian-friendly as well as woman-centred space. Thus, while large numbers of liberal feminists were focusing on equalizing opportunities for girls and women, a smaller group of radical feminists were trying to transform the very nature of competitive sport.

These two distinct political agendas have important implications for a discussion of compulsive exercise and eating disorders. By placing top priority on equalizing opportunities for female athletes, coaches, and administrators, liberal feminists were not necessarily concerned with challenging existing structures and ethics in sport. And so, in the rush to promote equal sporting opportunities for girls and women, many women were uncritical of the traditional male-defined model of competitive sport with its overwhelming emphasis on winning. They paid little attention to the negative impact on athletes' health and well-being posed by the competitive model, or to the problem of male coaches' abuse of power and authority. Nor did they consider the dilemma of the female athlete who worried that the level of muscular development required for her sport would jeopardize her femininity, and hence resorted to dangerous eating behaviours in order to stay thin.

It is unfortunate, but not too surprising, that most feminists with no sporting background have been singularly uninterested in sex equality in sport. Perhaps they see no great merit in producing a female Ben Johnson or John McEnroe, or in becoming part of a system that commodifies and controls the bodies of high-performance athletes. However, if feminist transformation of sport is to occur, either from within or from outside the current system, feminists need to acknowledge that some women simply want access to the same opportunities as men — that is, some women see this as a human rights issue — while others share the goal of transforming sport to make it more humane and more enjoyable for all participants.

WOMEN'S BODIES AND COMPETITIVE SPORT

Activities that we know as "sport" have long been defined and controlled by men, with male anatomy and physiology held up as the standard by which to judge all human performance. The Olympic goals — swifter, higher, stronger — define sporting excellence. Success in sports defined in this way is directly related to low body weight, high lean body mass, and optimal muscular development.

Partly as a challenge to these malestream definitions, women have been working towards greater public acceptance of sports that are evaluated on aesthetic appeal, where skill, grace, coordination, and flexibility are valued more than speed, strength, and endurance. It is therefore ironic that the pressure towards ultrathinness is especially strong for female athletes in these aesthetic activities, notably gymnastics, figure skating, synchronized swimming, and dance. Athletes who compete in these activities are evaluated for both technical and artistic merit. In terms of technique, thinness may enhance performance, because a lighter body can move through space more quickly, while the artistic component is evaluated by many judges in terms of the "thinness = heterosexual attractiveness" equation. Adolescent girls who are not athletes average 20–25 percent body fat, while girls in gymnastics, ballet, or figure skating are often urged to reduce body fat to less than 10 percent. Even outside of aesthetic sports, pressure to reduce to 10 percent is experienced by female nordic skiers and distance runners ("The 10 Percent Dilemma" 1987).

Females as a group have a higher percentage of body fat than males. A difference in body fat of approximately 9 percent is also found between male and female athletes within a particular sport. In addition to differences related to the sex of the athlete and the nature of the sport, ethnicity and age have been identified as variables in fatness and fat patterning. The association of certain body types with certain racial/ethnic groups means, for example, that people from one background tend to be tall and muscular, while those from another tend to be short and sturdy. In terms of maturation, the onset of puberty affects fat patterning: for example, young women develop breasts and hips, and a higher body-fat level overall. There is, however, a wide variation for both sexes across all sports. For example, female and male field athletes (in throwing events such as discus, javelin, and shot put) have 23.9 percent and 15.6 percent body fat, respectively — levels that are close to those of the average nonathlete — while the figures for distance runners are 15.7 percent and 5 percent (Drinkwater 1984; Mueller, Shoup, and Malina 1982; Sady and Freedman 1984).

The high body-fat levels in female distance swimmers aid in buoyancy and thermoregulation (regulation of body temperature), especially in open-water distance swimming where the body has to contend with cold water for long periods of time. The low body-fat level of female distance runners, on the other hand, is an important factor in a sport that requires moving the body through space. Thus, body composition is a factor determining suitability for particular sports, and, conversely, participation in these sports may contribute to developing and maintaining a certain body fat level.

As well as body composition, somatotype (body type) may be a factor in selecting a sport, and participation in that sport may, in turn, influence body type. For example, athletic training may promote muscularity in a mesomorphic (muscular) body type. In the case of prepubescent female athletes, strenuous physical training may delay menarche (onset of puberty), and the limbs may grow longer during this extended growth period. (After puberty, growth in the long bones of the arms and legs stops.)

Research on body composition has tended to focus on high-performance athletes, and these studies have generated prescriptions for "ideal" body types and "ideal" fat levels for particular sports. The formula for the ideal distance runner, for example, is calculated in terms of height/weight ratio, and since height is fixed, weight reduction is the only option. In most female sports where speed is paramount, weight loss is a taken-for-granted route to improving one's time.

Even among elite athletes or dancers, however, there are exceptions: highly successful individuals whose physiques and fat levels differ from what is considered ideal for their activity. Therefore, a different body type need not be a deterrent, since it is only one of many factors contributing to athletic competence and enjoyment. More important, the overemphasis on the ideal body type for success in high-performance sport needs to be challenged. Clearly, the vast majority of girls and women are not on the road to becoming high-performance athletes, and they would be well advised to select sports that are compatible with their interests and priorities, as well as their physical abilities.

EATING DISORDERS AND SPORT

Girls and women who lack the "ideal" body for a particular sport or physical activity are at higher risk of developing eating disorders than are the small minority whose bodies are a close-to-perfect fit, according to current definitions. For example, in classical dance, the "ideal" physical requirements are very narrowly defined, and studies have shown that companies with early and stringent selection processes (and rejection and dropout rates of up to 95 percent) retained young women who, for a variety of genetic and physiological reasons, could maintain an "ideal" weight without resorting to dieting or dangerous eating behaviours (Hamilton et al. 1988).

Obviously, it could be argued that the sport rather than players needs to be changed if so few women are suited to it. Like figure skating, synchronized swimming, and gymnastics, dance is a spectacle sport that has evolved in accordance with audiences' and judges' subjective evaluations of "aesthetic excellence." In contrast, there are alternative modern dance troupes that value female dancers' skills in interpretation and expressiveness above the values of traditional dance. Women with a wider range of body types can successfully participate in these kinds of dance.

There is clearly a need to challenge traditional values in sport. To "win at all costs" is the prevailing ethic in the world of sport, as the recent Dubin Inquiry into steroid use among Olympic athletes clearly demonstrated. It could be argued that training regimens for high-performance sport both produce and reinforce obsessive/compulsive behaviour in the two related areas of eating and exercise. The social context of competitive sport is an ideal breeding ground for the development of eating-disordered behaviour. In this environment, the development of a lean body and control over caloric intake are actively encouraged by peers and authority figures, especially coaches. Self-deprivation — physical, social, and sexual — is valued and enforced, and it is not coincidental that similar self-depriving behaviours are exhibited by individuals with eating disorders. Severe limitations on athletes' social life and leisure time are imposed, and in many situations, high-performance athletes forfeit their individual freedoms for the alleged good of the team (Eberts and Kidd 1985; Smith 1980). All these factors contribute to the overall vulnerability of young women in competitive sport.

Furthermore, girls' and women's socialization into the sporting subculture, as well as heavy training schedules, isolate them from their nonathlete peers and thus limit the possibilities of consciousness-raising around women's issues or issues of worker exploitation. The world of competitive sport often frames their entire existence, and they have difficulty seeing themselves either as women or as workers in the sport industry. In Canada, for example, high-performance athletes receive a minimal subsidy from the federal government on which they are expected to survive financially; in turn, they forfeit a number of basic human rights when they become "carded" athletes. However, given the glamour associated with this level of sporting competition, it is difficult for these athletes to view themselves as workers, employed (and controlled and exploited) for the purpose of bringing home medals and enhancing Canada's reputation as a "winner" in the world of international sport.

WOMAN-CENTRED ALTERNATIVES

A number of research studies have demonstrated gender-related trends that have probably been obvious to many parents, physical educators, and recreation leaders for decades. There are significant gender differences in relation to priorities, interests, and values in sport. Girls and women tend to value fun and friendship, along with benefits to health and fitness, while boys and men focus on winning and improving their performance (Lenskyj 1993). This does not mean that there are no highly competitive girls and women, but it does suggest that the values and priorities of the average male coach may be dramatically different from those of the girls and women he coaches. Thus, female coaches with some feminist consciousness would be more appropriate for female athletes.

More important, in women's hands, women's sport could be transformed, But, as noted above, given the generally liberal perspective of those few women in sport who identify themselves as feminists, there appears to be a general acceptance of existing power relations and practices. There is a pressing need for women athletes and coaches to develop a critical consciousness of their oppression and exploitation as women and as workers in the sport industry. Developing such consciousness would better equip women who choose the route of competitive sport to challenge the win-at-all-costs ethos, to redefine what is sporting success, and to resist pressure towards dangerous eating behaviours.

EATING DISORDERS AND EXERCISE:

DEBATES IN THE RESEARCH

The first articles on the problem of eating disorders among female athletes appeared in medical journals and in the professional literature for physical educators and coaches in the late 1970s, but only in the last five years has the problem received widespread attention in these circles. Although the vast majority of athletes with eating disorders are girls and women, it should be noted that there is a serious problem among male college wrestlers, who are pressured to "make weight" in order to fit a particular weight category for wrestling competition. Few research studies take race and ethnicity into account; hence, it is important to note that, while eating disorders among the nonathletic population have, until recently, tended to be concentrated among white, middle-class females, the high representation of Black females in sports such as track and field is likely to affect this trend within the athletic population (Hamilton et al. 1986).

Research findings are diverse and contradictory. Studies have shown that female gymnasts, dancers, and distance runners are likely to engage in dangerous eating behaviours. However, these behaviours were also found among female athletes in sports such as field hockey, tennis, softball, volleyball, and track, where appearance is not evaluated, and where thinness bears less relation to athletic success (Black and Burckes-Miller 1988; Rosen and Hough 1988; Teskey 1986). It has also been reported that there is no higher incidence of dangerous eating behaviours or anorexia nervosa among a representative sample of female marathoners than among the general population. A study of three groups of adolescent females showed that although the athlete group and the student group showed anorexic-like behaviours (dieting and body dissatisfaction), both had significantly higher self-images than the eating-disordered group (Mallick, Whipple, and Huerta 1987; Weight and Noakes 1987).

A number of studies have shown that overestimation of body weight is a defining characteristic of individuals who are anorexic, and so this single measure has been used to differentiate anorexic and nonanorexic subjects. For example, one study of runners reported significant underestimation of body weight, leading the investigators to claim that these runners were not anorexic (Siegel, Stewart, and Barone 1990).

Conflicting findings have led researchers to question the reliability of the various self-image and body image scales, most of which were not designed specifically for an athlete population

(Campbell 1985). Many scales are also blatantly heterosexist in nature, with questions about attitudes and attraction to the opposite sex that fail to address the fact that at least 10 percent of those surveyed are lesbian or gay. There is a clear need for qualitative research in order to understand the complex interplay of factors at work.

There has been extensive debate over the hypothesis that certain sports attract athletes with so-called anorexic personalities, and that compulsive athletes, especially compulsive distance runners, display the same traits as individuals with anorexia nervosa: for example, preoccupation with food, body size and bodily functions, and ritualistic self-denial and self-discipline. A controversial article in the *New England Journal of Medicine* titled "Running: An Analogue of Anorexia Nervosa?" (Yates, Leehey, and Shisslak 1983) sparked dozens of studies designed to disprove this link. Some of the rebuttals made illuminating references to "normal" runners, as opposed to individuals with anorexia nervosa, thus disassociating runners from any taint of abnormality or "disease." Similarly, they spoke of "normal" training and obsessive exercise behaviour as if the two were poles apart (Blumenthal, O'Toole, and Chang 1984; Siegel, Stewart, and Barone 1990).

Any of the biographical accounts of everyday life as an Olympic athlete will dispel the notion that training for high-performance sport constitutes a "normal" life (e.g., Brill 1986; Clarke and Gywnne-Timothy 1988; Issajenko 1990). Profound self-deprivation and competitive drive characterized these women's sporting experiences, and the monitoring of their activities — eating, sleeping, training — was as much a function of self-policing as it was of external pressure by coaches and peers.

Some more reasoned discussions of eating disorders and compulsive exercise called for a distinction between exercise as an end in itself and exercise as a means to an end. Researchers noted that physical activity, while a valued social behaviour in many contexts, may become a symptom of anorexia nervosa when carried to extremes. Others contrasted "adaptative" behaviour, where endurance athletes restrict caloric intake to achieve "optimal body weight for maximal performance," with maladaptive behaviour where subsequent loss of lean body mass led to diminished performance. They admitted, however, that there was a "subtle boundary" between the two (Fleishmann and Siegel 1983; Moriarty and Moriarty 1986).

EXERCISE MOTIVATION AND BEHAVIOUR: A PROPOSED FEMINIST MODEL

In keeping with feminist analyses of women's eating behaviours, it is useful to consider a continuum as a way of making sense of a range of human behaviour and motivation regarding exercise. This approach avoids the normal/pathological dichotomy inherent in traditional disease-model approaches. Exercise behaviour can be placed on a continuum ranging from healthy to dangerous, with obsessive/compulsive behaviour at the dangerous extreme. Similarly, on the continuum of exercise motivation, reasons range from process-oriented (exercise for its own sake) to goal-oriented (exercise as a means to an end, e.g., weight reduction). Given societal pressure on women to be thin, in combination with guilt over perceived overweight, it is likely that stated reasons for exercise motivation may vary significantly from real reasons. The two continua can be viewed as intersecting rather than parallel. For example, goal-oriented exercise (improving one's running time) can be achieved by healthy exercise behaviour (a moderate program with flexible goals) or by unhealthy behaviour (training every day, regardless of injuries, weather, health).

Gymnastics is one of the aesthetic sports that poses particular hazards to girls and young women. With the advent of the Korbut/Komaneci style of Olympic gymnastics in the 1970s came a new image of the female gymnast: a prepubescent body, with no noticeable breasts or hips. Aside from the illicit methods allegedly used in some countries — puberty-delaying drugs, for example —

to keep gymnasts thin, there was a relatively simple means by which a coach could manipulate an androgynous body type. Extreme dieting would ensure that a girl's body weight and body fat remained below the level necessary for the onset of puberty, and thus would delay the development of a mature female body, with breasts, hips, and more body fat than the prepubescent girl (Hargreaves 1984).

The power differential between male coaches and female athletes gives rise to specific problems in relation to eating disorders. Male coaches, in their double role as instructor and male authority figure, exert considerable influence over female athletes' eating behaviours. The pressure to conform and the socially constructed desire to gain male approval may make young female athletes particularly vulnerable. Male coaches who publicly criticize girls and women for failing to stay within some arbitrary weight range, or even those who make casual references to weight, may precipitate dangerous weight control behaviours. Some coaches go far beyond casual references. Many girls and women experience abusive coaches who publicly ridicule and humiliate them by having public weigh-ins each week and maintaining a "fat list" of offenders posted on the gym wall. In our weight-preoccupied society, even the most assertive girls and women are vulnerable to these kinds of humiliating tactics. Of the large number of articles on athletes' eating disorders in the professional journals of the last decade reviewed here, only one drew attention to the problem of public weigh-ins and called for an end to this practice (Thompson 1987).

Research studies show that, while most coaches seemed concerned about the issue, only a few reported awareness of actual problems of eating disorders among the girls and women they coached, perhaps because they did not know what signs and symptoms to look for. Indeed, dieting is so commonplace among girls and women both inside and outside sport that coaches would probably perceive it as "normal" behaviour. Well-meaning but uninformed coaches should discontinue all practices that might trigger eating-disordered behaviours; for example, overemphasizing weight or body fat; telling athletes they will perform better if they are leaner; and assigning unrealistic weight goals (Kloss 1989). They need, first of all, to understand that pressures on girls and women — both inside and outside sport — may lead to dangerous eating behaviours. They need to provide sound nutritional advice for athletes, and to maintain strict confidentiality and sensitivity regarding athletes' weight, body shape, and possible eating problems. Most important, they need to advise athletes with eating disorders to seek out appropriate, woman-centred clinics and counseling services, since it is unlikely that coaches themselves will be adequately equipped to provide such counseling. However, those female coaches who are familiar with feminist analyses of eating disorders, and who themselves experience societal pressure to be thin, may have greater understanding and empathy than their male counterparts.

Increasingly, the professional literature calls for coaches to exercise constant vigilance over female athletes for purposes of early identification and intervention regarding eating disorders (Moriarty and Moriarty 1986; Stephenson 1991). Although intervention is undoubtedly important, this recommendation is not without problems. There is disturbing evidence that male coaches, like men who have power and authority over girls and women in other social settings, commit acts of sexual violence against female athletes. There is also evidence of more subtle controlling and psychologically abusive behaviour on the part of male coaches (Crosset 1990; Donnelly 1986; Lackey 1990). For these reasons, any recommendation that increases male power and authority over girls and young women should be viewed with extreme caution.

Some recommendations in the professional literature regarding coaches' surveillance of female athletes constitute clear breaches of privacy, regardless of the gender of the coach. For example, since amenorrhea (cessation of menstrual periods) is one symptom of anorexia nervosa, coaches are commonly advised to check up on the menstrual status of athletes whom they suspect are suffering from an eating disorder (Romeo 1984; Stephenson 1991, p. 134).

(Ironically, this very same kind of monitoring by physical educators was recommended in the 1920s as a way of ensuring that young women did not take part in any strenuous activity while they were suffering from their monthly "disability" [Lenskyj 1986].) While it is, of course, true that menstruation is a normal bodily function that should not arouse embarrassment, it is clearly inappropriate for the coach to investigate menstrual irregularities arising from eating disorders or from any other cause.

PHYSICAL ACTIVITY AND WEIGHT CONTROL

There are numerous studies of the benefits of exercise for women's health and for weight control. Although there is some disagreement, most mainstream scientific research asserts that obesity poses health risks: high blood pressure and high cholesterol levels increase risk of coronary heart disease, and high blood-sugar levels are associated with diabetes. However, there is evidence that larger women are at lower risk of cancer and osteoporosis, and some medical researchers are beginning to question long-standing assumptions of the dire health risks of large body size and existing methodologies for determining what is, in fact, healthy weight. Since it has been estimated that 80 percent of body size has genetic origins, a different approach to these issues is clearly needed (Stunkard et al. 1986).

Regular physical activity, in combination with caloric restriction, has long been recommended as a strategy for weight loss. Whether or not changes in body weight occur, there are other important beneficial results of exercise, including increased lean body mass (i.e., fat-free tissue), decreased blood pressure, and improved cardiovascular efficiency. Increases in lean body mass are not necessarily accompanied by weight loss, since increases in muscle mass may offset decreases in body fat. Equally important, regular physical activity can promote physical fitness and psychological well-being, and has been shown to have a significant effect in alleviating depression, and premenstrual and menopause-related problems (McCann and Holmes 1984; Prior and Vigna 1987).

PHYSICAL ACTIVITY AND LARGER WOMEN

The growth of the fitness industry in the 1980s has had a mixed impact on women who identify themselves as large or fat; this category is likely to include many women who currently have, or in the past have suffered from an eating disorder, notably bulimia. On the positive side, affordable exercise programs are now available for women with limited financial resources in most urban centres. On the negative side, the trend towards ultrathinness has often been reinforced by instructors' overemphasis on weight loss through aerobic exercise. As Bain and her colleagues point out, "if instructors or participants in an exercise class interpret a healthy lifestyle as a moral issue, they may judge the obese person as morally inferior," thus exacerbating the problem of "fat prejudice" (Bain, Wilson, and Chaikind 1989). The potentially devastating effects on women suffering from bulimia are obvious: their deficiencies are not only physical but also moral, according to this line of reasoning.

Factors contributing to fat women's continued participation in an exercise class include a nonjudgemental instructor and a climate of social support, achieved by stable group membership, opportunities for discussion, and protection from "spectators." Flexibility in individual daily goals and collaborative program planning involving professionals and clients were also important (Bain, Wilson, and Chaikind 1989; Jaffee, Lutter, and Straiton 1990; Robinson 1985). There are some pioneering woman-centred fitness programs in the United States and Canada, conducted by and for fat women, where the major emphasis is on fun, friendship, and the joy of movement. These initiatives are also sensitive to the special situation of Native women and women of colour, who are likely to suffer discrimination in the workplace and community, and may have limited financial resources. For example, a time is set aside when the facilities are only used by Muslim women and their children, and classes are free of charge. Small-group settings promote a self-help approach to problems of self-esteem, control, and body image, and aerobic exercise designed specifically for "overweight" women is an important component of this model (Lyons 1989).

These woman-centred programs for fat women have important implications for all fitness instructors. Approximately 25 percent of women with anorexia nervosa are extremely athletic and it has been estimated that 50 percent of women with eating disorders use exercise for weight loss purposes. The Canada Fitness Survey (1984) reported that 51 percent of all women and girls (over age ten) are physically active for the purpose of weight control (Leon 1984; Moriarty and Moriarty 1986). Therefore, it is certain that a fitness instructor will encounter significant numbers of women whose sole purpose for participating is weight loss, whether or not they suffer from an eating disorder.

Fitness leaders may be able to change these attitudes and behaviours by making it clear that the focus of the class is health and fun, not competitiveness and weight loss. Class discussions of nutrition and eating disorders, including debunking of the "thin = fit, fat = unfit" myths, are valuable. The leader herself can provide a positive example if she maintains a healthy weight rather than striving to be ultrathin. Similarly, in her appearance, clothing, and leadership style, she can actively challenge the "Barbie Doll" image of the fitness instructor promoted by televised fitness shows and the fitness fashion industry. Community-based recreation programs for women can also counter these commercial trends by implementing "affirmative action" hiring of fitness instructors: women who represent a range of body types and racial and ethnic backgrounds, rather than only women who are ultrathin, white, and heterosexually attractive.

CONCLUSION

The preceding discussion demonstrates how links between exercise, sport, and eating disorders are reinforced in a society that objectifies women's bodies and equates thinness with fitness and heterosexual attractiveness. Any recommendations addressing the problem of eating disorders among women who are competitive or recreational athletes need to take this social context into account.

The empowerment of girls and women is central; the purpose is not to enhance male coaches' power and authority. This process needs to start long before the young female athlete is socialized into the traditional sporting subculture, with its overemphasis on winning no matter what the cost to athletes' bodies and minds. Similarly, for the girls and women who use physical activity as a means to an end, namely, weight loss, the route to empowerment needs to emphasize the sheer pleasure of physical movement as an end in itself, and as a component of holistic self-actualization.

◆

¡DELICIOSA!
THE BODY, PASSION, AND PLEASURE

Farah M. Shroff

Feasting
Do you eat to live?
Do you live to eat?
Do you have sex to reproduce?
Do you have sex to make love?
Are you a good girl?
Are you a bad girl?
Do you exercise self-control when eating?
Do you act discreetly about your sexuality?
Say yes and you're a good girl ....

The body and its appetites for food and sex are regulated in all societies. Today's emphasis on slimness in the Western world requires that women control their appetite for food rather than enjoy it as a source of pleasure. It is interesting that this occurs at the same time as an apparent freeing of women's sexual appetites. Women's bodies, including their appetites, have typically been a battleground in patriarchal societies. This essay offers some thoughts on the regulation of women's bodies and ends by encouraging the celebration of women's bodies and the fulfilling of women's appetites and pleasures. *Deliciosa*, a Spanish word, expresses exultation of food, sensuous and sexual experiences, and women.

THE FEMALE BODY AS BATTLEGROUND

Women strive to meet standards for their bodies in terms of shape, size, amount of hair, scent, and skin colour. These norms vary by historical epoch and from place to place, but in most patriarchal cultures, women have many reasons to be dissatisfied with their bodies, as the "ideal" body is attainable by so few. In many African and South Asian cultures, an "ideal" woman is buxom and curvaceous. Her build is ample and voluptuous — in the "right" places. Hindi films depict heroines in this fashion, and thin women rarely obtain lead roles as they do not meet the socially defined norms of beauty. Additionally, women in countries such as India have to contend with colonized mentalities that dictate that fairer skin is more attractive than dark skin. Fair-skinned women are more desirable as brides, according to prevailing ideology, and finding a husband is the most important aspect of a woman's life, according to popularized norms. Indian folk songs praise the virtues of light-skinned women with dark hair. Bleaching of skin is fairly common in some parts of the world, as is bleaching of facial hair. Even women whose bodies are completely veiled most of the time are subjected to hair bleaching, waxing, and threading (a way of removing fine body hair.

In most agrarian societies of Europe, too, the ideal female body type has been a "substantial" and relatively fair-skinned one. Where food is scarce, a larger woman is sought after. When food is plentiful, a thinner woman seems to be sought after — one reason why anorexia nervosa and bulimia are more prevalent among women in the privileged worlds. Losing weight is their obsession, while gaining weight is a desire of many women in the colonized worlds. However, faced with multiple oppressions, those from the colonized worlds are unlikely to make weight gain for the sake of body image a priority over getting food on the table. Economic deprivation, fueled by classism and racism under capitalism and imperialism, are obviously more immediate struggles for some women. For working-class women in the privileged worlds, there is a concern both for getting enough high-quality, as opposed to inexpensive non-nutritious, food and for maintaining a thin body because being thin facilitates upward mobility for women.

The social regulation of women's body size and shape strongly affects the regulation of women's appetites for food, but it is not the only factor affecting such regulation. Fundamentally, the consumption of food is necessary for the survival of both the individual and the species, just as sex leading to reproduction is necessary for the survival of the species. However, all human societies govern the consuming of food and the practice of sex through rules, taboos, and mores, which are applied differentially to men and women. Appetites for food and sex are hence also socially regulated, and patriarchal societies tend to characterize women's appetites as dangerous and to act as suppressants of them. As a result, women's practices in relation to both eating and sex, and their sense of identity as gendered beings, are affected. For example, a woman in North America who has a hearty appetite for food is likely to seen as unfeminine.

In some patriarchal cultures, certain foods are denied to women through religious taboos. Often these are foods with high protein content that are saved for men (Asian and Pacific Women's Resource Collection Network 1989). Historically, in Europe and North America, the largest portion of the meat served at a meal was divided among the males and given to the females only if there was enough to go around. Both these practices run contrary to the fact that women in their reproductive years need to be strong and healthy to produce strong and healthy offspring.

In Western Europe and North America, an enormous dieting industry emerged during the post-industrial era. The dieting pundits and their kissing-cousins (the aerobics industry, cosmetic surgery, and the advertising industry) assist in creating anxieties for women, then supplying "solutions" to such socially constructed anxieties. Eating such foods as chocolate, ice cream, and other socially constructed "treats" induces guilt in women. The constant commercial bombarding of consumers with images depicting the deliciousness of these foods makes them into "temptations" that women are supposed to show strength and control by avoiding. Failure to avoid temptation and its consequent guilt is "paid for" through dieting. Food for women is thus sanctioned exclusively in relation to nutrition, growth, and sustenance. The dieting industry, reinforced by social agencies (Hollywood, some electronic and print media, and so on), benefits from the creation of several generations of female dieters who unwittingly support these huge capitalist interests.

Women who are singularly focused on weight loss do not have much time left over for struggling against the forces that oppress them. They are too busy complying with commercially created "needs" for certain dieting products. Patriarchal and capitalist control are maintained in this way. Even women in positions of relative authority are judged according to the way they look. For some women, the body is thus the last frontier of struggle against male domination.

Women's sexuality too has been mythologized and socially regulated. In traditional Judaeo-Christian mythology, women's appetites for food and sex are seen as temptations that need to be controlled. Biblical imagery of Eve eating the forbidden fruit and becoming aware of nudity and sexuality makes a well-known link between the appetites for food and sex. Popular notions of "wine, women, and song" communicate the idea of women as pleasures to be consumed by men, showing the contradictory position women find themselves in. Women are, on the one hand, a source of male pleasure and, on the other, "bad" when they tempt male appetites; in fact, they are seen as responsible for the unleashing of those appetites. In addition, women experience the contradictory aspects of power and powerlessness that their bodies bring. There are, at once, power and pleasure in tempting male appetites and extreme vulnerability in the inability to control the effects of such temptation. Simultaneously, women are expected to constrain their own appetites and pleasures.

In Western societies today, women are permitted, even encouraged, to enjoy non-reproductive sex, but not without a cost. Widespread marketing of the birth control pill and concomitant social changes during the 1960s freed some women by providing them with choice about pregnancy — let loose, enjoy, and take part in the "sexual revolution" was the message. However, the pill also made the female body more available to men by removing the possibility of pregnancy as an obstacle to male-female intimacy, leaving women with no "legitimate" reason to say "no" to sex.

Notions of "sex as sin" continue to make it difficult for women, heterosexual, lesbian or bisexual, to enjoy their sexuality and to admit to finding pleasure in it. Religious and other institutions endorse messages of shame about the female body, making it difficult for women to openly discuss issues regarding their bodies. Sexual expression is thus often associated with guilt. Like social control of the appetite for food, the contradictory aspects of the regulation of women's sexual appetite result in the traumatization and control of women and make it difficult to fight back.

Finally, the connections between heterosexual sex and violence are glamourized through movies, magazines, and television, while the lived violence of date rape, domestic battering of women by their male partners, incest, sexual assault, and other forms of sexualized violence against women is minimized. Women are encouraged to make themselves sexually attractive and vulnerable in a social context which is not sexually safe for women.

FEASTING

She doesn't eat to live.
She doesn't live to eat.

She eats to satisfy her body's physical needs, to put sweetness on her tongue, to feel warmth in her body, to feel coolness in her body, to be with others in a festive, sharing way.

She lives to celebrate, to dance, to think, to love, to
learn, to teach, to grow, to be connected....

THE FEMALE BODY AS BLISS

Decoding, demystifying, and deconstructing some of the characteristics of oppressive hierarchies may be useful ways of understanding
the world in which we live. What comes next? Feminism encourages women's empowerment through body-image liberation. It is
empowering for women to make decisions about their bodies and
appetites that are based on their own needs.

A woman who accepts her own body, whatever size, shape, or
colour it is, is a woman who is resisting some of aspects of patriarchy, heterosexism, racism, and capitalism. For instance, it means
not being a compliant consumer of packaged images and products,
and not being afraid of taking up space in a "skinny" society. It
means allowing herself the power and pleasure of her own desires
and appetites.

This kind of liberation cannot be realized in a political vacuum.
Social structures that feed off women's subordination must be
changed. This is not to say that it is impossible for individual
women to feel content in their bodies before "the revolution."
There are many pathways to feeling better about the body.
Counseling, therapy, journal writing, visual art, dance, long walks,
and dream interpretation are a few of the ways which women may
choose to help themselves. These may be vehicles through which
women express their pain and come to some reconciliation about
their feelings regarding their bodies.

As a woman of South Asian descent, I feel that part of the
political project of freeing the body is related to decolonizing the
mind, in concert with others, and beginning to value aspects of our
heritage and its world-views. For example, seeing the body as separate from the mind and spirit, as has been typical in Western thinking, has led to separations of human and the earth, of man and
woman. A richer more integrated approach to understanding the
body is possible, as is provided by Indian science.

A holistic world-view is evidenced in Ayurvedic medicine, a system of Indian medicine with a 6,000 year history; yoga; and meditation. Yoga literally means "to join." Joining the mind, body, and spirit is a major goal of these practices. One fundamental premise upon which they operate is that the human being is a microcosm of the universe. In Ayurveda, the concept of *panchamahbutas* states that everything in the universe is composed of five elements: earth, fire, air, water, and ether. Different combinations of these elements form the basic building blocks of all life. All beings are thus connected to each other and to the earth/sky/waters, as the same elements make up our bodies, and *kalapas* (tiny subatomic particles — conceptualized in Vipassana meditation theory) are vibrating within each of us.

Such a "joining" or holistic world-view helps open the way for experiences of body deliciousness in women's lives. Through various practices of Ayurveda, yoga, or meditation, it is possible to achieve a state of balance. In this state of equilibrium and equanimity, it is possible to feel positive about the deliciousness of the body, and about the food that nourishes it.

Erotic art, tantric yoga, and the *Kama Sutra* are positive ways in which sexuality has been expressed, although they have been interpreted using patriarchal and heterosexual lenses. Erotic portraits of passionate love can be a positive alternative to images of female brutalization in pornography, commercial advertising, and other impressions of the female body. Lesbian love is also portrayed in some erotic art. Ancient carvings display polyerotic sexual expressions of women — women love, vibrant ecstatic love scenes, and love-making in many different positions. The *Kama Sutra* offers helpful suggestions to lovers, advising numerous ways to kiss, to hold, and to reach orgasm. Reclaiming those life-enhancing ways of feeling the body can be a part of body liberation. Each woman may look into her own background, and that of others, to find ways of synthesizing a political and holistic vision of the body which suits her, to feel truly embodied.

A critical analysis of the ways in which women's bodies are regulated is a powerful step towards body-image liberation. Another step is to implement creative, bold ideas to replace those that currently prevail.

Pleasure, passion and joy are possible! Feminist anti-racist struggle necessitates a vision of the possible. Change is possible now, in the personal and social arenas. Women are not only victims: we can resist the forces that oppress us, the voices that tell us to eat in certain ways and love in certain ways. It is possible to affirm what feels right, to enjoy polyerotic expressions, in the unique and diverse ways each woman experiences the power, pleasure, and passion of her appetites.

THE SYSTEM

It drains distorts distends distresses dis-eases discourages
disembodies
Transnational corporations, the work force, the media
It all works to undermine those of us under
its claws.

We must resist
by fighting
By thriving

Not in spite
But out of our own place
Of ourselves

Connection
With our bodies
With our spirits
With kindred spirits
With the earth

With all life
Rhythms of life
Rhythms of our bodies

Feeling our moon time
The waves of orgasm(s)
The waves of hunger
Gestation time
Girl to elder
The rhythms of our lives

Rhythms of the earth
The seasons roll
The earth's fertility
The tides
Young forest mature forest climax forest new forest

The rhythms of our bodies
The rhythms of the earth
Are audible tastable touchable feelable
Listen! Taste! Touch! Feel!
The deliciousness of womanhood

✦

· II ·

COUNSELING

INTRODUCTION

FEMINIST THERAPY:
POWER, ETHICS, AND CONTROL

Catrina Brown

Today many feminist writings explore why most women are preoccupied with their weight and why some become anorexic and bulimic; however, very little instruction exists for those who wish to take a feminist approach to working with women with eating disorders. Even those who have already adopted a feminist, or woman-centred approach need to consider what it means to do specifically feminist clinical work within the continuum of weight preoccupation issues women experience. As is usually the case with feminist therapy, issues of power and control are pivotal. In the case of eating disorders, feeling out of control is a central aspect of the problem. Thus, a feminist approach to working with weight-preoccupation issues must be committed to the belief that women need to feel in control of when and how they give up their eating disorder. In that feminist therapy must emphasize women controlling and directing their own changes, it then focuses on empowerment and self-direction.

THE EMERGENCE OF A FEMINIST MODEL OF INTERVENTION

In the 1970s feminists began to think about how a feminist understanding of women's issues translated into a feminist practice. Feminists have explored the possibilities of incorporating feminist process in all areas of feminist practice, including conducting meetings, running organizations, teaching, research methodology, ethics, and therapy. Feminist therapy, or woman-centred counseling, evolved in response to feminist critiques of traditional modes of treating women's experiences and problems as diseases and pathology. Feminism challenged the dominance of the psychiatric paradigm and the medical model as reflecting the interests of a male-dominant status quo and reinforcing the existing asymmetrical power relations between men and women. Hence, the medical or disease model typically employed by psychiatry was rejected as an oppressive way to deal with women's problems. Through critiques of the psychiatric paradigm, women-centred analyses of women's problems began to emerge. In 1972, Phyllis Chesler's now classic book *Women and Madness* lent support and documentation to feminist concerns about the control and subjugation of women through the labeling of their experiences and problems as mental disorders. Later feminist inquiries into this subject, such as Dorothy Smith and Sarah David's *I'm Not Mad, I'm Angry: Women Look at Psychiatry* (1975) and Susan Penfold and Gillian Walker's *Women and the Psychiatric Paradox* (1983), continued to object to the psychiatrization of women. Medical sociologists and other critics challenged traditional notions of madness, arguing that defining behaviours as psychiatric disorders is often a social response to "deviance" and acts as an oppressive form of social control. Drawing upon these critiques, feminist therapy, which emphasizes empowerment and social change, emerged to provide alternative services to women.[1]

Rather than examining the social origins of women's problems in a patriarchal society, the disease model focuses on what is wrong with the individual, often prescribing drugs or institutionalization, without regard for the underlying causes of the problem. Feminists have criticized the medical model for not addressing women's real concerns, not hearing what women really had to say. Its solutions were seen to silence and pacify women, to submerge our anger and protest, and rarely to effect change in women's situations or actual lives. Women's anger and protests were too often defined as depression, manic depression, schizophrenia, or borderline personality disorder. Traditionally, a great deal of emphasis is placed on the labeling and diagnosis of diseases through the application of the diagnostic criteria of the American Psychiatric Association's *Diagnostic and Statistical Manual of Mental Disorders (DSM-III-R)*. This focus has permitted the male-dominated spheres of psychiatry and mental-health services in general to manage and control women's behaviour. Women began to organize and speak out against the mental-health services they received. Indeed, many women felt that their problems were exacerbated by the help they tried to get; moreover, some have felt that they have been revictimized by the "mental-health" system.

The principles of feminist therapy need not be reviewed here in detail, but I would like to suggest that they centre on two things in particular: issues of power and control, and recognition of women's diverse experiences of oppression within patriarchal society. By placing women's experiences in this context, we move away from a model that blames the "victim" and focuses on individual pathology and disease. Instead, we attempt to understand women's pain and problems through the knowledge that the "personal is political." Women often develop creative ways of coping with psychological distress and their feelings of powerlessness in society. Rather than emphasizing or focusing on changing the "symptoms," feminist therapy tries to hear the voice that speaks through the symptoms. And, through this approach, feminist therapy accepts and normalizes the problem: it avoids judging, trivializing, or sensationalizing the symptoms. The feminist therapist strives to establish empathy with the client and, where it is felt to be helpful, will disclosure as a way of communicating the commonalities of women's lives and to help alleviate feelings of aloneness. Where traditional therapy ignores issues of power, conflict, and control, operating to maintain the status quo by adjusting the individual to fit society, a feminist model of therapy advocates social change, aiming to attain more power for women, individually and collectively. Women are encouraged to take an active role in determining and structuring their own therapy: thus, the client determines the goals, agenda, and pacing with the therapist's support. This not only helps to demystify and clarify the therapy process, it provides the woman with greater control in the therapy dynamic, which assists in the overall achievement of empowerment and heightened self-esteem.

In the 1970s we began to observe a dramatic increase in the numbers of women who developed anorexia and bulimia. When these problems first surfaced, the response among families and the helping professions was panic, which was exacerbated by the flurry of media attention eating disorders received in the late 1970s and early 1980s. Anorexic and bulimic women were portrayed either as freaks or, as the problems become better known, as having glamorous diseases of the rich and famous. Anorexia and bulimia were, without exception, presented as diseases, as psychiatric disorders that were irrational and needed to be controlled and managed by psychiatrists. Initially, anorexic women were coercively hospitalized and treated with simplistic behavioural programs that forced them to eat under the threat of isolation and intravenous- or tube-feeding systems. More commonly, they were simply told what they must eat every day, and were policed until they did so. Anorexic women were supervised to be sure they would not hide food or flush it down the toilet, and bulimic women to ensure they did not purge. Rarely was any individual psychotherapy provided. Women were routinely kept in the hospital until they complied with the objectives of gaining weight or getting their eating under control. Those objectives and the speed of recovery were determined by the helpers, not by the women themselves.

There were virtually no choices available in terms of treatment approaches. Partly because of the panic, felt among the helping professions and by the families of the women with eating disorders, that these women would die, therapy was unnecessarily controlling, rigid, inhumane, and coercive. The anorexic and bulimic woman had no control whatsoever over the process, except to comply enough to be released from hospital. Although women were expected to be passive and compliant to the program requirements, they would often lose the weight they had gained or continue with bingeing and purging after they went home. Other women committed suicide. Recovery was almost completely defined by increased weight, cessation of bingeing and purging, and demonstration of an ability to eat three prescribed meals a day. Women were told that these treatment approaches were in their own best interests. But were these women heard? Did anyone really understand what their problems were? Were the problems resolved? Were these women helped in any lasting way? Or did the treatment strategies used compound the difficulties these women already had?

THE DEVELOPMENT OF A FEMINIST APPROACH

TO EATING DISORDERS

Although it took some time for eating disorders to gain significant recognition within the women's movement, feminists began to question why so many women were becoming anorexic or bulimic. After writers such as Susie Orbach (1986, 1978), Janice Cauwells (1983), Marilyn Lawrence (1984), Marcia Millman (1980), Marlene Boskind-White and William White (1983), and Kim Chernin (1981) produced popular feminist books on "eating disorders," these issues began to be given more serious consideration. More recently authors Susan Kano (1985), Marcia Hutchinson (1985), Éva Székely (1988a), and Naomi Wolf (1990) have contributed to a feminist understanding of weight preoccupation. It was predominantly feminists who asked the commonly overlooked yet obviously important question: Why were 95 percent of anorexics and bulimics women? Generally, it was concluded that we needed to understand how being a woman in our society predisposed one to develop these problems.

Feminist activists in the area began to focus on the social obsession with weight that was holding women prisoners of their own bodies and appetites. They began to challenge the necessity for women to be thin, and pointed out that 95 percent of all diets failed. They wondered what women were communicating about their lives with their bodies, what women get out of dieting or being anorexic and bulimic. Many noted that controlling the body had become an accessible and viable way for women to achieve some measure of control in their lives (Brown 1991, 1990a, 1990b, 1987a, 1987b; Brown and Forgay 1987; Lawrence 1984, 1979; Lawrence and Lowenstein 1979; Orbach 1986). It seemed that being thin, and controlling one's food intake, offered two important things — greater self-esteem and an increased sense of control — that seemed to be desperately needed by many women.

Yet, despite growing interest in explaining the social obsession with thinness, very little discussion developed around what a feminist therapy approach to eating disorders would consist of.[2] A feminist understanding of the problem does not guarantee a feminist way of working with the problem. It is essential that we extend our feminist analysis of eating disorders to begin conceptualizing ways of working that empower women.

In 1979, when I was struggling with my own eating disorders, I found the literature on eating disorders, like the prevailing treatment, deeply offensive and profoundly disconnected from women's experiences of eating and their bodies. My reactions to these accounts led me to think about how a feminist understanding would translate in practice and therapy. Later in 1983, as I was beginning to conceptualize a feminist way of working with anorexia and bulimia, I decided to start a program for weight preoccupation at the Winnipeg Women's Health Clinic.[3] I came to the understanding that the only really effective way of providing help to women who are anorexic or bulimic is to guarantee them that not only do they have the right to control their bodies and therapy, but that it is crucial to the success of the therapy process that they do so. As feeling out of control is central to the experience of anorexia and bulimia, therapy that takes control away only exacerbates the problem.

A feminist approach to working with anorexia and bulimia must begin with an understanding of these problems as extensions of the common experiences most women have with their bodies and eating (Lawrence and Lowenstein 1979). Further, it is critical that we not separate anorexia and bulimia from the experiences of most women: we cannot view anorexia and bulimia as pathology and condone the weight-preoccupied behaviour of women in general. Understanding weight preoccupation as a continuum is essential to a feminist perspective, which attempts to avoid a medicalized and individualized view of the problem and instead facilitates placing it within a social context (Brown and Forgay 1987). Thus, the principles outlined for therapy with anorexic and bulimic women generally apply to work with all women on this continuum.

Therapists need to be aware of their fat prejudices and biases and how these impact on their work. It is important for the helper to think about her own experiences with weight, shape, and eating to determine how these experiences will influence her work. Further, the therapist needs to be aware of the myths and fallacies our society propagates about weight control and dieting and must be careful not to perpetuate them herself. Although we should not advocate weight gain for anorexic women or weight loss and dieting for fat women, we can help women explore body-image issues, the social pressures to be thin, the stigma experienced when fat, personal meanings of fat and thin, dieting histories, eating behaviour, self-esteem, family background, personal emotional histories and abuse, and provide support for dealing with current crises and difficulties.

At a time when virtually no one questioned the legitimacy of hospital programs for treating eating disorders, one critique affected me profoundly. The following statement by Marilyn Lawrence and Celia Lowenstein (1979, p. 42) established for me the necessity for feminist therapy to recognize the centrality of the issue of control for women with eating disorders and the importance of nonviolating and noncoercive help:

> In our experience the kinds of issues anorexic women bring to therapy concern their attitudes and feeling toward themselves. These are entirely negative, and range from feelings of self disgust to denial of body ownership.... Related to this is the anorexic's overwhelming feeling of helplessness and loss of control in every aspect of life. These negative self images are reinforced by the usual methods of treatment which anorexics receive. They are forced into passivity and treated as bodies rather than complete people. All decisions about day to day living are made for them. Their fears of loss of control are, in fact, realized as all control is taken away from them. Thus the treatment of anorexia can be seen as an example of the kind of "treatment" women can expect to receive in all areas of their lives; passivity is rewarded as is surrender and abdication of control. Self-respect and independence are discouraged. It seems that this kind of treatment would be damaging to any woman, but is particularly so to anorexics as their existing conflicts are magnified.

How effective are treatment programs that control, manage, and define women's needs for them, when the structuring of the anorexic and bulimic woman's needs by and for others in her life is often part of the problem? As Lawrence and Lowenstein (1979) suggest, this is a little like treating sexual problems with rape. Rigidly structured inpatient and outpatient programs too frequently emphasize changing the symptoms; the goals are gaining weight for anorexic women and cessation of bingeing and purging for bulimic women. They tend not to hear what the anorexia and bulimia communicate, and, as a consequence, often miss the central issues. Indeed, such programs are often so far off base in understanding these problems that the treatment remains superficial, never really discovering what the real issues are. What they do is manage the problems, rather than resolve or change them in the long term.

Most women who are anorexic or bulimic will desperately cling to these methods of coping and gaining a sense of control over their lives when their sense of being out of control escalates. The more treatment programs, punish, control, and manage women's behaviour, the more likely women are going to feel increasingly out of control. A power struggle often develops between the helper and client. In these power struggles the helper and the woman fight for control over the woman's body and her life. This struggle is reframed as the woman's problem: she will be seen as difficult, manipulative, and — worse — disordered. She cannot win in these situations, because whatever form her expression of her difficulties or concerns with the program itself takes, it will be viewed as further evidence of her disturbance, rather than as a problem with the treatment itself.

The body is an arena through which women's struggles and conflicts are often expressed in Western society today. Women are speaking with their bodies, and until this voice is heard, most women will continue to need to speak through the body and eating. Clearly, therapy needs to enable women to find more direct ways of expressing their pain, while respecting the symptoms presented. Many anorexic and bulimic women who are first seeking help are unaware of the sorts of things anorexia and bulimia express for them. Feminist therapy is a means for a woman to be supported and facilitated through a process of understanding her own pain and how it is expressed through her eating and her body. Not only do others need to hear her, she too must hear her voice, often for the first time.

Anorexia and bulimia are expressions of the contradictory expectations and experiences women have in their lives. The voice of struggle and inner conflict is often centred on such issues as self-esteem, self-definition, self-direction, and the need for recognition and validation of one's own emotional needs and feelings.

Feminist therapy stresses to women the importance of their own needs. When working with eating disorders we must regularly check out how women are feeling, and what they want. This is true partly because women are socialized in our culture to be quiet, passive, and restrained about expressing their needs and feelings. Furthermore, women are often unlikely to say what they really feel, need, or dislike in therapy unless they feel safe and reasonably certain they will be heard. This is even more of a problem when women are dealing with therapists and doctors, people whose authority women are taught not to question.

In therapy women must be able to control what is happening to their weight, bodies, and eating. Any intervention that undermines this control will likely be destructive and unhelpful in the long run. This is a difficult issue for many therapists as they themselves often feel threatened, powerless, and unsafe, particularly when working with very low weight anorexic women. But the therapist must remember that when she tries to "help" her clients by asking them to gain weight, see a doctor, or be weighed, she may really be doing this for her own peace of mind or her need to be in control. Indeed, such an approach may be antithetical to her client's needs.

Many therapists routinely weigh their clients, and many women resent or fear this. Weighing women presents many problems, not the least of which is that it often overemphasizes the importance of weight. It implicitly, if not explicitly, suggests there is a correct weight that a woman should be. The truth of the matter is anorexic women are going to gain weight when they are ready and able to do so. The scale in no way facilitates that readiness; it simply offers a sense of control and security to the therapist. Some have argued that it teaches women not to be afraid of being weighed or of the numbers on the scale. But it is rather like throwing someone who is terrified of water in the deep end of the pool. Instead of a controlling and unnecessary intervention, a psychoeducational approach, consistent with the fat liberation movement, which emphasizes throwing away the scales, is more productive.

Most clients weigh themselves at home and are aware of changes in their body weight. Since changes in body weight can signify emotional changes for the client, they should be discussed, but it is important to avoid making discussion of women's weight the centre of therapy. It is essential when discussing weight and weight changes with a client that the therapist be nonjudgemental in exploring the meaning weight has for the client, and its relation to her immediate life. While I have never found it necessary to weigh women in therapy, I do not believe categorically that doing so would never be useful in any way. However, it is important to realize that it is the meaning of changes in body weight that are important, rather than the number on the scale. Therapists can contract with their clients about how they are going to handle the question of weighing, and weight. Such contracting is useful to women who gradually want to stop weighing themselves.

Feminist therapists also need to beware of imposing therapy strategies, such as body work and visualization, on their clients. There are several reasons why these strategies are not helpful to some women, particularly those who have been sexually abused. While both strategies can be immensely useful, I think we need to be cautious that our own enthusiasm for these techniques does not obscure their limitations. We need to be very sure that we are not violating clients' boundaries, that the client is really giving informed consent and fully understands, is comfortable with, and is ready for them. In no way should a client be given the message that she is wrong to not want to participate, as she needs to be able to trust her own sense of her boundaries and to determine what feels violating to her.

For anorexic and bulimic women, for whom controlling the body is paramount, visualization or body work can be terrifying, and even damaging. They may consent to these techniques and then discover their panic and fear. Many women who have been abused have trouble protecting their own boundaries; others have very closed boundaries as protection. For those women who have yet to develop a sense of their own emotional and physical boundaries, such interventions can prove to be quite harmful, and may become one more way in which women are revictimized. Extreme sensitivity is needed when doing visualizations or body work to ensure that it is what a particular woman wants and needs. These techniques may not work for everyone, and care must be taken that they not become routine parts of programs, thereby compelling women to participate, despite their apprehension.

Therapists always have more power than their clients in the therapy relationship. The use of power in feminist therapy is a central ethical issue in our work. Ethics of feminist therapy, stress the importance of equalizing or minimizing power differences. We need to be constantly aware of what is going on in terms of power and control in the therapy relationship and take responsibility for not employing power over interventions. Weighing clients, telling them what to weigh, how to eat, how fast to make changes, or determining the changes they must make, are examples of the therapist using her power in a way that further disempowers the client. The objective is to help empower women and this means that clients must be encouraged to be actively involved with the therapist in determining the therapy process.

Feminist ethics also stress the recognition of diversity in women's lives and experiences. Women's social location in terms of age, marital status, sexual orientation, race, class, cultural background, and so on will shape and influence her values and standpoint. As therapists and helpers, it is critical that we be aware of our own location and our own biases, so that we do not impose them on others. Women's backgrounds will affect how they feel about their bodies, eating, sex roles, and social expectations, for instance, and must be taken into account in our work.

This section of the book explores issues frequently encountered in counseling women preoccupied with weight. Robyn Zimberg connects food, needs, and entitlement in her exploration of emotional eating among women. Central to Robyn's argument is the recognition that all people eat for emotional reasons, and that food is inextricably connected to one's personal history and to its larger cultural meaning. Nonetheless, as she points out, people of all body sizes and shapes can develop experiences with food that are extremely painful and problematic to them. It is from this perspective that she goes on to address the emotional hunger paradox in which women attempt and fail to satisfy central emotional needs through feeding themselves.

Addressing the lost dreams of thinness, a critical aspect of body-image therapy, is based on encouraging self-acceptance and adopts an anti-dieting philosophy. Andria Siegler shares her insights into the grief process associated with giving up one's dreams of thinness, and demonstrates how this process is a necessary step for women who seek to move on to body acceptance.

Niva Piran and Karin Jasper examine the importance of countertransference issues in feminist therapy; in sharing some countertransference situations that have come out of work with women with eating disorders, they show how the feelings that emerge in the therapist are a central aspect of the therapy relationship, and they expand on how awareness of these feelings can be instructive and used successfully to strengthen the therapy process.

Contracting is a way of negotiating issues of power and control within the therapy relationship. It minimizes the therapist's power over clients and maximizes women's empowerment in therapy. Catrina Brown explores the use of feminist contracting as a way to combine behavioural change and insight work in therapy. Contracting is a process of establishing an explicit set of expectations and goals agreed to by the helper and client, that are reviewed continually and changed as needed. Because both the helper and the client determine the goals and expectations, contracting enables a greater balance of power, mutual decision making, clearly agreed-upon expectations, open communication, demystification of the therapy process, and sensitivity to issues of control. In this way, therapy process, and sensitivity to issues of control. In this way, contracting establishes focus and direction and produces an experience of therapy in which women remain in control of the process.

Karin Jasper explores how women develop body image problems and provides some strategies for helping women begin to accept and like their bodies. She illuminates what feeling fat really means by looking at how women's feelings and experiences are displaced onto the body. Karin describes how five central themes — body-image history, replacing displacement, self and body care, shame and change — are addressed in the body-image group she facilitates.

Therapists have observed for some time the prevalence of sexual abuse and sexual violence in the lives of women who become preoccupied with their bodies and weight. As the body has been the site of violence for many women, it can also become the focus of displaced feelings of self-hatred, powerlessness, and a lack of control and safety. Patti McGillicuddy and Sasha Maze write about the issues and needs of women dealing with sexual violence.

In addition to histories of sexual violence and the childhood trauma of sexual abuse among women who use food repeatedly as a way to cope, survive, and meet their emotional needs, alcoholic family backgrounds occur frequently. Connie Coniglio makes the connection between eating problems and alcoholic families, outlining many of the salient features of these homes that can produce a sense of chaos and lack of control later expressed through women's relationship to food.

Ellen Driscoll explores the politics of recovery, offering both a critique of the recovery movement and an examination of its role in providing a place for women's resistance and empowerment. Connie Coniglio, Patti McGillicuddy and Sasha Maze suggest that many women who struggle with their bodies have histories of alcohol or chemical dependency, sexual abuse, or other trauma. Ellen Driscoll observes that many of these women enter into the twelve step programs that have become so popular, but she challenges the commonly accepted notion that people can be or are addicted to food. Her assessment of the recovery movement includes a consideration of its pathologization of the individual and its neglect of the social context of women's emotional difficulties.

Women with eating problems sometimes use "self-harm" as an additional way to express their pain, and as a way to achieve emotional release. Not unlike the bulimic cycle of bingeing and purgeing, self-harm paradoxically provides an outlet for anger, pain, and needs. Maxene Adler discusses the use of metaphors as a way of working with these problems in therapy.

Feminist groups offer a positive alternative and or a supportive supplement to individual counseling. Groups are a very effective therapy approach to body-image and eating problems as women are able to both share with and learn from other women. Sandy Friedman describes some of the benefits of this kind of group work from a feminist perspective, and provides examples of some features of groups that reflect a feminist approach.

Some women who have eating disorders are living within very difficult family situations. These situations are often a part of the problem, and need to be addressed. Jan Lackstrom explores how feminist family therapy can be a helpful strategy for counseling women with their eating problems. She emphasizes a sensitivity to gender roles, power differences, and the needs of all family members. While Lackstrom focuses on the young woman living with her family of origin, the principles she outlines are also useful to addressing the interaction of eating disorders and other family situations. Family therapy with a feminist orientation may also be of use to the adult woman with a lover, husband, or children of her own.

It can be difficult to use feminist-therapy approaches when working within institutional settings, as such settings commonly adopt a disease or medical model. Niva Piran examines whether it is possible to do feminist therapy within traditional institutional settings and contrasts these structures with alternative work environments. She examines some of the possibilities for feminist work

There are often gaps between feminist ideology, feminist experience, and feminist practice. Éva Székely and Patricia De Fazio identify some of these gaps and urge us to explore them, suggesting that therapists need to be able to be honest about their real experiences. By recognizing these gaps, therapists create an opening for further discussion. However, if we assume women's experiences are homogenous, or if we begin legislating too narrow or correct an approach to these issues, we risk silencing women.

◆

NOTES

1. Among well known and important works critiquing psychiatry and the medical model are; Burstow and Weitz 1988; Ehrenreich and English 1973; Goffman 1961; Illich 1981; Rosenhan 1973; Ryan 1971; Scheff 1968; Szasz 1974, 1971, 1970, 1968; Canadian Mental Health Association Women and Mental Health Committee 1987; and Zola 1981. Some feminist writers and practitioners who have made a significant contribution to the development of feminist alternatives to practice include Brown and Root (1990), Burstow (1992), Gilligan (1982), Greenspan (1983), Laidlaw et al. (1990), Levine (1981), Baker Miller (1986), and Robbins and Siegel (1985). Very recently (1992) a report entitled *Missing the Mark: Women's Services Examine Mental Health Programs for Women in Toronto* was prepared by the Coalition for Feminist Health Services. Many additional women have written feminist therapy books in specialized areas such as sexual abuse, battery, self-esteem, sexuality, and addiction, providing useful ideas about non-oppressive ways of working with women.

2. While feminist writing on eating disorders has often been theory
   rather than practice-focused, some writers have offered ideas about
   feminist practice: see Brown 1991, 1990a, 1990b, 1987a, 1987b;
   Brown and Forgay 1987; Brown 1987, 1985; Boskind-White
   1983; Dana and Lawrence 1988; Hutchinson 1985; Kano 1985;
   Kearney-Cooke 1988; Lawrence 1984; Lawrence and Dana 1990;
   Lawrence and Lowenstein 1979; Orbach 1986, 1982, 1978;
   Women and Therapy 8 (3) 1989; Wooley and Kearney-Cooke,
   1986; Wooley and Wooley, 1985.

3. See Brown and Zimberg, this volume, for an account of the develop
   ment, structure, and philosophy of the Women's Health Clinic
   program.

FOOD, NEEDS, AND ENTITLEMENT: WOMEN'S EXPERIENCE OF EMOTIONAL EATING

Robyn Zimberg

When I was first asked to write this essay, I was pleased that the issue of emotional eating had been included in a collection like this. All too often, women's experiences with emotional eating have been neglected, trivialized, and misunderstood. These experiences have been dismissed as "just weight problems," and considered less significant than the "real" eating disorders. As a woman and a feminist social worker, I have come to recognize that emotional eating is a painful issue that touches the lives of many women and is worthy of our consideration and understanding. In this essay my intention is to share with you some insights into the area of emotional eating that I have gained from the women with whom I have had the privilege to work, as well as to offer some possible intervention strategies.

WE ALL EAT FOR EMOTIONAL REASONS

Food surrounds us and is an intricate part of our celebrations and our mourning, of our rituals and our holidays. It means different things to different people in different cultures and with different religions. Food and eating are filled with meaning. Food can be sensuous, soothing, social, a stimulant, and a depressant. Clearly, when we eat, it is often for reasons other than pure physiological hunger.

We celebrate and socialize with food; we eat according to the capitalist lunch bell instead of our internal hunger cues; we eat/don't eat to please; we eat/don't eat to rebel; we eat/don't eat to punish; we eat/don't eat to reward.

As very young children we often learn and internalize these meanings. We learn how to please when we are praised for being "good little girls" when our plates have been cleaned, and are subsequently rewarded with dessert. We learn that saying no to food is a first and powerful way to rebel against our primary caretaker (most often mother or a female mother substitute). We learn that being denied food is punishment for doing something wrong, and are soothed with food when we are hurt.

When we have grown up in a family where food was scarce, its meaning is different from that in families where food was abundant. Several women with whom I have worked have shared their intense need to keep their cupboards full in response to their fear of not having enough food, as was the case during their childhood. Similarly, when we have grown up in a home where mealtimes were chaotic or potentially violent, food has a different meaning than it does for those whose family mealtimes were peaceful. Many women who use food for comfort describe their experience with food in their families as more positive than do those who severely restrict their intake of food or who punish themselves with food.

As a mother of a two-year-old, I am constantly reminded of the underlying significance of food and eating. I often find myself reaching into my bag for containers of cereal and raisins to keep my son happy (or, to be entirely honest, quiet while out in public), all the while questioning the message I am passing on to him. I am deeply aware of my feelings of utter frustration and incompetence when he refuses to eat something I have prepared especially for him, and my feelings of pure pleasure as I watch him joyously eating the very same thing the very next day. In accepting or rejecting the food, it somewhat feels as if he is accepting or rejecting me, or at least a part of me. These feelings are, of course, quite under-standable. Given the reality that we live in a capitalist society, which implies that we are primarily defined and valued by the work we do, and if we recognize that women are still primarily responsi-ble for the care of the family, which includes food preparation, food logically becomes much more than a substance to be ingested for survival. It is a product, a creation, an extension of ourselves as caregivers, lovers, and women. Children cannot help but be aware of this connection.

Our first experience of food is through the breast or the bottle. This type of feeding is a means of providing both sustenance and comfort. The comfort received cannot be denied, nor does it miraculously disappear. Certainly, babies learn and develop alterna-tive comfort measures, but even as we grow older this connection between putting something in our mouths and feeling good con-tinues.

It is virtually impossible to eat outside of the emotional web woven at infancy, and outside of the social meanings of food. We all eat for emotional reasons at one time or another. We all eat for reasons other than pure physiological hunger. So why do we need to examine emotional eating if it is both natural and common? Largely because it has been made to become a problem, particularly for women.

WHY IS EMOTIONAL EATING PRIMARILY
A WOMEN'S PROBLEM?

Although men are affected by issues related to food and eating, research and my experience suggest that emotional eating is still predominantly a women's issue. Women's relationship with food is, in part, shaped by their role as nurturers. Through feeding others, women learn that food is a way to give to and take care of others; in this way, food can become a logical way to give back to oneself.

Mary described her emotional eating in this way: "By the end of the day, after cooking, cleaning, bathing, listening, playing, chauffeuring, I was just all tapped out.... I had nothing left inside of me to give. Curling upon the couch with a bowl full of ice cream and whatever left-over dessert remained was the only real thing I could use to fill myself up again and do just for me."

Women are also fundamentally identified with their bodies (Greenspan 1983). It is through the body that they gain access to power in this society. Women's bodies have the power to reproduce and to attract a man (still an important indicator of status in our heterosexist society). As well, women's bodies have the power to feed and nurture an infant. Moreover, for women the body is a socially acceptable means of self-expression. However, society propagates a contradictory message: women's bodies are to be feared, hated, and mistrusted. This view has been expressed throughout history and is evident in various religious teachings, mythologies, and today's multimillion-dollar pornography business. This contradictory message places women in the position of having to control their bodies and, at the same of time, recognizing that their bodies are their power.

To further complicate matters for women, not just any body will do. Throughout history, women have been presented with different cultural standards of beauty and have been psychologically coerced into sculpting themselves to fit a variety of moulds; the quest to conform to the ideal has led women to foot-binding, lip stretching, corseting, and modern-day weight preoccupation and eating disorders. Women's identification with and contradictory feelings towards their bodies have left them vulnerable to such psychological coercion.

One might question whether emotional eating would be a problem for women if this pressure to be excessively thin did not exist alongside society's overt fat prejudice. For many women, even a minimal amount of emotional eating, under prevailing social strictures, is both guilt-producing and feared. Without the ideals Western society provides for them to mirror, women would probably not choose to constantly set themselves up to binge eat, by going on self-deprivating weight-loss regimens. However, the realities of contemporary society are such that most women are uncomfortable living inside their own bodies.

THE CONTINUUM OF EMOTIONAL EATING

When women come for help and support with the issue of emotional eating, they often express a desire to eat "normally." Women hope to learn to eat only to fuel the body; however, as we have discussed, no one eats only for sustenance. Emotional eating exists on a continuum — from those who rarely engage in emotional eating to those who constantly and compulsively eat for emotional reasons. Importantly, I do recognize that there is a difference between sharing a piece of birthday cake at a party and having the cheesecake in the fridge call out your name hour after hour, night after night or frantically searching the cupboard for something ... anything to fill the void. However, what must be understood is that all points on the continuum reflect the use of food to meet needs and serve purposes beyond physiological ones. Therefore if we all eat for emotional reasons, emotional eating, by definition, cannot be inherently negative.

One of my concerns is that, even within feminist literature, emotional eating is, in fact, considered to be intrinsically "bad," something one ought to work towards not doing (Orbach 1978; Roth 1989). This premise negates the existence of a continuum of emotional eating and advocates abstinence, which is both an unnecessary and an unreasonable expectation. Since we all eat for emotional reasons, suggesting abstinence to someone experiencing difficulty in this area seems unhelpful and unfair. Why should we encourage our clients to feel unentitled to eat simply because their bodies maintain a particular level of fatness? Why should the natural and pleasurable experience of emotional eating be only acceptable for the few whose bodies naturally conform to the current thin ideal. Furthermore, what is so terribly wrong with women's self-feeding? What is so terribly wrong with women nurturing and pleasing themselves with food?

For too long women have been taught to control their bodies and appetites, both sexually and with food. Our appetites have been described as something outside of ourselves that has tremendous and dangerous possibilities. The thought of fulfilling these appetites, for the pure pleasure they can bring, has been largely discouraged. Women have been taught that both sex and food are primarily for the other people in their lives to enjoy, certainly not for them. Only recently, have women struggled for the right to explore their own sexuality. However, the fear of women's appetite for food remains strong. The message is clear, if women do not control their appetites, horrible things will transpire.

The idea of trusting our bodies is something that evokes tremendous fear for most women. Whenever I speak with a group of women, I talk about the importance of giving up dieting and the whole diet mentality (Kano 1985). I encourage women to learn to listen to their bodies and feed themselves what they want, not what they think they ought to want. The looks of sheer panic set in quickly. There is this sense that, if they give into their "desires of the flesh," their appetites will be insatiable and uncontrollable: "If I start to eat what I want I will never be able to stop...."; "Chocolate is my weakness...."; "I could never stop with just one...."; "If we care what we look like we need to have some self-control." I try to assure them that, if they truly listen to their bodies, chocolate would not be their main staple, and that they would, in fact, be able to stop eating when they chose to.

I also share with them my experience that, when a woman first gives up dieting she may go through a period of what I have affectionately come to call "fuck you" (or, for those who may prefer, rebellious) eating. This eating is a response to all the years of deprivation. It is often a time when "forbidden food" is enjoyed. It is a way to say no to all of the social pressure to conform to an unrealistic socially constructed ideal. It is a way to say no to all the oppressive rules which result in self-denial and deprivation.

For some women this time can be quite liberating. As Mary enthusiastically described: "For the first time in my life I can actually go to a restaurant and order what I really want ... no anxiety attacks two hours before ... terrified that the menu will not have something that I can eat. I cannot express how free I feel."

For others, this type of eating can be very frightening. Weight gain may occur, which can lead to feeling out of control. It is precisely for this reason that I feel it is critical to let women know that this may happen, but reassure them that this part of the healing process does not last forever. When we truly listen to our bodies and treat our bodies, and therefore ourselves, with the love and respect that we deserve, then the food with which we nourish ourselves becomes a part of self-care. Let's be honest: if we ate only chocolate, we could not possibly feel very good for very long.

Women must begin to challenge the notion that a woman's body left unmonitored is a threat, and somehow less moral. We must reclaim and reappropriate our desires and needs. Women are entitled to delight in and savour the tastes and the feelings of food. Women must seek to gain equal rights in relation to food and stop suppressing their appetites in the mistaken belief that such self-sacrifice is part of ensuring that others' needs are fulfilled. At the beginning of one workshop I facilitated, one woman asked how we can develop the strength to say no to food. I respond that, for me, the central question was how we can develop the strength to say yes to ourselves.

THE EMOTIONAL HUNGER PARADOX

In emphasizing that emotional eating is part of all women's lives, I am not suggesting that exploring and working on one's emotional eating is not necessary. I am quite aware of the profound pain that can be interwoven in a pattern of emotional eating. What I am proposing is an awareness of the "emotional hunger paradox" (a concept that Catrina Brown and I developed at a workshop on emotional hunger). On the one hand, I firmly believe we deserve to and are entitled to eat, regardless of our body size, gender, or reason for eating. We have the right to nurture ourselves in whatever way works and is available to us. On the other hand, eating can be a way of suppressing feelings and needs. Consequently, at times women may feel as though they are taking care of themselves and their needs through food, but may ultimately be engaging in a form of self-denial. In such cases, needs are merely controlled; they are not actually acknowledged or fulfilled. Nothing changes.

Therapists must acknowledge and respect women's choice to use food in this manner. At the same time, they must assist women to understand this paradox so that they can truly make an informed choice about their eating. Women need to become aware of the possibility that their use of food may be repressive and oppressive, keeping them emotionally out of touch with their needs. At such times, constructive and gentle confrontation is often necessary. This task is particularly challenging for therapists; they must sensitively walk a tightrope, balancing women's needs and choices in relation to emotional eating with encouragement to see that such needs will never be fully met in this way. The therapist then needs to facilitate the recognition that emotional eating, at times, can result in a denial of self.

The women I have counseled have shared a multitude of reasons for their emotional eating. These include feeling angry, depressed, dissatisfied, out of control, lonely, bored, empty, afraid, and even happy. The use of food has been described, time and time again, as a way to escape from or numb these feelings. Laura described it this way: "I would wait all day, biting my tongue, smiling appropriately, trying to ignore the rude comments, anticipating the relief at home ... safe ... eating and eating, stuffing myself until there was no room left ... not for food ... not for my feelings ... not for me.... Sleep was all I wanted.... exhaustion would set in ... another day had passed."

Clearly, Laura's use of food was on some level helping her manage her feelings, but at a great cost — a cost that she determined was too high to go on paying. Laura came to realize that her feelings were a significant part of her and that, when she denied and silenced them, she denied and silenced herself; she was not fully living.

WEIGHT LOSS AND FEMINIST THERAPY

Many experts in the field offer the promise of weight loss once emotional eating is under control. It appears that two controversial assumptions underlie such promises: that fat people eat more than thin people do and that fat people eat for emotional reasons and hence are responsible for their fat bodies. It is well documented that fat people do not eat more than their thin counterparts (Dyrenforth, Wooley, and Wooley 1980). As well, genetics have been found to play a significant role in determining one's level of fatness (Bennett and Gurin 1982).

It is, however, equally critical that therapists not ignore the realities of a woman's life. In my work with women, and in my own personal life, I am aware that, during those times in which one is actively using emotional eating as a coping strategy, one may be consuming more food than usual, and consequently may be at a higher weight. Thus, when/if one chooses to find alternative coping mechanisms, one may eventually and slowly lose weight (usually, however, not to the point where one fits the unrealistic cultural ideal of slenderness). It is important for therapists to be aware of the research in the area, yet, at the same time, be opened to the possibility that an individual woman's experience may contradict the data. Therapists must consciously strive not to make assumptions about their clients based upon their clients' body size, and then truly listen to what women have to say about their own experiences with food and weight.

Susan was a participant in a support group and identified herself as a compulsive eater. Over the previous five years she had lost and gained more that a hundred pounds, and, at the time she entered the group, she had seen three doctors, one nutritionist, two therapists, and of course had joined several formal weight-loss programs. Susan described her experience this way:

> No one ever really listened to me. I felt as if I was banging my
> head against a wall. One person would treat me like a misbehaving

child for cheating on my diet; the next would say that the problem is fat oppression. I was given scores of conflicting information explaining how I was not responsible for my fat, how I could change my lifestyle to decrease my fat, and that my fat was protecting me from my sexuality. I am not a stupid person. I know that my problems run very deep, but I also know that staying home day after day, night after night only to enter the real world to go grocery shopping is not "normal," and not the way that I want to live. I know that I will never be thin, and that is okay ... but I also know that the way that I eat is really hurting me ... but I just can't seem to stop.

Susan was clearly searching for some acknowledgement that her pain was significant. She was open to exploring the underlying purpose of her weight preoccupation, but at the same time was desperate to begin to make some changes in her relationship with food. The task of therapy was to balance insight work with behavioural change. Working together to develop small and doable changes helped her feel listened to, and that there was hope that she could make significant changes in her life.

Susan's story illustrates how important it is to simply listen to the experiences of our clients. This may seem a trivial point to make; however, I often encounter colleagues challenging the idea of exploring a woman's emotional eating. I have been told that such exploration is anti-fat and often have been referred to the studies which maintain that fat people do not eat more than thin people do. Clearly, such thinking is not helpful or responsive to the reality of women's lives. A woman may or may not be eating more than is usual for her, and only the woman herself can know this. Only the woman herself can tell you.

As a feminist, I am also deeply concerned about the implications of offering thinness as an ultimate goal. Feminist therapy must be anti-dieting, and it must not be weight preoccupied. If the client is weight preoccupied and uses emotional eating as a coping strategy to control her feelings and needs, the goal of weight loss in therapy may solidify her reliance on that strategy. When weight loss is the goal of therapy, the underlying issues that contributed to the development of the weight preoccupation in the first place may never be addressed.

Furthermore, by presenting thinness as a goal, the therapist, consciously or not, serves to perpetuate the oppressive and restrictive pressure to be thin. The message that thinness is psychologically healthier and more attractive than fatness must be avoided. Advancing myths about weight and ignoring the diversity in women's body sizes perpetuates the oppressive pressure to be thin and fat oppression. We need to be aware of the politics of this "tyranny of slenderness" (Chernin 1981).

Eating or not eating has also been described as a way to make the body larger or smaller as a protection from sexuality. A number of women I have worked with have shared their experiences of being both fat and "excessively" thin as a way to feel safe and free from their own sexuality. Some women have described themselves as feeling less like a woman, being so thin that menstruation ceases, or having layers of fat that make the female genitalia appear relatively small and less obvious. This can serve the purpose of removing them from the sexual arena. They feel less likely to be viewed and pursued, more protected and safe — a logical response given that we live in a misogynist society which condones violence against women. However, one must not assume that such is the case for all women. Some women are naturally thinner, and some are naturally fatter. Once again, the bottom line is to not make assumptions. We must not trivialize or overanalyze women's experiences by assuming that all women are X because of Y. We are not mathematical equations that are easy to figure out once we identify the variables. We are complex individuals who deserve the right to be understood as such. Certainly, some may fit into one formula or another, and it is helpful to be aware of them, but let us not lose sight of the individual by simplistically attempting to fit all women into a single mould.

THE MANY FACES OF CHANGE

Women who choose to come for therapy are often seeking peace and freedom from a life of preoccupation with weight and food. They are often at a point on the continuum where emotional eating is adversely impacting on their lives. It has been my experience that they want to make changes. However, change is a very scary proposition. Often, a great deal of ambivalence surrounds it, especially given the reality that the use of food as a coping strategy has been successful on some level. Thus, change must occur slowly, at a pace directed and controlled by the woman herself.

It is important to remember that change does not mean the same thing for every woman. For some women, it might mean learning to accept that they are entitled to use this coping strategy and form of self-nurturance, without guilt. In such cases, the problem identified is not self-feeding per se, but the self-hate that often accompanies it. One woman that I worked with spoke about the guilt she experienced after eating as a bad aftertaste, "hardly worth doing it, if you are left with that in your mouth." It is interesting to note that some women have discovered that one purpose of their emotional eating is to experience the guilt and punish themselves. Laura remembers: "I always thought that food was my greatest lover ... always there for me ... to comfort and take care of me ... with no demands ... but then I finally became aware of all of the guilt and self-hate.... The ugly and destructive things I said to myself after I ate were far worse than the words anyone else had said to me. Why was I setting myself up for all of this self-abuse?" Consequently, when such guilt is removed, or at least challenged, eating no longer serves its purpose; with the cycle broken it becomes possible to explore this need to punish.

Change for other women might mean beginning to identify which feelings trigger the need for emotional eating. The identification of the feelings leads to having a choice as to how to deal with them. For example, a woman might choose to experience them, journalize them, discuss them with someone, take a bath, or eat. What is important is that eating always remains an option. I never suggest that a woman eliminate it from her repertoire of self-nurturing and coping skills. There are times in our lives when we simply cannot experience every single feeling that emerges. It may be that our attention must be focused elsewhere or that the feeling is too painful. It may be that other avenues of self-nurturance are obstructed or denied, as is common in societies in which the traditional ideal of the "good and selfless" woman is upheld, and violence against women is a reality. Whatever the reason, for some women, at some times, emotional eating may be the best way to care for themselves. The issue is having a choice. Women can develop skills and an awareness that enable them to identify and experience their feelings, or choose not to. In this way, they take control and eliminate the perception that food and eating control them.

Emotional eating can also be used as a way to be in touch with what is happening emotionally. If, for instance, I find that I am eating more than usual, I sit down and ask myself what this is all about. How am I feeling? What is going on in my life? I use it as an indicator of conditions in my emotional life. Here, too, eating is no longer the controller. In fact, I am able to harness the positive potential of emotional eating.

Clearly emotional eating is often about much more that eating: it is about feelings, needs and entitlement, control and power (Brown 1985). Feminist therapy must politicize this issue by challenging the current pressure to be thin, questioning the myths and biases surrounding food and weight, as well as understanding women's experiences within the contexts of their lives. This issue is extremely complex and filled with what might appear to be contradictions. A feminist approach to working in the area of emotional eating is truly a balancing act. We must be cautious about making assumptions regarding women and weight and, at the same time, be responsive and respectful to the experiences of women. We need to appreciate that we all eat for emotional reasons, and simultaneously recognize that, for some, this eating may interfere, on some level and at some times, with their lives. An awareness of the emotional hunger paradox is essential. We must respect women's choices regarding emotional eating, empowering women to feel entitled to fulfil their appetites while encouraging and facilitating the more direct expression of feelings and needs. Oppression occurs when we deny our emotional selves. For too long women have subjugated their feelings and needs to those of others. Women have experienced violations too painful to acknowledge and feel. Hence, feminist therapy needs to encourage women. It needs to provide women with the opportunity to fight against the denial of self, without contributing to their self-hate and pain by neglecting to understand and fully appreciate women's emotional eating.

◆

GRIEVING THE LOST DREAMS
OF THINNESS

Andria Siegler

Ruth B., a woman in her mid-forties, is a partner in a prominent Toronto law firm. She is married and is the mother of two bright, healthy children. In her family of origin she was considered the "smart one," while her sister was the "pretty one." Even as a young girl, Ruth was not satisfied with the shape of her body, as she saw herself as "fat, short, and bottom-heavy." By adolescence, her body image became intolerable to her, and Ruth began thirty years of chronic yo-yo dieting. Ruth's mother was also a dieter, and dieting became both a connection and a competition for them. After her mother died, Ruth continued to frequent weight loss programs, "diet doctors," and nutritionists in her quest for permanent thinness. Nothing worked and Ruth became increasingly depressed. To add insult to injury, Ruth's husband began to complain about her size, especially as she grew heavier with age, pregnancies, and dieting. Almost out of desperation, Ruth began to seek out information on the harmful effects and ineffectiveness of dieting and weight preoccupation. She discovered she was, indeed, ready to explore her own food and weight issues, her relationships, and alternatives to the deprivation and the torture she had been inflicting on herself for so many years. With the help of counseling Ruth began to acknowledge and appreciate her body. Her grief for the thin body that "might have been" was alleviated only by her new sense of self and purpose. She gave up dieting and began the long process of "normalizing" her eating. Physical activity became a part of Ruth's life as she learned self-care and self-nurture rather than restriction. She also began slowly to educate her family, especially her husband, who has come to understand both the struggle and the healing of Ruth's process.

There is a growing community of women like Ruth who are giving up dieting and attempting to free themselves from their preoccupation with food, weight, and shape. The transition from dieter to nondieter can be painful and difficult, with a sense of loss and concomitant grief being the most consistently reported features of the process. In order to examine this grief process and its distinct issues, one first has to ask why Ruth or any woman would choose to explore an alternative to what has been a secure, familiar, and socially condoned practice. Why, in this diet-obsessed society, with axioms like "thin is beautiful " and "thin is healthier," are women beginning to consider this option and to take the first step on this long journey towards self-acceptance?

There are several reasons. First, there is mounting scientific evidence to suggest that dieting is potentially physically and psychologically harmful. It is also becoming clear that dieting is an ineffective strategy for long-term weight loss, and that repeated weight fluctuations may be more of a health risk than a higher, stable weight. Second, the size-acceptance movement has begun to make its mark in the media. For the first time in decades, body-image myths are being debunked, and the message that size and shape are neither within one's personal control nor a measure of self-worth is being heard. For some women, nondieting is a last resort for dealing with the pain of repeated dieting and possibly even surgical failures. Still others attempt to stop dieting because they secretly believe, or have been led to believe, that their fat will simply disappear when they shift their focus to the "real issues" in their lives.

Feminist theorists and counselors have long encouraged women to listen and pay attention to the experience of their own bodies. And women have long suspected that their bodies were fighting the torture and deprivation of diets. Only recently, however, by giving up dieting, have women like Ruth acted on that belief.

Whatever motivates a woman to work towards ending her food, weight, and shape obsession, she is likely to be ambivalent, confused, and scared. Whether on her own, in individual counseling, or in a group experience, she must prepare herself for inner conflict and a tumultuous process. Giving up dieting, especially for fat women, is not without consequences, for it can be synonomous with letting go of the dream, the hope, the fantasy of someday living life as a thin person.

It is impossible to talk about the loss of the dream without first understanding the nature of the dream itself. Just as with a death, life must be discerned before grieving can begin. Although dreams of thinness may mean different things to different people, thinness itself is only the penultimate goal. The ultimate goal is whatever thinness promises to bring to the dieter. The thinness "package" usually contains any number of positive attributes, such as beauty, good health, success, glamour, fitness, intelligence, acceptance, sexiness, and of course, a mutually satisfying long-term love relationship! It is the perceived loss of the dream of this "package," not thinness per se, that is mourned so deeply by those becoming nondieters.

For the past several years I have been working with chronic dieters in my private counseling practice as well as in the "Beyond Dieting" program (see Ciliska, this volume). Based on my clinical observations of literally hundreds of "overweight" food-, weight-, and shape-preoccupied women and my own personal struggles with the issues, the loss of thin dreams and the subsequent grief process are the most broadly shared among these women's experiences. I am not aware of any formal studies relating the grief process to giving up dieting, but the clinical evidence speaks for itself. Not only does grieving play an important part in the transition, but it

appears that true resolution of the loss resulting in positive attitudinal and behavioural change cannot be accomplished without some
pause to grieve the loss.

What is grief, and what is its relationship to dieting? Grief is
defined as intense emotional suffering caused by loss or misfortune.
The responses to loss and expressions of suffering have many variations and no set time schedule. The various stages of grief have
been identified most clearly by Elisabeth Kübler-Ross in her classic
study *On Death and Dying*, (1969). The stages are: (1) denial and
isolation; (2) anger; (3) bargaining; (4) depression; and (5) acceptance.

I prefer to look at the grief process as consisting of overlapping
phases that are not used as rules or standards by which to judge the
effectiveness of grieving. The "stages " are useful because they help
to point to similarities in human grief. Awareness of these similarities and shared experiences do much to promote inner healing as
well as empathy for others. Loss is expressed uniquely, however, and
the differences deserve to be given credence and respect.

Grief is not new to the chronic dieter. Anyone who has been
through the diet cycle at least once, which includes the majority of
North American women, is familiar with this kind of emotional
pain. The diet process lends itself to pain because the
restriction/binge cycle is a relentless rollercoaster ride. For even a
first-time dieter, the pain can take the form of low self-esteem,
anger, guilt, anxiety, frustration, apathy, self-hate, and, unquestion-
ably, loss. Each time lost weight is regained, often plus interest, a
sense of loss prevails. Whether it is because the two minutes, two
weeks, or two years at a "goal" weight are over, or because the long-
held belief in personal control of one's physical fate is fractured, a
mourning reaction occurs. For the seasoned yo-yo dieter, feelings of
defeat and failure continue until the enthusiasm for and commitment to a fabulous new diet puts the final grieving process on hold
one more time.

When women seriously consider stopping dieting, they are generally ready to take in the scientific information about set-point

theory, metabolic adaptation to dieting, and genetic links to body size and shape. This knowledge often plunges them into denial, which is the first stage of grief.

> Karen F. is an intelligent and intuitive woman in her mid-twenties. She has traveled extensively and has had a few different jobs since her graduation from college, but is having difficulty finding a direction in life. Karen presented in the assessment with severe food, weight, and shape preoccupation, having been a yo-yo dieter for at least ten years. It became clear after a detailed diet and weight history as well as a psychosocial history that Karen was suffering from depression, probably due to separation and individuation issues and a lack of emotional connectedness with her family. Her weight issues were serving as coping strategies and a means to perpetuate her negative feelings about herself. In this way Karen could also avoid her ambivalent feelings toward her "perfect" family. These insights were revelations for Karen and she felt ready to tackle the family issues as well as her eating problems. After reading some suggested books and articles and discussing them with me, Karen seemed to have a good understanding of the sociocultural issues and the scientific arguments against dieting. Despite this knowledge, Karen continuously posed the question, "Well, okay, so now how do I get thin?"

This investment in denial is one of the ways women numb themselves after the initial loss experience. In Karen's case, her denial served as a shield from the intensity of her many new awarenesses. The combined losses of the fantasy of a "perfect" family and of thinness would have been too much too face at one time.

"Why me?" is usually the next question asked by women struggling with grief around thinness. The question encompasses their anger, both free-floating and specifically directed, as well as the longing for the resuscitation of their dreams of permanent weight loss. The free-floating anger is about the helplessness and powerlessness to change what used to seem like an easily alterable situation. What has finally come to be known as oppression evokes anger towards society in general, the media, and, often, men. The focused anger is a constructive attempt to shift the blame from themselves to specific people in their lives who supported their dieting rather than helping them to love and accept themselves. These people typically include friends and family, especially mothers, teachers, physicians, and other health-care professionals. Frequently, anger is directed towards the bearer of the new information. I am often the target of the anger in groups or individual counseling in a "kill the messenger" fashion. Of course, self-directed anger abounds for getting on the rollercoaster in the first place, and buying into the myths. This is often expressed as "How could I have been so stupid to have ever started dieting?" or "If only I knew then what I know now."

This quickly leads to bargaining. "If I promise never to diet again, will I stop gaining weight?" "If I start eating breakfast daily, will I lose weight?" "If I stop dieting and start exercising, can I get thin?" The hope is to try to fool Mother Nature — by set-point manipulation, or by avoiding metabolic adaptation to dieting through only minimal restriction of intake. Women at this point in the grief process often find it intolerable to be with dieters, or even thin people. Both the anger and the bargaining stages are characterized by frustration and envy, information seeking and yearning, and continued low self-esteem.

Eventually the dream disintegrates, hope is abandoned, and the reality of the loss sets in. Just as the "thin" fantasy and dieting provided security, the "fat" reality and nondieting can lead to disorganization and despair. Weight gain can occur during this phase, often as a result of a binge response to the depression, which brings further guilt, shame, and self-hate.

> Barbara W. came from very far away to attend her weekly "Beyond Dieting" group. Whatever the weather, she never missed a session. She actively participated and was considered the "life of the party" by the other participants because of her terrific sense of humour and her openness. Barbara was in the "regain" part of the diet cycle when the group began, and she was hoping

that this alternative approach would nip her weight gain in the bud this time. Despite her attempts at "normalizing" her eating and increasing her physical activity, Barbara's weight continued to climb as usual, along with her anxiety and depression. The group noticed a dramatic change in her presentation. She would weep openly during the group constantly referring to herself as "fugly" (a contraction of "fat" and "ugly"). She was tormented by the idea of giving up dieting and dreams of thinness. She felt stuck while she stayed in the depression phase for many months. She struggled to redefine herself and to create new dreams instead of returning to dieting, but this struggle left her overwhelmed with sadness.

However long the sadness lasts, and it varies from woman to woman, a resolution in some form will follow in time. Many women will return to dieting during this phase in order to relieve the pain and to keep themselves from being "screened out" as sexual, beautiful, or even smart persons. In my clinical experience this is the choice most often made by women whose mourning process has not been supported. My own personal experience and the experiences of many women with whom I've worked have been to move relatively smoothly into acceptance, which is not necessarily a happy state. It is the place in grief where women must ultimately accept the unacceptable and reestablish their identity. No longer do they ask "Why me?", but "How do I respond to this new reality?" Barbara eventually came to this place, as did Ruth.

The shifts that occur during this juncture are pivotal. The dichotomous thinking so common in dieters begins to decrease as women gain perspective. Moralistic views of "good" and "bad" foods diminish as women give themselves permission to eat when hungry, to be physically active, and to pay attention to their health and their appearance, whatever their size. They begin to take their lives off "hold." That fine line between healthy, free living and body preoccupation becomes more clearly defined, despite the disturbing trend towards obsessing over good health and "staying alive." The "good old days" of weight cycling and intermittent thinness begin to be recalled as the "bad old days" of deprivation and guilt. Women previously at war with their bodies prepare to do battle with society instead, and to take on well-meaning family and friends.

The reorganization of this acceptance stage of grief gradually means positive realization rather than dejected resignation. Karen's initial denial dissipated as acknowledgement of her family issues filtered in, leading her to work with her family towards healing. Indeed, her grief for many losses was resolving as she took action and made changes in her life. By this point in the grief process it is unlikely that fat people will be shamed or frightened into going back to dieting. They have much too much work to do. And that work revolves around coming to the end of mourning, assimilating the loss, and healing the wounds.

The loss can never be fully assimilated in this culture, of course, and the internal struggles, however fleeting, never really end. Healing, therefore, translates into women reclaiming themselves, often with a renewed life force. Awareness of the fact that there is no turning back, no return to what they were before, brings a kind of peace. Goals that are within a large woman's reach, such as sensible nutrition practices, self-care, and moderate exercise, replace the elusive goal of weight loss. Women's relationship to themselves, to others, and to the community transforms as well, with less emphasis on food and size and more emphasis on human connections. Accepting their fat as part of themselves rather than as pathology, or personal deficiency, helps women to take affirmative steps. This combination of acceptance, concrete behavioural changes, and "letting go" of the dream spells victory for women on the road to healing.

Counseling women plagued by food, weight, and shape issues has been one of the most challenging and gratifying experiences of my professional life. I am constantly challenged to fully understand the depth and the breadth of these issues for each individual and to discover and implement appropriate techniques and methods to foster their self-exploration and their healing. I am gratified to be trusted, and privileged to accompany so many women on their very private and personal journeys. I am also gratified to have contributed to their increasing sense of power, autonomy, and self-acceptance. How I, as the therapist, am perceived can be important to the process. For the most part, I am seen as someone who has felt the pain and faced the same dilemmas, yet who appears to have survived without compromising integrity. Occasionally I am perceived as simply trying to rationalize my own size with this work. This, of course, needs some discussion, but can be a positive beginning to treatment. Clearly, whatever the therapist's size, it is a treatment issue for chronic dieters.

One message that needs to be given by therapists working with women struggling to give up dieting is that grieving is not pathological, but a natural and integral part of the process. What is pathological is the prevailing attitude towards fat. It is imperative that a feminist therapist convey a fundamental understanding of the role of society in creating the attitudes and feelings inhibiting to women's self-realization. It might be helpful if the counseling contract contained an agreement to explore the sociocultural issues pertaining to food and weight.

The contract must also make clear that this process does not in any way guarantee weight loss, nor should weight loss be considered one of the treatment objectives. It is important, however, to acknowledge, in a nonjudgemental way, a woman's secret wish and expectation that this process will result in weight loss for her.

Another message a feminist counselor needs to transmit is that it is not reasonable to expect women to live happily and healthily while they are enemies of their own bodies, and that their despair is completely understandable. But the process of befriending their bodies must be supported, as their bodies have been ascribed negative value and have been a source of pain on many levels.

Permission to mourn, in whatever form it is expressed, is crucial to the process. In fact, probably the single most important thing a counselor can do for women working on giving up dieting is to support their grieving experience.

Healing and grief resolution are difficult to measure clinically. Women's experiences, feelings, and behaviour manifest the integration that has actually taken place. Most women, however, regardless of the depth of their healing process, would still jump at the chance to take a side effect–free, effective, magic permanent-weight-loss pill. Why? Simply because it would be easier being thin in this culture at this time. It might also be easier being rich or tall or talented in this culture. But most of the women who have been through this process spend little or no time agonizing over any of these things. Like Ruth, Karen, and Barbara, they are much too busy living their lives in liberation and taking good care of themselves.

◆

COUNTERTRANSFERENCE EXPERIENCES

Niva Piran and Karin Jasper

The concept of "countertransference" has undergone important transformations since its introduction by Freud in 1910. Women authors have had a particular role in changing the perception of countertransference from that of a hindrance, to that of a facilitator of psychotherapy.

Freud (1910, 1915) identified countertransference phenomena as the reactions — images, feelings, impulses — of the therapist to the client. He characterized them as being rooted in the therapist's own conflict-laden experiences, and therefore as impediments to his ideal of therapist neutrality. This pejorative view of counter-transference experiences led to the requirement that psychoanalysts undertake a "training analysis" aimed at reducing their counter-transference reactions. Racker (1968) has noted how prohibitive this understanding of countertransference phenomena was to mak-ing them a more common field of inquiry and understanding, at least until the early 1950s. One exception to this suppression was an article by Helene Deutsch (1926) suggesting that the counter-transference phenomena had potential value. She specified two types of countertransference experiences: one reflecting the thera-pist's unconscious identification with an aspect of the client's own experience, and another representing the therapist's identification with a significant other in the client's life (a complementary attitude). These identifications were seen as the basis for intuitive empathy.

The development of Object Relations theory within the psychoanalytic framework and, in particular, the introduction of the concept of "projective identification" by Melanie Klein (1946), allowed for an enriched understanding of countertransference experiences. Projective identification describes a process in which different aspects of the patient's experience of self and others are split off from one another and then the split-off part is projected onto another person and identified with. While with the client, the therapist becomes the recipient of these projections.

Working within the British Object Relations school, Paula Heinmann (1950) published a ground-breaking article which questioned the idealized neutral stance of the therapist. She described the process of the therapist getting to know aspects of the client's internal experience through her lived and felt experiences when with the client, induced through this process of projective identification. Margaret Little (1951) stressed the importance of a therapist's openness to own her impulses and experiences when with clients and recommended sharing them so that clients' experiences would be validated and a genuine human connection would be formed. Tower (1956) shared several of her clinical experiences and concluded that the emotional upheaval in which both therapist and patient are involved enables the therapist to emotionally understand the patient, and may even give the patient a sense that the therapist is, indeed, engaged. The process of working one's way out of the upheaval is important. In a later paper, Hanna Segal (1975) vividly described the experience of being subjected to difficult projections by two clients who induced in her the traumatic experiences and feelings they had as children, while the clients assumed the role of the traumatizing parent. These and other seminal contributors, such as Heinrich Racker (1957), Leon Grinberg (1979), W. R. Bion (1963), and Christopher Bollas (1987), highlighted the importance of the therapist staying highly responsive to client projections and to her own internal states. Otherwise, an emotional barrier between client and therapist may be created, and unknown experiences of the client remain unknown. These authors spoke about a split within the therapist between a part that becomes "situationally distressed" by the client's projections and another part that contains the projections, metabolizes them, and uses them constructively in the interaction through a back-and-forth process.

Other authors (Strupp and Binder 1984; Gill 1982; Sandler 1976), working mainly within the current psychoanalytic stream, which focuses on the interactive dimension of psychotherapy, have highlighted another important aspect of countertransference — the therapist's unconscious participation in the enactment of a specific role assigned to her or him by the client. In other words, unconscious changes in the therapist's actual behaviour relate to a particular unconscious "pull" by the client, so that the therapist ends up being cast in a particular role in relation to the client who, in turn, may then be cast in a complementary role (Sandler 1976). An example of that would be the therapist becoming frightened, silent, and passive (like the client felt as a child) while the client becomes aggressive and abusive (like the parent was), or vice versa, or both sides playing both roles at different times. Sandler (1976) termed this phenomenon "role responsiveness." A counselor's past and present experiences will necessarily affect her or his reactions to the client including client-induced affective states or role-enactment pulls.

While the psychoanalytic framework highlighted the relevance of past conflictual material and of training to countertransference experiences (e.g., Racker 1968), it failed to consider the crucial role of cultural factors in the counselor's response to the client. Gender issues compose an important category of cultural factors affecting the counseling relationship. Teresa Bernardez (1987) addressed the important topic of gender-based countertransference, especially of female therapists in psychotherapy with women. She mentioned the "errors of commission or omission" in the counseling interaction that relate to shared cultural beliefs, societal mores, and biased assumptions about gender-role behaviour. For example, a counselor may not assist and may actually suppress an exploration of a culturally syntonic characteristic, such as a female client's dependency or submissiveness. Bernardez recommended that the woman counselor increase her awareness of her own cultural transferences and deal with her own reactions of grief, anger, powerlessness, or negative female identification formed in response to the social and political reality women face.

In this essay, we use the broad definition of countertransference phenomena, namely: all the experiences stirred up in the counselor through her interaction with the client. These include reactions to the client as a person in a real relationship, reactions to the client related to cultural norms and prejudices and their effect on our growth processes, reactions related to personal conflictual experiences, reactions to experiences induced in us, and roles we take on as a component of the intensive interaction with the client.

We view countertransference phenomena as one important dimension of relatedness and understanding in the counseling process. When a counselor is working with clients with eating disorders and weight preoccupation, such an understanding of countertransference phenomena may allow her and the client to avoid defensive or acting-out reactions. Such reactions may involve, among other things, withdrawal, distancing, hostility, or imposing control. Moreover, dominant gender-based values transmitted in our Western culture, including attitudes towards a woman's body, may further impell the counselor in the directions of devaluation and control. The counselor of clients with eating disorders can expect to feel the whole array of human experiences, at times traumatic and difficult experiences. We prefer to view each countertransference experience as unique to a particular counselor-client dyad rather than to describe "typical" countertransference phenomena in counseling this group of clients.

The essay includes several case vignettes, describing the uses of the empathic approach to countertransference experiences in the treatment of eating-disordered clients. In these vignettes, we focus on the counselor's experience and exclude almost all historical material related to the client for the purpose of preserving clients' confidentiality. Each vignette is written by one or other of the authors. Clients have read, discussed, and contributed to the sections pertaining to themselves, and have agreed to have the relevant material printed here. All these experiences occurred within a woman-counselor/woman-client dyad. The vignettes purposefully focus mainly on body-related experiences since these experiences are more relevant to the counseling of eating-disordered clients. Feelings about the body are acquired within an interpersonal and social context. Countertransference experiences, as an aspect of an intensive interpersonal interaction, may have particular importance in revealing feelings about one's body.

A MOTHER-DAUGHTER EXPERIENCE
IN THE COUNSELING RELATIONSHIP

A few times during the first phase of counseling with an anorexic client, I noticed her looking at my body, and especially my stomach, with an expression that made me feel like I was revolting and scary. Yet, my invitations to include these experiences in the subject of counseling (e.g., by commenting on my being heavier than her and asking how this made her feel) were not productive.

A turning-point came when I arrived at a session following some dermatological surgery which had left my face bandaged at a few spots and somewhat swollen. The client's overt response to my appearance was that of polite concern (e.g., how was I doing?), yet her facial expressions were those of anxiety and aversion. I vividly remember the cluster of feelings I had at that time. I felt that I had actually harmed her by coming to the session looking the way I did. Showing up seemed a self-centred act based on my idea of caring, which was to show up consistently, rather than on her idea of it, which was not to show up if not in good shape. I was not well enough to get close or relate to her. There was also a strong sense of thin boundaries — it was as if my affliction would rub off on her and that, by being damaged and getting close, I would damage her, with her having no protection. While overtly she idealized my action of following through on the session (especially presenting myself in public when "looking like that"), I felt that she experienced me as potentially destructive to her, and I sensed her experience of threat and her anger.

The countertransference feelings were invaluable in enabling us to connect intensely with crucial experiences the client had had with her mother. First, they revealed a field of experience the client was not aware of at the time, yet had been deeply affected by. Second, my countertransference experiences enhanced my empathic understanding of her experiences, which allowed for further empathic shared exploration. Third, the countertransference experiences sensitized me to new learning that needed to occur within the counseling relationship.

Decisions about interventions are always complex and affected by many factors. In that particular instance, I decided to share my countertransference experience directly with the client since she seemed to be in emotional pain while consciously caring for me and idealizing my actions. Also, the moment seemed to be both unique and complex emotionally, and we had established a strong rapport. I therefore commented that I felt like I may have actually burdened her by coming to the session this way rather than rescheduling it. Her response came from a very pained space, and she kept repeating that she was not wanting to take care of me. The experiences she related, some again understood through further countertransference experiences, revealed how weak she felt in relation to her mother's unhealthy body, having to psychologically "carry" her mother (sustain her), and how scary and threatening this experience was. She needed to flee this experience and it made her angry. Having an unhealthy body was also associated for her with having a heavy body, having a subordinate role and being helpless.

Awareness of and connection with countertransference brought key experiences of the client to the foreground and gave me a first-hand experience of the client's sense of burden and fear. In terms of the importance of new learning, the client was relieved to find that my medical condition that day did not affect our connection. It was important that she could unlearn negative relational associations with a "pained" body. New learning in the counseling relationship is as important as the recovery of powerful experiences.

A Patriarchal Experience of the Body
in the Counseling Relationship

In this instance, a client was describing having attended a social event with her male mate. At this social function, he seemed to get excited by and be attracted to women who were both extremely thin and fashionably dressed. He was neglecting her, and she was feeling lost and depreciated. As she was describing in detail the events at the party, her tone became more self-critical. She was evaluating herself and her looks "from the outside": Was she fun? Was she good looking? As she was speaking, she was restlessly glancing at herself, tidying up her clothes and checking her belt, and, at other times, looking at me, my hair and attire. I felt like I myself was being subjected to an evaluation from "the outside."

My own experience at the time was that of being subjected to harsh scrutiny and competition. I also remember the experience of alienation that came with this external evaluation, compared with the deep connection experienced during many of our counseling sessions. At that moment we seemed miles apart, connected only through being subjected to the same harsh treatment in the same room. Another experience was a sense of loss, loss of the important things that had transpired in the sessions and at that moment seemed to have been eradicated and invalidated. I was thinking, for example, about other experiences of her body she had shared in the sessions, which had seemed so connected with her authentic self:

the experiences of health, stamina, vitality, strength, and power, as well as her pleasure in her intimate relationship. Another reaction in me was that of protest and anger for all that was lost, and could be lost, in the presence of binding patriarchal standards of attractiveness. I felt let down since my way of being with this client, which represented support for and acceptance of her authentic identity, power, and size, was at that moment being penalized. I also felt what a woman helper cannot avoid feeling at times (just like mothers of daughters): stuck in a no-win situation whereby the "room" we advocate that women take inevitably imposes on them new and difficult social challenges.

The connection to my countertransference experiences was invaluable in different ways. First, my experience paralleled hers. I felt penalized for what I represented, and felt the threat of losing all the gains that had been made. She was being penalized for being a less "perfect," object and the threat of losing in that competition made her wish to disconnect from all aspects of herself that stood in the way of the competition. I was able to connect with her deeply from this place of threat and loss through comments like: "It is so hard to feel that all that you are cannot be valued. It also leaves you in a dilemma about which part of you to keep or how you can feel good about the rest of your experiences."

Another aspect of the countertransference experience at the time was a vivid remembering, on my part, of the client's experiences of joy, power, and competence, including those anchored in her body. While the client was experiencing a rift separating her from her body, her self, me, and our shared experiences, since those seemed too incongruent with the "demands" of a "victorious" functioning in the real patriarchal world, I was maintaining a strong connection with all aspects of the client's self through my countertransference experiences. One could therefore view the counselor's connection to varied countertransference experiences as a way of containing or holding, for the client, experiences that seem too difficult or incompatible for her at the time. I could therefore draw upon those "incompatible" experiences as they became relevant in the session. Different themes came up, but, most importantly, the client carried out of the session a respect for her "whole" self and her struggle around owning the whole gamut of her experiences, including incompatible ones, and a poignant sense of how the objectified norms of appearance and behaviour can destroy that experience of wholeness.

SEXUAL ABUSE AND COUNTERTRANSFERENCES

Sexual abuse harms in a major way one's connection with one's body, with one's self, and with others. The character of counter-transference experiences that emerge in counseling can shed light on the existence of past sexual abuse and on the experience of the abuse itself, and can also guide the counselor in relating to the client.

I remember my experience with a severely emaciated client who was referred to me. My strongest sense was that, every time I spoke or moved, my actions were putting her in jeopardy. Even asking how she had gotten to see me seemed aggressive, intrusive, and a violation of her safety. In fact, there was no sense of interpersonal safety whatsoever. It made me freeze and compulsively check how I was moving, speaking, and behaving. Yet the sense of fear, of inevitability of harm, remained. This experience and way of coping, I found out later, corresponded to the client's experience and strong compulsive tendencies. My feelings continuously vacillated between those of a frightened victim and those of a torturer. Considering this most extreme experience, I was not surprised to hear a long term history of complete social isolation.

The initial countertransference experience guided me in giving her as much safe space as she needed (for example, by not asking and just repeating, by not suggesting, and by not offering more of myself than she wanted). Related to her severe emaciation, I talked about the importance of her safety and therefore suggested an ongoing monitoring of her health by a gentle woman colleague of mine. Yet, I did not suggest that she stop her hours of exercise or change her diet. Her need for control of her body and herself was her only way to live. It took a long time to uncover a history of early and severe physical and sexual abuse. Safety remained a major theme in the counseling of this client.

The particular nature of the abuse and its interpersonal context can be reflected through differing countertransference experiences. For example, compare my experience during the initial interview described above with the following. This client smiled a lot and invited me to listen to her experiences, which she always presented as appealing, interesting, and benign. Gradually what she was presenting turned into horror, but always before I, as the listener, could prepare for the change in content. This pattern of seduction and horror was quite repetitive. Indeed, her history of sexual abuse revealed that the perpetrator was quite seductive with her, promoting himself to her, inviting her to partake in his charm and his special adventures, but always at the price of some "dues." The client's description was most important; the countertransference experience added a strong sense of the interpersonal and internal experience associated with the abuse. Later on in the counseling process, the countertransference experience of seduction and lack of warning of future harm became an important observation in the prevention of revictimization.

CONNECTION AND DISCONNECTION

This client had been bulimic off and on for more than ten years and had been in counseling with me for a year. Approximately two years earlier, she developed physical symptoms that made it difficult for her to work more than part time and impossible to be physically active. Since she had both enjoyed sports and used activity as a weight-control method, the physical limitation was extremely difficult for her to accommodate to. In addition, she had suffered cyclical depression for many years. When depressed, she would feel hopeless and inclined to give up trying to improve her life. Her experience had been that things would not get better and stay better — they would get better for a while and then come crashing down again. When she was at the bottom of this cycle, her bulimic symptoms would increase and she might cancel an appointment, or speak at length in therapy about the pointlessness of continuing.

This client's depressions seemed truly debilitating, but she had never initiated the idea of using antidepressants, as some clients do. When I raised the issue, she declined my proposal that we seek a consultation on the possible benefits of an antidepressant to her. I noticed that I made the proposal for such a consultation when I was feeling helpless, in the face of her repeated expressions of hopelessness.

One day she arrived at my office and, before she had even sat down, began by saying that she almost hadn't come. She went on to describe her depressed feelings. She mentioned that her physical symptoms had become so severe that she was going to have to leave work altogether until a diagnosis could be reached and suitable treatment found. She talked about her feelings of hopelessness and the pointlessness of therapy without looking at me and without pausing.

My countertransference experience was of feeling there was no place for me to respond to what she was expressing and of being submerged in her feelings. I noticed also a feeling of powerlessness as I felt unable to help her emerge from her darkness. I began doubting my own abilities and thought that I should be referring her to someone more skilled. I found myself wondering again about the value of antidepressant medication.

I didn't want to respond out of any of these feelings, however, and focused on my countertransference experience. It occurred to me that the more my client got into her depression in this way, the more cut off from her I felt. She would cease talking about herself in a way that allowed a connection between us and begin talking in a way that left both of us isolated. I decided to describe this experience of disconnection from her as a kind of wall coming up and said that it was a wall that I wished to see over or through. She paused for a moment, looked up at me, and then began talking about her own feeling of separateness in a way that once again permitted an empathic connection.

In the sessions that followed, this client spoke about how she had always withdrawn from relationships when depressed because she was afraid to let the other person see her depressed side. She expected this side of herself to overwhelm the other person or to cause him or her to reject her. My suggestion of antidepressant medication was a kind of repetition of this pattern: she risked revealing how depressed she felt and I responded by suggesting something that would change her feelings. This response simply reinforced her belief that her real feelings were too much for others to accept. When I resisted responding this way, but indicated that I really wanted to know her feelings, we avoided another repetition and opened the door to new developments.

Over time, she also saw that increasing bingeing and purging during times of depression gave her a rationale for staying away from people. For her, it felt safer to stay on the periphery of relationships, where she felt less vulnerable to hurting others and being hurt by them. Obsessing over her body size and numbing herself through bingeing and purging also helped her to manage her fears about acceptance, rejection, and expectations in relationships. Making these observations allowed her to begin reevaluating the ways of relating she had learned in her family of origin. She also began considering supplementing individual therapy with a group in which she might be able to try out new ways of relating to others, in a relatively safe environment.

AN EXPERIENCE OF "FEELING FAT"

In this instance, I was working with a client who was concerned about having gained weight over a two-year period. She was eating more than she had been accustomed to eating, but was not bingeing. Although she had always been over average weight, she felt very dissatisfied about her current weight. Over the year she had been coming to counseling, she had become less weight preoccupied and felt proud of improving the way she was handling difficult situations at work.

During one session, she described a telephone call that had left her feeling very distraught. She was on the phone with a man she had broken off a relationship with (they had agreed to remain friends) and during the conversation asked him if he was seeing anyone new. She later described asking this question as "opening a door I hoped he wouldn't walk through." He did walk through, however, and told her about a woman he was interested in, but was afraid to approach, because of her stature in her field. My client began offering him advice, ideas, and encouragement. At times she felt resentful about helping him handle his relationship with another woman and wanted to hang up, but she didn't. After the conversation was over, she realized she felt jealous and began thinking it may have been a mistake to leave the relationship with this man. She also started feeling fat, a feeling that in general had been bothering her a lot less.

My experience in listening to her on this occasion was of being transported back to an earlier time in her therapy, hearing themes that had been fading out playing loudly once more. I also felt discouraged at what seemed to be a step backwards, and she felt discouraged too. Situations that trigger old feelings (and usually also discouragement) can be very useful. The client often has enough distance to allow her a more objective view than she would have had at the beginning of therapy, but the feelings connect her directly to significant experiences. I suggested we explore what had happened in the telephone conversation to cause such an overwhelming recurrence of the old themes: feeling fat and regret at having left the relationship. She was able to use the perspective I was suggesting to move from feeling stuck to feeling curious about what had happened. In stepping aside from her reactions and looking with interest at her experience, she realized that hearing her former boyfriend talk about being with this woman made her feel that she was not "special." She wasn't in a relationship and she wasn't progressing as quickly as she would have liked in her own career. Suddenly it seemed important to be thinner and desirable to be back with this man, both things she felt would make her feel special again. It is a culturally conditioned response that women react to feeling bad, e.g. not special, by wanting to be thinner, to lose weight and/or to be with a man.

My countertransference experience as she spoke was of being jarred; the things she was putting together did not fit with my recollection of how things had really been. There was a discrepancy between her current wish to feel special by being with this man again and my sense of what she had reported feeling when she had actually been in the relationship with him. She had often felt that he was unable to meet her needs and that there were significant ways in which she could not respect him. I wondered out loud about the discrepancy and added that my impression was that she had felt far more special in a previous relationship.

That relationship had been very enlivening, and my client felt she had shut down an important part of herself when she ended it to keep peace with her parents. The man was a member of a visible minority and her parents threatened to stop speaking to her if she continued to see him. At the time, she was not ready to test this threat and closed off the relationship instead. It was a great loss to her. She felt oppressed by her parents' expectations. If she were to follow her own inclinations in taking her career seriously, they predicted that she would never have a satisfying family life, that she would not be loved. Further, her choice of partner had to be tolerable to them or they threatened to cut off their love and support. It was too difficult for her to pursue both of her wishes at once, but abandoning either one left her feeling bereft.

Her relationship with the man we were discussing was far less satisfying. This man was not a stimulating person for her to be with, the things she most liked about herself were not the things he liked about her, and she found she didn't really respect him. However, her family was not threatened by him, and there were some things she did like about him. Being in the relationship helped her fend off the fear (generated by her mother's warnings) that she would not find love and might end up with a career but with no family of her own. The relationship lasted two years, during which she ate more than usual and gained weight. While remembering these events, my client was struck by the degree to which she had resigned herself to disappointment after ending the first relationship and the degree to which she had compromised her own ideals and desires in the second one. While her life had the form she wanted it to have (career and partner), it did not have the spark she wanted or the room she needed to express her passion. These issues were hidden while she was distracted by her weight gain into thinking that being thinner would make her feel special again. She observed later that her eating increased amounts of food seemed like a compensation for what she had lost in her life. Her body seemed to be taking up more space at a time when she strongly felt a requirement to constrict her self.

In this situation, attention to the countertransference experience of shared discouragement and of being jarred by things not fitting together allowed my client and I to get underneath the culturally sanctioned understanding of why a woman might feel fat and want to lose weight. This opened the door for her to start taking steps and risks in a direction that could allow for real self-expression and satisfaction in her life.

CONCLUSION

Attention to countertransference poses particular challenges to the counselor. It requires that she engage in an ongoing process of self-examination, self-understanding, and growth. An openness to her own experiences as a female in her culture, her own past experiences, and her experience with her client is the material from which she can draw a strengthened empathetic connection with her client.

◆

Feminist Contracting: Power and Empowerment in Therapy

Catrina Brown

Feminist contracting is a way of negotiating issues of power and control between the therapist and client. This system of ongoing mutual negotiation and communication about the client's needs integrates emotional issues and behavioural change without subordinating one to the other. The emphasis is on empowerment and self-determination for the client in an atmosphere of safety and trust. A heightened awareness of, and responsible use of power in the therapy relationship is central to the process of feminist therapy and to feminist ways of working. Contracting as a way of working involves a commitment on the part of the therapist to relinquishing some of the power her role ordinarily invests her with and to a belief that it is of fundamental importance that women be in control of themselves and their own bodies during therapy. The latter is of primary importance when working with anorexic and bulimic women as controlling the body is often the only sure way available to them to gain some sense of control over their lives. One of the chief contributions feminist therapy has made is its approach to the analysis and treatment of issues of power and control in women's lives within patriarchal society. The value of feminist contracting is its ability to make the negotiation of power and control between therapist and client an open process.

When power, safety, and control are not negotiated, therapy is often disempowering. Feminist contracting is a process of establishing, reviewing, and changing as necessary an explicit set of expectations and goals agreed to by the helper and client. Because the helper and the client collaborate in determining the goals, expectations, and pace of therapy, contracting encourages the minimization of therapists' power over clients and the maximization of women's empowerment in therapy and leads to a balance of power, mutual decision making, clearly agreed-upon expectations, open communication, demystification of the therapy process, sensitivity to issues of control, a climate of safety, an integration of emotional insight work, and behavioural change. Further, it establishes focus and direction of the therapy. Contracting is particularly effective in crisis situations, and its use in such situations is a good illustration of its essential features. Contracting enables the interaction of behavioural change and insight work in therapy in a climate in which the client feels safe and in control of the process.

DISEMPOWERMENT AND EMPOWERMENT IN THERAPY

Conventional therapy's failure to address issues of power and control as they relate to anorexia and bulimia and the actual meaning of these eating disorders in women's lives reflects a lack of understanding of women's experiences and produces therapy methods that often exacerbate their problems. Frequently, conventional treatment of eating disorders reflects a profoundly disconnected understanding of women's experience of eating, their bodies, and their lives. The emphasis on controlling and managing symptoms creates a therapy climate based upon the client's compliance and surrendering of control. Therapy often proceeds by using "power over" and control of the client to produce change, reinforcing in the client a sense of powerlessness.

Conventional therapy often disempowers women because the structure, pace, and direction are determined by the therapist. Expectations and goals are commonly defined by the therapist, which encourages clients to be passive recipients rather than active participants in therapy. For example, outpatient programs for treating eating disorders are designed and structured to meet objectives determined by professionals to which women are expected to conform. Women are told when they must eat, their food choices are limited, and they are weighed. Rarely are women asked what they would like or not like, or what would be the most helpful to them. The focus tends to be on behavioural change, on gaining weight, eating more or eating less, or stopping bingeing and purging. Inpatient and outpatient treatment programs often require women who starve themselves, binge/purge, or eat "compulsively" to simply change or stop these behaviours.

In many instances, the focus on changing behaviour results in a critical lack of attention to the role and meaning of these behaviours in women's lives and the positive functions they serve as coping mechanisms in day-to-day life. The impact on the emotional well-being of women who are asked to abandon their coping strategies without an alternative in place is too commonly neglected and reflects a deeply insensitive and thoughtless approach to therapy. Any therapy intervention that removes women's choices concerning their own bodies is both violating and disempowering. It is understandable that therapy measures which seek to control a woman's body are likely to produce poor results. Moreover, it is doubtful that such therapy can be effective, especially when the client's problems are in themselves reflections of a disempowered self.

The need for a greater sense of control and power over their lives is perhaps the most vital force behind anorexic and bulimic women's relationship to their bodies and eating. We must find ways of working that will help to establish a sense of empowerment rather than take away the tenuous control that has been achieved through the body.

Contracting emphasizes a greater balance of power between the client and helper through mutual decision making, clearly agreed-upon expectations, open communication, demystification of the therapy process, and sensitivity to issues of control. The client and therapist work together in setting the focus, direction, structure, and pace of the work. When women are actively involved in planning and structuring therapy they have a sense of greater control over the process. As important, feminist contracting respects the need to combine insight work with behavioural change, encouraging a sense of accomplishment for both the therapist and the client. Although not a goal to which all else is subordinated, behavioural change can often accompany the development of insight into a woman's feelings, social situation, and the larger social context of her life. This emphasis, I believe, allows for the attainment of empowerment.

PRINCIPLES OF CONTRACTING

As feminist contracting requires openness from the therapist as well as the client, the therapist should outline her perspective, style, and approach to therapy, thereby helping to demystify the process. Doing so encourages the client, as consumer, to decide for herself whether she wants to work with this particular helper. Thus the client's right to self-determination is emphasized at the outset, through choosing the therapist and the style of therapy she is most comfortable with.

Because women's experience with the helping professions has typically meant subordination to the knowledge and power of the expert, the equality that characterizes contracting may seem odd and uncomfortable. However, the fact that the therapist's role bestows extra power should be acknowledged by the therapist. It is therapeutic in and of itself to encourage women to be active and self-determining in therapy since such empowerment may encourage similar life changes.

Feminist contracting is an important way to avoid usurping the client's position of control. The most important contract established between the client and the helper will guarantee that power, safety, and control will not be taken away from the client. Experiencing a sense of control over the therapeutic process is a good starting-place for developing a sense of control in her life. Although an anorexic woman feels completely out of control on one level, she feels very in control through self-starvation. This is the "control paradox" central to anorexia and bulimia (Brown 1990a, 1990b; Lawrence 1979). I stress that if the client is not emotionally ready to give up anorexic or bulimic behaviour as a way of coping, she must not be made to do so. I believe this area of agreement between the helper and the client is essential. In a contract around the issue of control, the therapist must promise the client that the anorexia, bulimia, emotional eating, or compulsive exercise will not be taken away from her. She needs to know she isn't going to have to do anything she doesn't want to do. Contracting around control pays careful attention to what she is needing and feeling. Through constant attention to her needs, she may be able to develop confidence in her own ability to deal with her feelings and needs, and thus progress towards a greater sense of self-esteem and empowerment.

Anorexic and bulimic women are often labeled manipulative by therapists. When helpers view clients as manipulative, they may be exhibiting a lack of understanding and empathy for the women's experience. Too often, if the therapist personalizes the women's actions it becomes difficult to understand the reasons women may feel they need to conceal the truth about their behaviours or feelings. Contracted goals are likely to be more realistic and acceptable than those simply imposed by a therapist. There should be no reason for a client to find it necessary to be deceptive or to "manipulate" in a therapeutic relationship that is respectful of her needs and feelings. It is my sense that clients "manipulate" when they feel they are powerless to do what they would choose to do, when manipulaton is their only recourse for establishing some sense of control over the situation. Sometimes, when therapists feel they have inadequate control over the situation, they can harmfully impose control over the client. Contracts around control and safety can eliminate these problems, for both the therapist and the client.

Power struggles between the anorexic or bulimic client and her therapist are disastrous. Such struggles may force a woman who already feels very vulnerable, unsafe, and out of control to cling even more desperately to the only control she feels she has — that over her body. The more the therapist tries to take power away from the client, the more her "symptoms" or behaviours are likely to escalate. For some, this escalation will be manifest in her continuing to starve herself and become even more emaciated, since doing so is the only thread of power left to her. Therefore, by entering into power struggles, the therapist exacerbates the control paradox. Through their own fear of anorexia and bulimia, many therapists try to control these behaviours and are thus unable to hear the messages of despair contained within the symptoms.

Therapy that communicates to women that they are unable to deal with making choices or having power only reinforces a sense of worthlessness, helplessness, and powerlessness. Therapy should not become another situation where women feel trapped and incapable of taking action to change their lives. We can validate women's experiences and develop awareness about the real structural constraints women have in their lives and the oppression that women live under without reinforcing their helplessness and powerlessness. We can combine understanding, insight work, and consciousness raising with work on the ways women can be effective in changing their lives.

Contracting is an empowerment tool. Change and a sense of accomplishment create a sense of personal effectiveness, which, in turn, encourages women to move to the next step. Insight without action may exacerbate a sense of helplessness. Feminist therapy has often emphasized empathy and understanding, but the extension of insight and understanding to action and change is a central issue in therapy. This is particularly true for women who come to therapy feeling helpless and yet desiring change around distressing behaviour.

Women grow impatient with an endless path of insight work when they themselves cannot see any changes in how they feel or in behaviours that are causing them difficulties. Women come to therapy for change of one type or another, which successful therapy must facilitate. For women who feel that therapy has been directionless for them in the past, contracting can be a great help. Thus, in the initial stages of therapy, contracting can be useful for both the therapist and the client. Ongoing contracting is a means by which woman can attain a sense of accomplishment and empowerment, as interim goals, are achieved. Through contracting, the therapist and client can together set a balance between emotional insight work and behavioural change.

Many women with eating disorders experience understandable ambivalence about giving up bingeing, purging, or compulsive exercise. Recognizing the positive "functions" of bingeing, purging, and compulsive exercise is usually more difficult than identifying their negative aspects. Contracting around behaviour change will require sensitivity to the woman's ambivalence about letting go of her coping mechanism. In particular, the contracting work should identify the tensions, contradictions, and struggles around change and set a pace for change that is both safe and challenging. This is particularly important if the goals of the contract are to be realistic and offer any possibility of success. Contracting around ambivalence is valuable as it demonstrates an understanding of the difficulty of change. It is essential that a woman work through her ambivalence about issues before change can occur in associated behaviours.

A feminist contracting approach is useful in pacing emotional work when women are frightened, ambivalent about change, and feeling out of control. For women who feel very vulnerable and unsafe confronting their previous and current emotional experiences, contracting provides a structure that allows for a greater sense of control and thus safety within the process of therapy. It allows the client to set the pace at which therapy approaches issues, and in doing so mitigates feelings of being controlled by the therapeutic process itself. Contracting around the speed or pace of change is more likely to ensure that a woman is comfortable with changes in her body, eating behaviour, and life. Therapists and clients can contract around weight and eating, reducing severity and number of binges and purges, introducing new foods, and learning how to be aware of emotional hunger when bingeing. This approach provides a sensitivity to women's individual needs that is not evident when woman are simply expected to comply to the therapy rules or objectives determined by their helpers.

Contracting is also a helpful therapy tool in crisis situations, and during suicidal periods. The negotiation that characterizes contracting is essential during a crisis as it ensures that interventions meet the real needs of the client. It provides some structure for women who self-harm, and provides emotional and physical safety in general. It is not, for instance, realistic to simply ask a woman not to self-harm, but it is possible to talk about how she will do this, how much, when, and what other options may be available to her. Similarly, women of a low body weight who are in physical crisis can be contracted with around restoring health to a level the helper and the client agree is acceptable.

Issues such as sexual abuse — increasingly associated with eating disorders — need to be acknowledged and dealt with in a climate of safety and trust. Again contracting is a useful approach. It might, for instance, be decided between the woman and the helper that they are going to begin to work on sexual abuse before working on body image or on changes in eating behaviour. In general, how and when certain issues become the focus in the work needs to be mutually agreed upon.

My own way of contracting for eating disorders is based on a way of working together — a partnership. It combines goals for behaviour change around self-starvation, bingeing, or purging with a mutually agreed-upon direction to the work. During our first session I outline for the client my perspective and how I work. I attempt to find out what kind of therapy experience a woman has had and what influence such experiences may have on the way she approaches therapy. I explore what a woman feels might work best in therapy. For example, some people are much more concerned about seeing concrete change and are very happy to be setting therapy goals for themselves. Others are very interested in exploring their emotional issues in an in-depth way and are less interested in contracting goals around behaviour. I try to adopt a style of working the client is comfortable with.

I usually ask a client a number of questions about what she wants from therapy, what she doesn't want, what concerns she has, what role she sees each of us playing, and what kinds of things she anticipates may get in the way of her therapy. A woman will often think about these questions during and after the first session, and we discuss them further in the follow-up session. These questions can be written down and given to her as a "handout"or simply talked about. These kinds of questions begin to form a contract about how the helper and client agree to work together. We may discuss some of the possible modes of working together, such as visualizations. We decide together where and how we would like to start. Clearly, contracting is not limited to dealing with behavioural issues. My approach to contracting centres on the belief that feelings, behaviours, and situations are always interconnected.

WORKING WITH CRISIS AND HEALTH PROBLEMS

Many women experience a great deal of worry and anxiety around their health. Contracting around health issues allows both the helper and the client to feel more comfortable and safe should significant health risks arise. Therapists often use contracting in crisis situations with clients because it affords lots of safety checks, helping the client to feel safer at a very vulnerable time. Crisis counseling around sexual abuse, severe depression, suicidal feelings, selfharm, or very low body weight and a precarious health status is common when working with anorexic or bulimic women.

I contract around weight and eating from the beginning with low-weight anorexic women. I include a clearly stated discussion of the issue of a woman's right to control her own body, and offer assurances that I will not take that right away. We agree that she will set the pace. I talk about the importance of "baby steps," as many women don't acknowledge the difficulty of even small changes. We discuss the possible meanings of the anorexia or bulimia, and stress that they play an important role in her life. Unlike the medical model, the system I employ stresses that we need to respect the "symptoms": they are there for a reason; further, they will likely continue to exist as long as there is a need for them. I suggest to women that an important aspect of our work together will be to discover the full extent of what the anorexia, bulimia, emotional eating, chronic dieting, or compulsive exercise means to them. We explore these issues in conjunction with behavioural change. Both emotional and behavioural work is done when women are feeling ready and safe enough, not before. Sometimes we focus more on feelings, or on understanding situations; at other times, we examine the behaviour itself. However, they are never really separate.

Body weight is a critical factor for some helpers in determining whether anorexic women must be hospitalized. Marilyn Lawrence and Hilde Bruch, for instance, who have reported success in working with women on an outpatient basis, will work only with women who weigh at least 95 pounds (Lawrence 1984). I would suggest that body weight should not be used as a way to determine whether a woman may need hospitalization as, in itself, it does not indicate the degree of psychological distress experienced, or the extent to which women are likely to incur health problems. By using contracting, I have been able to work with anorexic women with weight as low as 60 pounds on an outpatient basis. I usually initiate discussion with a client on outpatient verses hospital-based care. If there is a need, I express calm concern for her physical well-being. We contract around her maintaining a stable, if low, body weight and an agreed-upon reasonable health status so we can work together outside the hospital.

The medicalization of eating disorders is often justified by the belief that anorexia and bulimia pose a constant health threat. I have found that health practitioners are often sceptical of the ability of a feminist model of intervention to adequately address crisis in women's physical health. I believe it is essential that the helper and the client are both satisfied that a minimum level of health exists. However, experience has taught me there is very little need to panic, and that it is, indeed, anti-therapeutic to allow such panic to shape therapy. When therapy focuses on the management and control of behaviour, it usually does so at the expense of what the woman really needs. I believe that the principles I have outlined above about the need for women to be in control of their own bodies and lives become in many ways even more significant the more in crisis a woman is. One can safely assume that when behaviours such as self-starvation, bingeing or purging become increasingly desperate, chaotic, and health threatening, the client is feeling vulnerable, powerless, and out of control.

A well-intentioned helper may decide to take control in a crisis situation in order to rescue a client. However, what the client actually needs is for someone to help her feel more in control. When a woman's need to seek a greater sense of control over her life through losing even more weight gets to the point of seriously risking her health, she is desperately feeling out of control. The helper cannot take control away from a woman who already feels she has none, since her "symptoms" are likely to escalate. The result is that as the helper attempts to impose some control on the situation, the woman in crisis feels an even greater need to use her body as a way for her to feel some control. More damage than good can be done through this process as the client is thrown into a tailspin. Instead, the situation needs to be stabilized by helping the client to gain a greater sense of control. The therapist feels increasingly powerless when she feels nothing she is doing helps. At such times, therapists run the risk of becoming increasingly heavy handed and coercive. When a power struggle emerges in therapy, in particular with an anorexic or bulimic woman, the onus is on the therapist/helper to defuse it. She should have no investment in winning the power struggle, or in taking power away from a client trying to build power for herself.

It is helpful to have established an effective and respectful working relationship, based on trust between therapist and client before a medical crisis arises. Clearly, it is quite a bit more difficult to start to try to build this relationship when the client is already in crisis. Therefore, suggestions about working with women in medical crisis are predicated on the hope that a strong therapy/helping relationship has already been established. However, the same principles can be applied, although with difficulty, in situations in which such a relationship has not been developed. If such a relationship has already been established, the woman has learned or is beginning to learn that she will not be violated or coerced, that her boundaries will be respected, and that her sense of safety and control is central in therapy. She will know that her needs are valid and important, that change will be defined by her, and accomplished at a speed that she is able to endure without undo panic and fear.

Helpers who are not physicians will find it helpful to have access to one who does not disaffirm the work that is being done in therapy. In a collaboration of therapist and doctor, there needs to be consistency and agreement in approach in order for an effective team — comprising the client, health practitioner, and therapist — to be able to work together if a serious medical problem arises.

For example, one anorexic woman I worked with who weighed 62 pounds was severely dehydrated and showed signs of potential kidney failure. The seriousness of the problem was made clear to her in a calm and reasonable way. Through negotiation and discussion, we were able to agree that she would try to drink as much water as she found possible, and reduce her daily use of the sauna, if possible stopping it altogether. As follow-up, regular (twice weekly) blood tests and urinalysis were undertaken during this period of health crisis. As a result, the client managed to become hydrated enough to avoid the need for hospitalization.

Contracting with a client to see a doctor does not, however, mean forcing her to go. I have never had a woman I have worked with refuse to see a doctor when she was in bad physical shape. In the nine years I have worked with these issues clinically, I have learned women usually make positive and creative choices in helping themselves when they have dependable emotional support. None of the women I have worked with has been hospitalized for problems related to anorexia or bulimia during our work together as we have been able to agree on alternative solutions through contracting. The medical-model approach of quickly taking over control reflects a lack of confidence in women's ability to manage themselves. When women are given support and autonomy, they are usually able to manage well outside the hospital.

Body weight itself is not an adequate measure of health in either a low-weight anorexic woman or a fat woman. Neither needs to be weighed, and a anorexic woman does not need to be weighed even in a crisis. The therapist can express concern about having observed that an anorexic woman seems to have lost further body weight and is looking physically vulnerable (there is no benefit in not expressing what you have noticed; after all extreme low weight functions to communicate that a client is in trouble). She may tell the therapist how much weight she has lost, or how much she weighs at this point. Even in severe circumstances, one cannot focus solely on weight and eating. At such times, women are likely feeling very out of control, afraid, panicky, and vulnerable, and these are the issues that must be addressed. When behaviours or symptoms escalate, the reasons should be explored. Often problematic eating behaviour will intensify when clients are engaged in critical emotional work. A woman beginning to work with sexual-abuse issues, for instance, may suddenly find herself bingeing and purging. We have to expect some struggle in the process of all emotional work. The client needs to feel that a balance exists between working on emotional issues and direct behavioural change. However, emotions and behaviours are invariably intertwined so that when therapy explores eating behaviour, the relationship between women's emotional lives and eating is investigated.

Feminist contracting in therapy de-emphasizes weight and focuses on feelings and needs. When it is discussed, weight is evaluated in terms of what is going on in the client's life. It is crucial that therapy not reinforce a woman's tendency to reframe her problems and needs as dissatisfaction with the body. However, while discussing weight should not be the focus of therapy, it should not be ignored. When weight is discussed respectfully and with the acknowledgement of its greater meaning in her life, the client is more likely to take the helper's concern with her increasingly low body weight seriously. It is important that the helper present concern, not alarm and panic. It is also important that she express her concern quite firmly and seriously. Once again, assuming a good relationship has been established, and weight has not been the overall focus of the work, a client is more likely to take a helper's concern seriously. Assuming that the work previously done has attempted to connect feelings and experiences in her life with behaviour, in a crisis situation this approach should be maintained. The therapist should ask her client why she thinks she has been losing more weight and how she feels about it. She should talk to her about what is going on emotionally in connection to the further weight loss. And the therapist should express her concern about her client's physical well-being, about potential heart, liver, or kidney damage, and work with the client to create an atmosphere of emotional safety in which she would be willing and able to see a doctor. However, one must use one's judgement, developed through interaction with women with very low body weight. Although a woman's body weight may be very low, she is not necessarily in a serious health crisis. Indeed, physical problems such as dizziness, fainting, dehydration, and extreme fatigue may or may not occur at a range of body weights. Thus, body weight has no direct or unambiguous relationship with physical crisis.

Contracting was a very helpful tool in my work with a woman who, in her thirties, was diabetic and blind and had a problem with binge eating. Her situation was complicated by the fact that she also had serious heart and kidney problems resulting from her diabetes. Over the years, a range of experts, including diabetes specialists and nutritionists, had instructed her to follow a prescribed diet, as it was argued that her diabetes and overall health would continue to worsen if her insulin levels weren't better controlled. Her diabetes put her at risk from heart or kidney failure. Despite the health threats and the harassment by experts to stick to her diet, she was never able to.

Together we began to put together a plan that was realistic, and flexible, unlike the rigid diets usually prescribed. While the diets she was expected to follow were not weight-loss diets per se, they had the same psychological impact. She was expected to live a life of constant denial, deprivation, and control. Naturally this set her up to want to binge. It was simply not going to be possible for her to follow the rigid diet expectations of the traditional practitioners. Therefore, we set goals that allowed her some control over her eating so that she could control her insulin levels, and yet remained sufficiently flexible that they were less likely to drive her to binge eat. This balance was tricky, and took lots of experimenting. By setting up more realistic diet expectations for herself, she was able to establish greater control of her insulin levels in an attempt to stabilize her health. Because compliance with the medical-model treatment approach was unrealistic, we decided to do what was actually possible for her: we paid a lot of attention to what felt good to her, what she liked to eat, and when she liked to eat. In addition, we did educational work around the limitations of dieting.

The emotional context of her eating was explored and we discovered that she was often rebelling against the demand that she strictly monitor her eating. She had phenomenal anger at the diabetes itself, and felt very out of control of her body. Her need for emotional nurturance through food were more powerful and more immediate than her fears of the diabetes' effects. Although she was very depressed, and had been for years, this issue had never been addressed by her doctors. We hoped that, by doing emotional work, she would decrease the urgency of her need to binge and gradually would gain more control of her insulin levels. The previous medical interventions she had received had failed to attend to the psychological and social reality of her life or her diabetes. Her needs, desires, and feelings were effectively treated as irrelevant.

She was able to establish much greater control over her insulin levels once she obtained an insulin "pen" which injects premeasured doses of insulin. After repeated requests to her diabetes specialist, she was finally able to carry the insulin pen with her and was then able to give herself an injection based on her assessment of what she had been eating; this allowed her far more control over her body, health, and eating behaviour. While many diabetic women who binge eat can alter their insulin injections accordingly, this woman's blindness required that she first learn how to use the pen. Finally, we met with a team of the people she worked with, including a sympathetic feminist medical doctor, and discussed why things had not been working and explained the approach we had decided to take. The use of contracting in this therapy relationship allowed the client to find solutions that worked for her. She was able to have far more control over her own body by being encouraged to explore what she wanted.

INTEGRATING BEHAVIOURAL CHANGE

Therapy for eating disorders cannot simply focus on behavioural change; instead, there needs to be an integration of emotional work and behavioural change. Feminist therapy explores the actual meaning of anorexia, bulimia, emotional eating, and compulsive exercise in women's lives, recognizing that eating disorders, however paradoxically and problematically, provide an avenue for women to express and cope with their difficulties and conflicts. Feminist therapy can encourage and enable women to find more direct ways of expressing their needs and their pain, while respecting the symptoms presented. As many anorexic or bulimic women, when initially seeking help, are unaware of the sorts of things anorexia and bulimia express for them, therapy needs to explore what roles these behaviours have in their lives.

Focusing on the connection between women's current and past life experiences and the eating problem prevents the therapist from reinforcing the existing displacement of a client's emotional struggles onto the body and obscuring the larger and more substantial issues. To address the real issues or problems in women's lives, helpers must assist women in discovering why they focus on weight and eating. Feminist therapy can use contracting as a means for women to be supported and facilitated through a process of understanding their own pain and how it is expressed through their eating and their bodies. Through the process of therapy, or of self-discovery, a client often begins to be aware, for the first time, of her own needs, desires, and feelings. Through this awareness, she can begin a process of slowly letting go of her need to express herself through her body in this way. By consistently valuing the client's feelings and needs, and emphasizing her right to control her body and life, feminist contracting can mitigate the control paradox and ultimately facilitate empowerment. Through contracting, the balance accomplished between insight work and action permits the attainment of a more substantive and grounded sense of control in women's lives rather than the precarious control established through control of their bodies.

Contracting allows an anorexic woman to establish a sense of control over the pacing of behavioural and emotional change. An anorexic woman may suggest that she could eat half an apple more per day for a week. She will try this and work with the feelings that arise as she implements this change. Her behavioural changes may be very slow, but each one should be acknowledged, and it should be recognized that this "baby step" may have been very difficult to accomplish. Despite the difficulty she experiences with making small changes, a client may minimize their importance. It is useful, therefore, for the therapist to explore with her how she feels about the changes she makes, and to discuss their significance. At the same time that these behavioural changes are being contracted, emotional insight work is ongoing. Therapists must be careful to monitor their own impatience to ensure they are not pushing clients at a pace they find threatening. Encouraging clients to set realistic goals for themselves prevents them from setting themselves up for "failure." If a contract is not realistic, or is too difficult too stick to, it should be renegotiated.

A woman who is bingeing and purging many times a day may set up a contract to work on the emotional parts of the behaviour and for actual behavioural change. She may explore her history of dieting; her current eating behaviour and whether it sets her up to binge; her past and present life experiences; her body image and how to improve it; and her emotional needs, desires, and conflicts. She may begin her effort at behavioural change by simply trying to hold off her binge for one minute — just sitting with the feelings that arise and becoming more aware of them. Then, if she feels she still needs to eat, she gives herself permission to do so. Accomplishing this is an important step, for she has turned a behaviour which was automatic and "unconscious" into a conscious, however ambivalent, decision to eat. Not only has she made it her conscious choice to eat or purge, as the case may be, she has also made some connections about why she may be needing to do so at that moment. She has attained some control, however limited, over the process. Over time, she may be able to wait for longer periods of time, sitting with her emotions, before she eats. Eventually she may get to the point where she chooses to hold off on bingeing completely. She may then set new goals for herself around how often she is going to binge and purge. For example, she may try to binge and purge four times instead of five times a week. Other times she may practise bingeing without purging. To do this she may also contract to deliberately eat food which feels safe enough to keep in. Often these foods are fruit and vegetables, as they do not pose the threat of weight gain.

Employing a contracting approach with clients with eating disorders does not mean that it is necessary to talk about eating, weight, or contracts continuously. The client and helper strike a

balance that works for them about how they can effectively negotiate the process of therapy. The use of contracting needs to be flexible, and responsive on an individual basis. Through being in touch
with the significant issues and experiences in the client's life, the
therapist can help facilitate behavioural contracting that is both safe
and challenging. Contracting must be respectful of what a woman
can or can't do. It needs to reflect where she is in the process of
working with the emotional aspects of the anorexia, bulimia, or
compulsive eating. And it reinforces that she needs to set up expectations for herself that are comfortable and reasonable, rather than
complying with someone else's agenda. Some differences exist in
working with anorexia, bulimia, and emotional eating, but there
are even greater similarities. The contracting principles work the
same way in all instances.

I have outlined some ideas for structuring a feminist approach
to eating disorders, with a particular emphasis on feminist contracting. Feminist therapy for eating disorders needs to honour the myriad ways women resist with their bodies — through body acceptance, refusing to diet, anorexia, or bulimia. These are creative
responses to the psychological distress in women's lives within a
culture obsessed with thinness. We cannot hope to alleviate these
problems with methods which exacerbate women's distress by
futher disempowering them. Contracting is an empowering alternative.

◆

OUT FROM UNDER BODY-IMAGE DISPARAGEMENT

Karin Jasper

Imagine that you are driving your car along the street. It is an old Lincoln Continental. Friends, relatives, and strangers criticize you for driving this car. It's huge and awkward to park and, worst of all, it guzzles gas. Whereas at one time driving it enhanced your reputation — people assumed you to be a well-to-do and upstanding citizen — it now reflects badly on your moral character. People assume you don't care about the environment or anything else besides yourself.

You decide to buy a new car, perhaps one of those being advertised as "built for the human race." It is much smaller, gets far better gas mileage, and transforms your character in the eyes of friends, relatives, and strangers. Once again you are embraced by the human race. It feels good.

Just one thing, though: you can't seem to get the hang of driving the thing around. Despite the fact that you are in this much more compact car, you drive it as if it were the size of your old Lincoln Continental. You drive right past parking spots that would easily accommodate the new car, but would never have taken the Lincoln. When you do park, you notice that you leave enough space between your car and the next one to fit the difference.

Furthermore, adrenaline is released and your heart pounds when, as you are passing another car, just for a moment you lose touch with the boundaries of your new car, connect with those of the old Lincoln, and panic that you are going to be too close to make it safely. You relax as you reconnect with car you are actually in.

It takes time to accommodate to driving a car with significantly different dimensions from one that you have been used to. During the in-between stage your "car-body image" is distorted. It's not, however, a perceptual distortion, but more like a kinaesthetic one. If you were to step out of the car and look at it, you wouldn't perceive it to be bigger or smaller than it actually is, but you might behave as if it were while driving it.

Now imagine a woman who has succeeded in losing weight. Her character has been transformed in the eyes of her friends, relatives, and strangers. Compliments on her "accomplishment" abound. She is pleased. It feels good. Except, just like the person who *feels* like she's still in the Lincoln Continental, this woman still *feels* fat. Depending on how frequently this feeling occurs and how disturbing she finds it, she may try to lose more weight in order to restore her equilibrium.

WHAT IS BODY IMAGE?

Notice that the term "body image," which is highly suggestive of the visual, actually picks out a very complex experience. At any given time, a person's body image might include several of many elements. Imagine following a person coming back to civilization after a week in the woods. Upon encountering a mirror, the person looks at her image and exclaims, "Is that me?!" This event nicely illustrates a perceptual aspect of body image. She may continue obliging us by expressing feelings and judgements (read: affective and evaluative elements) about what she sees when she says: "That better not be me!" Coming to terms with reality and focusing now on the cognitive aspect, she sighs and says: "Yes, I do believe it is me, after all." Now, walking away from the mirror, she remarks on a kinaesthetic [1] aspect of body experience as she says to her friend, "You know, on that last mile, every step felt like I was moving myself through muck, but now that it's over I feel almost like I'm floating." It is not as easy to find a good label for the next and last element, but it is something like sensed body integrity. It includes experiences ranging from feeling solid or impenetrable to feeling one's body boundaries as almost permeable as in, for example, "Yes, I feel almost ghostly — as if someone could walk right through me and not bump into anything."

In these examples, physical changes are what give rise to the phenomena described, but similar body experiences can arise from emotional states. A person who is feeling shame, for instance, may notice an experience of heaviness or stuckness and of being excruciatingly aware of every inch of her body. Looking in the mirror, while in this state, may bring painful awareness of every "flaw" ever documented in a fashion magazine. In contrast, the same person, sometime later and in the initial stages of requited romantic love, may feel a kind of weightlessness or buoyancy as she moves through her day. Furthermore, when looking in the mirror, she is surprised: she has never before noticed how attractive she is.

Most North American women are very familiar with feeling fat, whether they *are* fat or not. The feeling comes and goes. Some women feel fat even when emaciated or malnourished as a result of severe food restriction or binge-purge behaviour. The immense disparity between what we see — a very thin starving body — and what we hear — "I'm fat" or "I feel fat" — is what we focus on, and the explanation we have gravitated towards is that the person in question doesn't see or judge herself accurately — she is experiencing a perceptual and evaluative distortion. But perceptual distortions of any magnitude seem to be rare, even among women who are anorexic. Perhaps the anorexic woman notices the disparity and is as shocked and dismayed by it as we are. Imagine, after all, denying yourself food day after day but finding that you continue to feel fat even though you can see your body has become thinner.

You might wonder: What is it going to take? How much do I have to not eat for this feeling to go away? As long as the feeling is still there, it doesn't matter how thin the image in the mirror is, because it is not thin enough to make you feel thin. The criterion for how thin is thin enough seems to be whether the experience of feeling fat has disappeared or not. Well, what is this experience of feeling fat? When a person "feels fat" she may actually be displacing[2] some feelings about herself onto her body.

DISPLACEMENT

Displacement is a simple process that can be seen in the way babies and small children use special objects, for example, blankets ("blankies") or teddy bears. A small child may have a blanket or teddy that is very special to her, that she will not part with, even for washing. She will need the object most when she is unhappy or is separated from her parents, and it is very useful, because it allows the child to cope with upsetting feelings without needing the parent nearby. We might say that the child has taken the positive feelings of comfort and protection that originally arose in relation to the parent and displaced them onto the blanket or teddy. This allows the child to stay connected with feelings of security associated with that parent, simply by snuggling with the object. The displacement provides a very natural and adaptive way for the child to cope with a range of difficulties.

With regard to body image, the process of displacement actually works within an individual. So, a woman may take feelings that first arise in relation to an aspect of herself and displace them onto her body. The grounding for such displacement is, again, cultural. In our society, women's bodies are (among other things) objects that are displayed for and scrutinized by others. In order to participate in this displaying and being scrutinized, women have to see their bodies as objects. The result is an alienation of the person from her body, and this alienation is what makes displacement possible.

Then, suppose that, as a result of having been emotionally abused, a person feels self-loathing, or that, having had a very depressed or alcoholic parent, she has learned to deny and distrust her own needs. She may feel unlovable or out of control, but have little idea how to change this. She may *displace* these intolerable feelings about *herself* onto her *body*, and experience this as "feeling fat." Since fatness is culturally associated with a plethora of negative characteristics, including shame, inadequacy, neediness, and lack of control, it is a likely candidate for this displacement. Identifying her body as the problem, through displacement, may initially help her in several ways: (1) it may diminish the power of the very negative feeling by localizing it; (2) it may allow her to avoid an overwhelmingly painful idea by changing its nature; (3) it may comfort her to believe she has a way of coping with the feeling. For, while it may be very difficult to find a way to deal with the feeling that she is unworthy as a person or that there is "something wrong" with her, it will seem relatively easy to deal with having a body that feels fat — in that case, she simply has to lose weight and exercise to reshape her body until it is satisfactory. It is likely that, as her body comes to resemble the ideal, people will say nice things about her and assume even better things about her. For a time she will feel lovable, worthy, and in control, all at the same time as she is reducing her needs. Eventually, however, the displacement will break down.

Even in our original example, displacement is not a foolproof tool to cope with distressing thoughts and feelings. Children who use teddies and "blankies" encounter situations in which their upsetting feelings really do require the presence of their parents for resolution, for example, when they get lost, or undergo trauma. The person who has tried to change her body in order to feel better about herself can experience a similar problem. Because it was her very self rather than her *body* that she originally felt ashamed of, fixing it won't make her feel better for very long. She is likely to get stuck in a cycle of: feeling fat; losing weight; feeling a little better for a little while; feeling fat again either because she regains weight or because something happens to make her feel ashamed, inadequate, ineffective or out of control; then trying to lose more weight to feel better again. Eventually, she will have lost so much weight that people no longer give her compliments, but express fear for her health and try to coerce her into gaining weight — a move that is likely to increase her feeling of being out of control. Or she may become stuck in a cycle of bingeing and purging, which will make her feel even worse about herself. At times, she may catch a glimpse of her own body and be taken aback by how thin it is, but she will be sure it isn't thin enough the very next time she feels fat. Breaking displacement is a key to resolving body-image disparagement and is one of the strategies used in the Body Image Group.

OUT FROM UNDER BODY-IMAGE DISPARAGEMENT: THE BODY IMAGE GROUP

While it is essential and unavoidable to address body-image issues in individual therapy, group work opens up possibilities that are not available in individual work. Groups of any sort offer participants the opportunity to learn from others who are struggling with similar issues, and the opportunity to contribute to the personal growth of others. In addition, however, a body-image group specifically allows women to create a counterculture (see Jasper and Maddocks 1992) in which beauty and thinness are not seen as equivalent, weight prejudice is challenged, and competitiveness around body size and shape is discouraged. Such a "weight-acceptance culture" helps women see more clearly the ways in which they have internalized cultural messages about women and body size, resulting in self-harming behaviours, and how they can begin to be more empathic[3] towards, and thus take better care of, their bodies.

What I describe here is based on my experience in clinical practice over the last five years — what I have noticed and what participants in the group have said about their experiences in it. Recently, in association with the Toronto Hospital, I have initiated research that will eventually provide more formal assessment of the value of the interventions that are part of the Body Image Group. Right now, based on feedback from participants, what is most valuable is simply being with a group of women who share body-image problems. There is much difference of opinion among participants about the usefulness of specific interventions that are part of the group's work. What I describe here is how I set up the group, the kinds of themes that come up, and some ways of facilitating the discussion of those themes.

When I first started doing the group, I relied substantially on specific exercises to help move the group members through a process of developing more positive attitudes towards their bodies and described the group as more of an extended workshop than a therapy group. Now I rely more on group process and use the exercises to help participants focus on specific body-image issues, at the time and in the order that seem to be needed. The group has thus become less workshop-like and more therapy-like. Five general areas cover most themes that come up or that I introduce in the groups: body-image history, replacing displacement, self and body care, shame, and change. In discussing these five general areas, I will describe the various ways in which each one is addressed in the group; however, it should be noted that not every group includes all of the things discussed here. One group may spend several weeks on body-image history; another group may spend more time on shame.

The body-image group meets for twelve weeks and is closed to new members once it has started. The group is designed for women who have had either an eating disorder or significant difficulties with food and weight. A woman can enter the group once she has made an inroad in normalizing her eating and as long as she is committed to non-dieting while working on body acceptance in the group. Those who are actively engaged in attempts to lose weight or in restrictive eating are not eligible to participate in this particular group. Often the group includes women with a wide range of shapes and weights; sometimes, the range happens to be narrower. In either case, group members are asked to notice the similarities in the feelings they have about their bodies, regardless of body size, and are asked to notice the differences between their beliefs about what life is like for thin women or fat women and the reality expressed by the women themselves. One area of difference for large women is specifically addressed: the fact that they do face social discrimination in such areas as jobs and job promotion, accommodation, and social harassment that average-sized or thinner women do not face.

During the first session, after a process that facilitates group members introducing themselves, group expectations are discussed, and a set of ground rules is proposed by the group leader. The ground rules are discussed again at the beginning of the fourth session, when group members have had a chance to live with them and may want to suggest alterations. Considerable emphasis is placed on attendance (this element is also underlined during assessment interviews — anyone who knows she will have to miss more than two sessions is asked to attend the group another time) because the group is both demanding and time-limited. Other ground rules include some general guidelines for group members' giving feedback to one another; permission to "pass" during group "go-rounds"; confidentiality; an agreement that, should a group member become engaged in restrictive-eating or weight-loss efforts during the twelve weeks of the group, she will inform the group; and an agreement that, should a group member become suicidal or overwhelmed by material taken up in the group, she will call her therapist, doctor, or group leader (whichever is most suitable). Generally, group members have no difficulty agreeing to these "rules," but it is not unusual for there to be a fairly lengthy discussion about the meaning of "engaged in restrictive-eating or weight-loss efforts" since most women attending the group are having their commitment to non-dieting and weight acceptance tested through a variety of life situations. Perhaps once a day, or once a week, or more, most group members will find themselves feeling strongly that being thinner would be better, doubting that it is okay to eat as much as they are eating, or slipping into exercising longer than usual. Material that comes up for discussion in the group may directly precipitate a "setback" of this sort.

Having setbacks is a theme that comes up fairly regularly in the group, whether in the form of renewed restrictive eating, bingeing and purging, compulsive eating, or weighing. When someone brings up having a setback, group members often raise their fear that they will never fully get over their eating problems. If no one else does, I will suggest a way of contextualizing setbacks that allows for both their occurrence and ultimate full recovery. It's a simple description of a spiral, where, in the process of going up the spiral, downward as well as upward movement occurs. When a person is in a downward place, it feels just like all the previous downward places all the way down the spiral. That it feels just like the place at the bottom of the spiral doesn't make it the bottom. Having a setback doesn't mean that everything learned has been unlearned, or that all progress is nullified. It just feels like it is. Stepping back from the feelings can help a person get perspective on what has happened, and can allow for new learning to take place: What precipitated this setback? What efforts did the person make to prevent the setback? What stopped the setback from continuing? New learning can be integrated and momentum generated for continued forward movement. Group members assist one another by sharing their own experiences of setbacks, sharing their ideas for preventing them, sharing phone numbers, and demonstrating with their own continued progress that setbacks aren't synonymous with "the end." Also, there are times when the setback will raise other important issues like perfectionism and meeting others' expectations. Those who have had no setbacks in the first months of recovery and then have one may find themselves hiding the truth from those around them, because, for example "I couldn't admit that I was having trouble" or "No one expected that I would have trouble this far down the road." By hiding the truth, women deny their own needs and their own experiences, effectively neutralizing their ability to respond. As several women have observed, just acknowledging to a supportive person that they are "in trouble" (feeling like restricting, bingeing, or purging) can be enough to prevent a setback.

BODY-IMAGE HISTORY

Group members are curious about how it happened that they got to be so unhappy about their bodies and so focused on weight loss as a way of feeling better. Making progress in identifying the many-layered answer to this question is important to them, both because it is a tool for change and because understanding is satisfying in itself.

Early on in the group, I use a slide show to introduce some of the sociocultural issues that I think are significant in relation to body-image disparagement and eating problems and to introduce the idea of displacement. I also use this opportunity to introduce subjects that group members may not have thought about or may not feel comfortable initiating in a group, e.g., issues related to abuse, sexual orientation, or the effects of racism on body image. Finally, I suggest, through the slide show, that a person's eating problem has meaning and may be interpreted as a message (or multiple messages) to the people around her. Most women have not thought about their eating problems this way, but, for the most part, they are intrigued by it and interested in trying to put words to their own "messages."

Through a written exercise after the slide show (or as homework), group members are invited to reflect on the ways in which the slide show did or didn't illuminate their own experience and to note important aspects of their own experience that were not addressed in the slide show. The idea of "internalizing" oppressive cultural messages is introduced and they are asked to monitor their own disparaging body and self talk for instances of such messages. The following week, discussion about what they noticed in this area is taken up.

Most women are very familiar with the idea that the mass media have communicated a body-image ideal that is completely unrealistic for women and is a contributing factor in the development of eating disorders. They are also resistant to a simple cause-effect analysis here, mainly because it does not fit their own experience. Contrary to theorists who argue that women with eating disorders tend to have bought into traditional female roles, the women I work with frequently see themselves as trying to avoid these roles. Taking the sociocultural analysis deeper is important for them to see how they have personally been influenced by it.

Personal body-image history is addressed through group discussion and/or a guided imagery exercise. Before the group gets into a discussion about events that have shaped their experience of their bodies, I present information about dealing with painful memories.[4] Not all members of the group will have to deal with traumatic memories related to emotional, physical, or sexual abuse, but most of the information is useful in relation to painful memories in general. Once I have presented this information, we work through a handout called "Your Body Image History," which includes sections on "how parents, relatives, and siblings reacted to your body"; "how your body changed over time"; "your experience of your physical self"; "your experience of your sexuality"; "physical abuse, neglect, and sexual abuse"; "accidents, illnesses, surgeries"; "your race/ethnicity"; "your economic class"; and "your gender." Discussion of these topics raises many important issues.

For instance, group members may remember feeling "watched." Their experiences range from being scrutinized and judged by a perfectionistic parent who treats the daughter as an extension of him or herself, to having their relationship sexualized by a parent who is pruriently interested in their body's development. These experiences seem to result in a compulsive controlling of appearance and a wish to hide. Group members almost universally remember the onset of menstruation as a shaming experience and as a point when their bodies began to feel like a burden to them. Some have described this as a time when they felt a real heaviness descend upon them, partly because of the sensations and care requirements related to menstruation, but mainly because, along with other developmental changes, it marked the beginning of unwelcome changes in their roles and responsibilities and in the expectations others had of them. Group members recall being told that unwanted sexual attention and preventing pregnancy was entirely their responsibility, but at the same time found that these things were often out of their control. Women who reached puberty earlier than their peers or who developed large breasts often report being cruelly ridiculed and harassed or assaulted by their peers. They tend to see their bodies as the source of the problem and look to changing their bodies as the solution. These changes, marked by the onset of puberty, leave girls few ways to relate positively towards their bodies. When they do not have the opportunity to recognize and develop their sexual feelings at their own pace, they lose the chance to experience their sexuality in a positive way. For a variety of reasons, puberty may represent the advent of loss rather than of any benefit or advantage. Talking about these issues helps women feel less isolated, assists them in learning to recognize what they did and did not have control over, and helps them to release themselves from blame. Some women experience a lifting of the heaviness at this time.

Discussing gender issues related to body-image history includes raising such questions as: Did your parents want a boy or a girl? Did you feel like a girl? Do you now feel like a woman? What were the advantages or disadvantages and expectations related to being a boy or a girl in your family and in society? Some women talk about having always felt that being a girl was a disappointment to one or the other of their parents, some talk about having been tomboys happily until adolescence when they were expected not to be tomboys anymore and experiencing tremendous loss about this. Some group members talk about having been wanted as a girl and having been favoured over other children in the family, making them feel special but also guilty. Others talk about seeing their brothers treated as the important members of the family and to whom the majority of the family resources were directed, resulting in feelings of inadequacy, inferiority, and neediness for the girls.

Nearly all women report watching their mothers model self-sacrifice and feeling strongly that they would not put themselves in the
same position. Group members will point out to one another occasions when they are being self-sacrificing or not taking care of their
needs, helping to raise one another's consciousness about this.

Abuse also affects body image. Whether it is perpetrated by a
mother, a father, or someone else, abuse tends to result in the
woman internalizing the abusive person's attitude towards herself.
So she may blame herself, and feel hatred or disgust towards herself.
The abuse itself may result in her experiencing her body as dirty or
as occupied. At the extreme she may consider herself and treat herself as not fully human. All of these attitudes will distance her farther from her own body so that it is less and less the place that she
lives.[5] Feeding it and caring for it will amount to betraying herself.
She will need time to learn that she has been injured rather than
that she is is diseased, and to offer herself the care that she would
offer any other injured being.

Sometimes women with traumatic histories start remembering
events they had not thought of for some time or had not ever
remembered before. Flashbacks, flooding, and a range of self-harming behaviours may begin (drinking, drug use, food restriction,
bingeing and purging, cutting, burning, and suicidality).[6] Two
aspects of the group help here: one is that group members have
been informed at the beginning that the group might trigger memories and that they are part of the recovery process; the other is that
group members have been provided with some suggestions for dealing with these memories. Neither is sufficient to prevent suffering,
but each provides a context for what is happening and gives a person some direction about how to handle it (this can take a while,
but at least the idea is there). Women have said that the point at
which they were able to see themselves as having been victimized
by the abuse rather than as having deserved or invited it was the
point at which remembering became useful to them rather than
simply retraumatizing. It's the point at which they can begin caring
for themselves once again, or for the first time. Sometimes women

in this situation are already working with an individual therapist, sometimes not. In the latter case, I work with them individually through the crisis, and help them find a suitable individual therapist.

Some women in the group have identified an illness or accident as marking a turning-point in the development of their body image. For instance, a prolonged illness during adolescence can both provide a young woman with attention and a feeling of specialness (that is otherwise lacking in her life) and delay her developing a sense of her own identity while her peers are busy developing theirs. Once she recovers, she is bereft of attention and identity and may look to "being thin" as a reliable and quick replacement. Women (including those who do not have a history of illness) talk about feeling despair when they realize how much time they have "wasted" with their eating and body-image problems, how far behind their peers they have fallen, and how they are still confused about what they would like to be or do. I have found group members to be very supportive of one another here, counseling each other to exercise a great deal of patience and to give themselves the freedom to experiment with various things until they find what they want.

In discussing race or ethnicity, issues of difference often predominate, whether they be the difference a women experiences as a member of a minority group or the difference she experiences within that group. For instance, women might talk about what it is like, as descendents of Eastern Europeans, to be naturally hairier or heavier than her peers, or what it is like to have a body shape that is common among First Nations women, but is not like the predominant body ideal for women in Western societies. Where the minority group is devalued in the society at large, women may struggle against disliking their bodies and internalizing a dislike for their group of origin. Or, even if their body shape is different from the dominant group's ideal, they may be able to derive some comfort from the fact that it is common within their group of origin. Difference *within* an ethnic or racial group raises other problems.

Oriental women who are large, for instance, may feel especially wrong or "at fault" because Oriental women supposedly aren't built that way. In the group we try to sort out these complexities so that each woman can re-contextualize her own experience of body-hatred and begin to externalize negative attitudes she has internalized.

Class issues also have implications for body image. Women who grew up in working class families sometimes talk about not having been able to afford the clothing and activities their peers in school were able to afford, and then responding to the resulting sense of being different and inferior by trying to be thin. Interestingly, women who grew up in upper class families report another kind of oppressive experience. In cases where their families had a strong investment in looking good all the time, women report having felt a tremendous pressure to keep a continuously perfect appearance. No trace of fat was acceptable, clothing had to be kept clean, and a smile was always required. In either situation and in a range of others in between, women talk about not having their needs and their value as individuals recognized and responded to. In the group we talk about how they have tried to voice their experience of oppression in these situations by changing their bodies.

REPLACING DISPLACEMENT

During the early stages of the group, I introduce the idea of displacement. I ask group members if they have noticed that body-image dissatisfaction, most often experienced as "feeling fat," usually occurs independently of actual changes in body weight. Some have already noticed this; others experience a kind of shock of recognition as we discuss it. I then encourage group members to start thinking in terms of displacement when they dislike their bodies, feel fat, feel heavy, or feel burdened by their bodies. This means simply asking themselves when the feeling started and trying to identify what triggered it. Sometimes we do a homework assignment on this topic, and debrief at the beginning of the next group meeting. Thinking in terms of displacement is a way of innoculating against setbacks.

I sometimes use a guided imagery exercise called "Body Scanning" (Hutchinson 1985, p.49) in which participants check out their sensed body boundaries kinaesthetically and locate various feeling states in their bodies (joy, fear, shame, anger, love). Towards the end of the exercise, they are asked to say aloud: "This is my body. This is where I, [her name], live." At the end of the guided imagery, I ask group members to draw a body map of the feeling states they identified. In group discussion, we look at connections between the areas of their bodies they dislike or hate and the locations of negative feeling states. This exercise is very rich. Often group members (of all sizes) notice that their body boundaries are closer in than they kinaesthetically sense them to be. This provides another way of seeing that "feeling fat" has little to do with actual size of one's body. The exercise also allows women to connect positive feelings like joy or love with their bodies and it is important for them to start making such positive connections. Women often notice that their body locations for anger or fear are places where they store tension. Noticing the tension may be easier than noticing the anger or fear and can then serve as a clue that anger or fear may be there. However, the exercise can also be very difficult for group members. Sometimes a woman will discover that her body boundaries are farther out than she kinaesthetically senses them to be and may be very distressed as a result. Most often this happens when a person has recently gained a considerable amount of weight over a short period of time and has simply not had time to adjust to the change. The exercise may also trigger painful or traumatic memories. So it is important for there to be plenty of time to process this exercise after it is done and to use it when the group seems prepared. Before the first time we try guided imagery, I let group members know that it is fine to open their eyes during the process if they don't want to go on with it or if they want a break from it.

Later on in the life of the group, I will introduce a guided imagery exercise called "Body Talk" (Hutchinson 1985, p.104) in which group members choose an area of their bodies that they victimize with negative thoughts, talk, and feelings, and have a conversation with that part of their bodies. The body part has a chance to talk back while the person listens. Eventually the two negotiate an improved way of relating. This exercise tends to bring the victimized body part to life, making it difficult for the person to continue relating to it in a completely unempathic way. The displacement pathway is blocked because displacement depends on alienation, and simultaneously a more caring approach to the body part is promoted. Women often choose their stomach or thighs to focus on and are shocked when stomach or thighs talk about what it feels like to hear the woman talk to them the way she does. This is a point at which some women recognize that they are talking to themselves the way abusive adults have talked to them in the past (demonstrating internalization of the abuser's attitude). For those women and for others, it is a time for recognizing the unfairness inherent in treating themselves in a way they would never consider treating anyone else. Recognizing this unfairness is enough to begin the process of change in some women. Others may need help at this point to see that there are no good reasons why they should be treated worse than everyone else. If, in fact, they were treated worse than everyone else in their family or their school (or wherever), seeing this can take a while. Many women vacillate between the two positions.

SELF AND BODY CARE

Fairly early on in the group, I introduce the idea that there are many ways that group members may not be taking care of their bodies, unrelated to eating.[7] I give a few examples, such as delaying going to the washroom, not resting when needing to rest, wearing shoes that hurt the feet, and then ask them to do a homework assignment in which they observe the ways they are not taking care of themselves. Often what happens is that group members come back and say that, although they had not noticed before, they are, in fact, doing these things. Usually one or two women will talk about other behaviours not on my example list, like exercising past the point of comfort, exhausting oneself through work or busyness, doing unsatisfying work, and carelessness that leads to bumps or cuts. Once any group member makes an addition to the list, other members start having recognition experiences. The whole process seems to make it easier for women to see their eating and body-image problems as part of a larger picture of not taking care of oneself, and this perspective seems to increase self-empathy. I generally follow this initial process with a few weeks of homework assignments where the object is either to avoid doing a self-harming behaviour or, to do something nice for themselves or their bodies that they wouldn't usually do, for example, going dancing, having a massage, or taking a relaxation class.

On the theme of self-care in relationships, I present information during the slide show on the ways women are socialized to approach relationships, the apparent differences between men's and women's needs in and for relationships, and the way in which women take responsibility for relationships' working (holding themselves responsible if a relationship doesn't work). I try to show how this approach to relationships limits our ability to be self-caring within them — if we are always responsible, we have to change ourselves for the benefit of the relationship, which often means denying our own needs, and ultimately losing the ability to identify them. For women whose personal histories have included a consistent lack of empathic response to their emotional (or other) needs, this effect is magnified. Group members help one another validate their needs and offer support and suggestions for negotiating conflicts betwen self-care and other-care in relationships.

A guided imagery exercise useful in developing this theme of self and body-care can be adapted from Susie Orbach's "Breaking into a Binge" (1982), in which we explore a recent time when the person either ate beyond the point of satisfaction or fullness or did not eat, even though she was hungry. This exercise allows group members to connect urges to overeat or to restrict food intake with moods, states, or feelings that are difficult to tolerate. Once the mood, state, or feeling is identified, group members help each other develop ideas about how to respond more effectively, including talking about the difficulty of just sitting with the mood, state, or feeling.

Theoretically, the work done in the group related to this theme will help group members become more aware of, more willing to, and better able to take care of themselves. Realistically, I think it gives group members a glimpse of how this can be and some practice with it.

SHAME

Another way of illuminating important aspects of body and self experience for women is through the concept of shame. To feel shame is "to feel seen in a painfully diminished sense" (Kaufman 1989, p. 17), and reactions to this feeling include the urge to hide, looking down, and an experience of paralysis. I present some information about the cultural sources of shame for women — most generally, that women are seen as inferior, and, more specifically, that when women's bodies don't match the ideal, they are seen as out of control (and therefore shameful in our culture). I discuss family dynamics that promote shame, for example, families in which rules must be perfectionistically adhered to and where relationships are always in jeopardy (Fossom and Mason 1989). Finally, I discuss interpersonal experiences that are shaming, including any abusive experience, but most generally any interaction where one person is used as an object by the other. In the group, women respond to these points by bringing up their own experiences and talking about the cumulative effect of many kinds of shame experience on their self and body image. Because feeling shame results in wanting to hide, it is easy to see how body shame might be responded to by covering oneself with loose clothing, making one's body smaller by dieting, or hiding oneself with fat. Talking about specific shame experiences in a supportive group environment and being able to identify their shame-specific responses seems helpful to many women. Again, recognizing and changing internalized or self-shaming attitudes is an important step to body-image satisfaction.

The guided imagery exercise "Body Talk" (described above) is useful in decreasing shame. The victimized body part can be seen as being shamed — that is, as being objectified and demeaned— by the person. Once the person can listen empathically to that body part, shame is reduced and the body part can be reowned.

I sometimes give a homework assignment that is adapted from an exercise called "Reclaiming Your Body" (Maltz 1991, p. 276); it was originally designed especially for survivors of sexual abuse, but is useful for most women who feel strongly disparaging of their bodies. This exercise asks women to experiment with various kinds of touch (but not touching their genitals or nipples) just to begin noticing how different areas of their bodies feel and what different kinds of touch feel like. As women feel less disgust (less shame) for their bodies, they will find this exercise easier to do. In general, I have found few women in the group who can make it all the way through this exercise. Most either stop part way through or don't do it at all. But nearly all of them struggle with it. In any case, I have found the group's discussion of the assignment and how members responded to it very helpful in opening up sexuality issues. Women often talk about the difficulties they have allowing their sexual partners to look at them while making love, their need to keep the lights off and the covers on — even when they know that their partners like their bodies. Other women talk about the difficulty they have even imagining being in a sexual relationship. Sometimes women leave the discussion feeling more courageous about trying the exercise again.

CHANGE

During the initial group session, I ask group members what topics they would like to cover in the group and what goals they would like to set for themselves. I also say a few things about the process of change. By the time they come to the body-image group, most women are very clear about how much their eating problems and body-image disparagement have cost them. They say they are very keen to start liking their bodies. They are fed up with having eating problems and excruciatingly aware of how much time they have lost. Most of them, however, have not thought about the ways in which their "problems" have helped them and continue to help them. So I just introduce the idea that "stuck" behaviours or attitudes are stuck for a good reason(s), and give a few examples. Later on, we do an exercise that makes this specific for each of them.

In between, we spend some time identifying negative self-talk or self-limiting thinking patterns. In addition to identifying patterns, like all-or-nothing thinking, personalization, filtering, "shoulds" thinking and so on, I ask group members to consider both how this kind of thinking is limiting in undesirable ways and how it may also have protected them or otherwise helped them get through difficulties. I think this helps them depathologize themselves. Most women who have been through the mental health system have learned to see themselves as sick or bad, and describe themselves that way. Although an illness metaphor may have helped get them started working towards change, it becomes a barrier to further positive development.

A guided imagery exercise called "Woman in a Trap" (Hutchinson 1985, p. 92) can be adapted to help women explore the positive and negative aspects of change and to develop strategies for accomplishing desired change. At the end of the exercise, I usually ask group members to draw a picture of what is inside and outside their "trap." Often women are surprised to notice the positive aspects of the insides of their traps and the threatening aspects of what is outside. Discussing their pictures with one another deepens their understanding of their own trap and allows them to explore what steps might be taken as a first approach to "escape."

The final meeting of the body-image group is set up the week before. Group members are given the following instructions.

> Please gather the following items and bring them to our group next week.

a) An item that represents some aspect of your eating and body image problems (or some other aspect of your life) that you are now ready and willing to let go of. This item will be left in the group room — you won't take it home with you. e.g. a toy, a photograph, a picture from a magazine, a song or poem, a piece of clothing, something you construct.

b) An item that represents what you are ready to work on next. You will take this item with you.

c) An item that expresses your acknowledgement of yourself and the group (*just one item, not one for everyone*).

Do not spend more than $2 on any item that you buy rather than make or find.

We spend the last group session having each group member talk about each of her items, explaining their meaning to her and why she chose them. We begin with each group member's item representing something she is willing to let go of. These items go into the garbage when they are done with, unless a group member requests otherwise, e.g. when she has brought clothing that no longer fits and is taking it to the Goodwill. Then we move on to the items representing what group members are ready to work on next, each group member keeping this item with her. Finally, after speaking about the items they have chosen to express their acknowledgements, each group member chooses one (not her own) of these items to take away with her as a keepsake of the group. Some group members put a lot of time and creativity into preparing their items. All are encouraged to be scrupulously honest in choosing their items and what they say about them. Sometimes women are not sure what they have gotten from the group or that there is anything that they are ready or willing to let go of. Others may be clear about that but very confused about what their next step is. We may have quite a long preparatory discussion related to the acknowledgement items, because women are often concerned about finding an item that is "good enough."

A couple of weeks following the last session, I have individual interviews with all of the women who attended the group. One group didn't feel ready to end, and I sensed that they had not come to a natural ending place, so we contracted for ten more meetings held every two weeks. There was a real sense of completion at that point, which we marked with a different ending ceremony.

The goal of the body-image group isn't to leave women completely free of body-image dissatisfaction, but to leave them clear about the issues such dissatisfaction may be masking and to give them some tools for dealing more effectively with those issues. Ultimately, finding ways to shift the culture without will be as important as making changes within.

◆

NOTES

1. Marcia Hutchinson (1985) introduced the importance of kinaesthetic aspects of body image.

2. I first developed the idea of displacement in relation to body-image dissatisfaction for a chapter entitled "Developing a Healthy Relationship with Your Body," in *The Road to Recovery: A Manual for Participants in the Psychoeducation Group for Bulimia Nervosa* (1989). The manual is used at Toronto General Hospital and is reprinted in *Group Psychotherapy for Eating Disorders*, ed. by Heather Harper-Guiffre and K. Roy MacKenzie (Washington, D. C.: American Psychiatric Press, 1992).

3. The idea of generating a more empathic relationship with one's body comes from Marcia Hutchinson (1985).

4. This information is drawn from three sources: a workshop by Clarissa Chandler called "The Care and Management of Flashbacks presented at the No More Secrets Conference sponsored by Community Resources and Initiatives, Toronto, May 1990; a presentation by Esther Cancella called "Surviving the Survival" made at the Ritual Abuse: Focus on Healing conference sponsored by Education Dissociation, Toronto, June 16, 1990; and my own experience working with abuse survivors.

5. See Hutchinson 1985, "Body Scanning," p. 49.

6. I recommend Bonnie Burstow's *Radical Feminist Therapy* (1992) as a source of direct practice suggestions in these areas.

7. Burstow 1992, p. 187.

WOMEN EMBODIED AND EMBOLDENED: DEALING WITH SEXUAL VIOLENCE

Patricia McGillicuddy and Sasha Maze

The truth about our childhood is stored up in our body and although we can repress it, we can never alter it. Our intellect can be deceived, our feelings manipulated, our perceptions confused and our body tricked with medication.

But someday the body will present its bill, for it is as incorruptible as a child who, still whole in spirit, will accept no compromises or excuses, and it will not stop tormenting us until we stop evading the truth.

— Alice Miller

A woman speaks:
I choose not to be silenced anymore. I allow my body to feel the pain it remembers in order to get through it, to be stronger, to want to fight, to eventually feel all those feelings which were always mine but were wrenched from me. I will not die. [1]

In pain, in strength, with boldness, with wilfulness, as women we live in our bodies and deal with the ongoing realities of physical, emotional, and sexual violence in our lives. Such violence has

effected the physical and emotional development of female children, the present day-to-day choices and restrictions women face,
our prospects and future plans. Counseling, advocacy, and activism
that address issues of sexual violence must be concerned with the
impact this violence has upon women's bodies. Work in the areas of
body image, body disparagement, eating patterns, physical illness,
chronic pain management, addictions, and weight preoccupation
must be concerned with the effects of sexual violence, and of the
threat of sexual violence, which is a normal part of women's and
children's lived experience.

Included here is a review of some of the theory, statistics, counseling interventions, and women's stories that have emerged from
anti-rape work with a particular focus on physical self and the need
to build connection with the self and with other women.

A review of the literature in the area of sexual assault reveals a
broad-based analysis of the impact of assault on individual women
and of the meaning of such a pervasive force within North
American society. This literature is classifiable into at least six general
areas (excluding assailant-related data): epidemiology; psychological-impact analysis; sex-role learning theory (including pornography-
impact studies); sociological analysis (including sociocultural variables and symbolic interaction theories); political and economic
theories; and most important, the stories and insights of women
who are survivors of violence.

In the area of fact-finding, epidemiological research and in-
depth interviews with women have been undertaken that indicate
that at least 50 to 60 percent of North American women will be
sexually assaulted at least once in their lifetime (*Badgley Report*
1984; Russell 1986). At least 34 percent of women and 34 percent
of their female children will be sexually assaulted before the age of
eighteen years (13 percent of male children will be sexually assaulted). Ninety-eight percent of the assailants will be male (*Badgley
Report* 1984). At least one in seven women will be raped by her

male partner (Russell 1982). At least one in five women will be physically assaulted by her male partner, at least once (Hamilton 1989).[2] Poor women are more likely to be raped both by known assailants and by strangers (Hamilton 1989, p. 35). Black women in North America are more likely to be suddenly attacked by strangers while traveling outside the home (ibid., p. 36). Lesbian women are more likely to be raped by male strangers than are other women in the same situation (ibid.). Women with physical or developmental disabilities are more likely to be physically and sexually assaulted, and the assailant will most likely be a caretaker, a doctor, a person known to them (Doucette 1986). Women domestic workers are physically, emotionally, and sexually assaulted by employers (Silvera 1988). The incidence of past and recent sexual assault increases to at least 70 to 80 percent of women if the women surveyed are in inpatient psychiatry units (Firsten 1991), are homeless, are working in prostitution or pornography, are in conflict with the law, are economically disadvantaged,[3] are newcomers as immigrants or refugees (Parades 1992), are First Nations women living in cities (Canadian Native Women's Association *Report on Child Sexual Abuse* 1989), or are physically or developmentally disabled (Doucette 1986). The women whom discrimination and systemic oppression make the most available to be raped *will* be raped within this "culture of violence" that uses the threat and the reality of sexual violence to legitimize and reinforce further violence and oppression.

The second area of research, psychological-impact analysis, draws on these staggering statistics to explain the interrelatedness of discrimination and violent victimization of women. An American writer, Jean Hamilton (1989, p. 40), notes that

> the key to understanding the more specific aspects of harm comes from recognizing the the internalization of social stereotypes and prejudices that devalue women, along with the subsequent activation of these attitudes by victimization ... internalized devaluation of oneself (and of one's group) and unworthiness is reinforced by the threat of violence and by the shattering of

the public/private split regarding sexuality. Although each small dose of discrimination may be tolerated, the overall effect — as with a poison — is cumulative ... discrimination can serve as a model for interpretation or a focus for the reactivation of abuse experiences and visa-versa.

Thus racism, classism, heterosexism, ableism, and sexism are mutually reinforcing sources of violence against women. Physical bodies hold women in time and space as open-territory women, as women available to be raped, as women who could be raped if members of the oppressing group chose to do so. Alienation from oneself and one's group, the reinforcement of unworthiness, the physical impact of pain, the traumatic crisis of being violated, the attack on sexual integrity — these effects of rape, compounded by the reactions of family, friends, social, and legal systems, most often result in a wrenching dissociation from the body, an overwhelming sense of psychic death and terror.

In addition to work that links the effects of systemic discrimination, a number of psychological-impact studies trace the effects of rape trauma on the physical, emotional, behavioural and cognitive aspects of women's reactions. Burgess and Holstrom (1979, p. 35) identified clusters of symptoms and a series of phases of trauma which they called "rape trauma syndrome." This conceptualization was based on their work with women who had been recently raped, and was used extensively by rape crisis workers in the 1970s and 1980s as a tool for assisting women in understanding their reactions. Other research linked symptoms of rape trauma syndrome to concepts of grief reaction — resolution of loss, sadness, mourning — and to post-traumatic stress disorder — a psychiatric diagnosis, now very popular, that was developed in studies on the effect of war on Vietnam army veterans in the United States and on victims of natural disasters. Women who have been raped, are critical of this schema, noting that rape is never impersonal or an "act of God" and neither can it be reduced to a set of stress responses which characterize the women as victim, minimize the criminal nature of the act itself, and decontextualize the nature of violence.

Learning theorists have examined the relationship between sex-role stereotyping and learned behaviour which condones rape. Complimentary, i.e., "rape-permissive," behaviours of girls and boys, and of men and women, are found to encourage female passivity and male aggression, female dependence and male independence (Bart 1986, p. 124). Images of sexual violence directed against women and children, in advertising and pornography, are viewed by some feminist learning theorists as pro-rape propaganda. Most studies of the effects of such pornography involve young, white male college students as subjects. Such studies conclude that exposure to sexually explicit pornography reduces men's sensitivity as to the harm of rape, increases their hostility towards the women's movement, and causes them to recommend shorter jail terms for sexual offenders. When exposed to prolonged viewing of filmed scenarios in which definite acts of criminal violence were being depicted, the men laughed more, saw less violence, increasingly identified with the assailant, and saw less harm done to raped women. One-third of the men studied said they would rape even in the most violent situations depicted if they could avoid being caught and charged (Zillman and Bryant 1982).

Feminist social scientists and anthropologists have taken concepts of learning theory one step farther to provide an analysis of North American white patriarchal culture as one in which the permission to rape women and children is enshrined. In such a culture, one group expropriates power and uses power to enforce sex on others. It is this pattern of expropriation of power and exercise of power and control that allows for sexual assault. So, in this view, the college students are not so much responding to the material as they are simply exercising their power. This pattern often dictates the women's experience with the legal system and with so-called helping professionals. Studies on social perceptions of rape victims suggest that family, friends, social agencies, and legal systems will all, to some degree, blame the women for the attacker's action (Brickman 1984; Foucault 1979). This is consistent with the nature of systemic discrimination in which victims of crime are held responsible, the crime is minimized, and the assailant is viewed as mentally ill.

Rape, then, acts as a symbol within the culture since it has a social meaning — as the acting out of male power, anger and sexuality — and it has a social purpose — as a mode of socially controlling women, and as an enhancement of male dominance (Plummer 1975, pp 42–46).

The power of this symbol and the pain and fear engendered by it are the subject of much of the writing of women about rape from the 1970s to the present (Criffin 1979). Pervasive assault and fear of assault are described as actually shaping women's consciousness of self and shaping their relationship with the world — with other women, with family, with work, with institutions. From the work of women survivors this pervasive symbol has come to be understood to effect the actual embodiment of women (Danica 1990; Vancouver Women's Research Collective (ed) 1989), and to effect the need to reshape the body to maximize safety or to become invisible, or to reinforce worthlessness. Concepts of claiming space, sexuality, individual body size and shape, creating new images of strength, finding strength in survival, and becoming warriors come from the learning of these women — learning which is intrinsically linked to liberation movements.

Political and economic theorists have used an analysis of historical data, race and class analysis, and economic-stratification data to examine the relationship between power (money and political control), patriarchy, class, sexuality, race, and gender. The social conditions that foster sexual violence are entrenched in issues of enfranchisement, equity, equal opportunity, rights and freedoms. Angela Davis, in addressing an audience on the issues of rape and racism, quotes a poem by June Jordon (1980), which speaks to the interrelatedness of these issues of body to mind to soul — to the world:

from "POEM ABOUT MY RIGHTS"

Even tonight and I need to take a walk and clear
my head about this poem about why I can't

go out without changing my clothes my shoes
my body posture my gender identify my age
my status as a woman alone in the evening/
alone on the streets/alone not being the point/
the point being that I can't do what I want
to do with my own body because I am the wrong
sex the wrong age the wrong skin and
suppose it was not here in the city but down on the beach/
or far into the woods and I wanted to go
there by myself thinking about God/or thinking
about children/ or thinking about the world/all of it
disclosed by stars and the silence:
I could not go and I could not think and I could not
stay there
alone
as I need to be
alone because I can't do what I want to do with my own
body and
who in the hell set things up
like this
and in France they say if the guy penetrates
but does not ejaculate then he did not rape me
... then I consented and there was
no rape because finally you understand finally
they fucked me over because I was wrong I was
wrong again to be me and being me where I was/wrong
to be who I am
which is exactly like South Africa
penetrating into Namibia penetrating into Angola ...
and if after all my kinsmen and women resist even to
self-immolation of the villages and if after that
we lose nevertheless what will the big boys
say will they claim my consent ... [5]

To be "wrong" in terms of gender, race, class, sexuality, power, ability, and age is to be physically wrong as well as psychologically wrong — it is to be visibly and noticeably wrong. To accommodate; to conform; to acculturate; to starve; to become preoccupied with body shape; to develop personae whose bodies differ in terms of age, feeling, function, to hold pain from memory; to develop control over breathing; to exercise relentlessly; to follow compelling patterns of thought or action — these are behaviours learned as children, learned in violence, learned in being sexual objects, which shape women's inner lives, our bodies, and our relationship with the world as surely as that relationship has shaped us. A downward spiral of alienation and disconnection from self and others escalates displacement of the physical, makes the body enemy, alien, other. Repeated violence and the continued threat of violence keep a child or an adult in continual crisis, create dilemmas regarding food and nourishment, reinforce the need for displacement and the need to identify visibly only as the assailant dictates. To comply connotes consent, or at least acknowledges function. To defy connotes arrogance, anger, visibility, and thus condones retaliation. Self-defence must be engineered with others, with identification beyond the abuser.

A woman speaks:
My body was like a chain linked to violence, rape and oppression. If I could starve my body or kill it, then I could break the chain. Food was evil, connected to life, blood, everything I hated, so life was hate. My body was dirty, ugly, visible.
Food is not like an addiction. The body needs food to stay alive but it does not seem like a necessity to me, like something positive or nurturing. It is as if I am consuming poison on a daily basis.

Women are defiant victims, defiant survivors — they let their bodies talk as best they can (Kasperowski 1991), boldly and persistently living in situations where they were not meant to survive at all. First Nations women know this strength in connection to life and community. Their strength was seen as very threatening by Jesuit conquerors who immediately set out to disempower these women, who were more than equal. These women are now working to heal the people again (Brooks 1991) from the abuse suffered in mission schools and under the Indian Act — they will not be displaced.

A woman speaks:
Food was connected to different parts of my self as a child and to what it was like around the dinner table. The dinner table was a place where emotional and physical violence took place, where we were forced to eat everything or deprived of meals, depending on the angry rules of the adults. This same kitchen table was the place I was raped and tortured at other times.

Counseling issues relevant to issues of body image and rape must consider the specific violence of acts of sexual assault upon the specific and particular lives of each child and woman with whom we work. We work in connection through crises and through witnessing and "standing with" the woman as she sees her life and permits herself to be seen,[6] standing with women in groups, in meetings, in court, in their families, at rallies. For, to come to our bodies, to take up space, to come back to our bodies, this is always radical and exciting work. There is power here to be held and felt and enjoyed, and used for change.

The connections to mind and heart are found here — for as the mind is not in the head, the heart is not in the chest. Feeling and thought, passion and pain are developed as the mind travels through the body, as our senses develop meaning and hold memory, as we touch and are touched.[7] The violation of rape is obvious; it is much more akin to attempted murder than to any other state-recognized crime — and is often accompanied by just that! The prolonged sexual assault and rape of children is more akin to the debilitating confinement of political prisoners in exile[8] than to any analogous exercise of power and control, use of sexual pain, use of isolation and enforced attachment to the guardian for survival, dissociation of the self.

A woman speaks:
Sometimes when I watch my eyes looking at me in the mirror, it all comes back and automatically I want to rip away my reflection and disappear. Everytime I've got to find a way of trying to believe my soul belongs to me, of not feeling other eyes staring and abusing me. This has taken a lot of work and time.

Often then, rape counseling first involves mourning the lost self, the self never found, the body never held, the body violated. This is essentially anti-oppression work. Cherie Morega (1983) writes about this work in a poem entitled "Amputation," in which she describes the feeling of remembered pain when the limb is severed or never wholly joined. The pain she evokes is women's pain, the pain of racism, homophobic oppression, the denial of children's lives, the pain of parent's memories (of the Holocaust, of concentration camps, of slavery, of our mother's shame). Always be ready to feel new limbs, new connections, changes in your body; never assume that the grieving or "re-membering" is completed, for we are always discovering more about who we are and what we can be.

Very often, as stated elsewhere here, women alter their physical appearance as a defence or a screen or an outward accommodation. After surviving rape, many women change their hairstyle or hair colour, how they dress, their body shape, their living situation (if they choose to and can afford to), and their friends.

Listen carefully to the details of the rape, to all the rapes the child held, the woman holds; notice with her the changes in her body, the way she seems to take up space, hold colour and shape; breathe more deeply as she talks, or draws, or acts, or sings, or works, or plays with a child. In this listening, seeing, and repeating, the true nature of experience, if felt, and emerges.

A woman speaks:
Control over my body was all I ever had. I could control what I put in it, how much, when I'd drink, how many pills I'd take,

whether I'd exercise, if I'd sleep.

There were times I wanted so badly to die. I held emptiness. I lived in darkness. I had smelled and known death too well for a child. Sometimes I waited for death. It would have ended the torture.

There are many crisis here: flashbacks, body memories, death sensations, despair, ruthless conflicts between parts of the self (between inner selves). The woman will often be experiencing "crisis" in her body as the norm, as that which is most familiar. This may take the form of vomiting, taking in food, gagging, feeling sick to one's stomach, diarrhoea, constipation, needing to clean her body out, binding her body, cutting or burning her body. She may be hypervigilant, watching for attack; monitoring her body, her mind, and her environment for danger; preparing for the predictable "next time." She may spend "much emotional energy actively despising and suffering over [her] body," as Sareh Allisen (1992) observes in a recent article on lesbian incest survivors. Allisen quotes (p. 26) one such survivor who describes this use of energy:

> "I like my hands and feet. I hate the rest of my body. I hate it all the time. Incest is totally and completely to blame. I feel like my body is not mine. I do not see it through my eyes. I see it through other men in my family's eyes.... I don't see it through my lover or anybody who would appreciate it ... it causes me more pain that any other thing in my life, my relationship with my body."

This sense of a painful relationship with the body can be even more profound if the assaults are ritualized torture, as in cult abuse, political torture, racist torture, where there is a systematic attempt to control the mind and heart by using the body as a vessel for pain, inflicting visions of death and permanent physical injury.

A woman speaks:
I believe that my physical problems were a result of the abuse. Endrometriosis, back and joint pain, bronchial problems.

Constant body pain kept me suspended in time, in torture. It's hard to live with my physical pain and heal from it when it's connected to humiliation, violation and repeated rape of my body and soul. Having a hysterectomy was the only way to relieve the pain and fragmentation.

Often women who are ritual-abuse survivors have very painful scarring of the vagina and the uterus, difficulties breathing, back pain, problems with circulation, and migraine headaches as a result of prolonged torture. Coming to the body then is an act of courage and faith, and to stay with the memory is to connect with the will, which was not broken. One of the founders of Breaking Ritual Abuse and Ending Violence (B.R.A.V.E.) states: "They tried to kill my spirit but I hid it far away. They tried to make my eyes look empty, hateful. Just like theirs. But my eyes are connected to my heart, feeling truth, wanting love."

A woman speaks:
My sexuality was not mine. My vagina belonged to the adults who used my body for pornography. Somewhere out there people have pictures of my naked child's body. My female self was ripped open and exposed. The camera made it feel like millions of eyes were watching me. Everytime somebody looks at me in one of those pictures they are raping me with their eyes.

Continuous threat, confinement, and sexual control are also characteristics of violence in relationships, violence against domestic workers, the realities of prison life or institutional life in a chronic-care facility. These institutions both reinforce past abuse and are abusive by nature of the control they exercise and the potential risk of further assault. Confinement causes women to outlive their hope of any sense of meaningful time and space — these are important considerations when counseling women, considerations that are often ignored in the in-patient treatment of young women with "eating disorders."

For a child who is repeatedly attacked and trained to view the inner self as split, or bad, or as female victim, or as sexually dis-eased, personae or multiple realities may develop that fit the roles available to girls and women, fit the roles projected by the assailant(s), and fit the stages of emotional and cognitive develop-ment of the child. Parts of the physical and emotional self will hold nothingness, and despair and feelings of death, which are not empty space but have sensations and memories of their own.

A woman speaks:
If I could make my body disappear then no one could hurt me. If my body was small maybe no one would see me.
Getting away from my body was the only way I knew to survive and hold on to my heart. My body screams inside. It shakes for release, for understanding, for safety. The children inside are still bleeding, crying "why?", begging "please don't hurt me", "don't make me die." Those little parts pretend to leave the body, to see the sun, to climb a tree in order to stay alive.
Or sometimes they hide deep inside. I try to believe that these parts of me might be held with warmth and tenderness. I don't think they'll ever know enough of it. I've never felt the fullness of my body.

Women may have several or many physical selves, and sensory memories that are quite different for one self than for another. Menstrual periods may be dictated by these perceptions: sense of height and weight, age, shape, maturity; perhaps race, class, gender, sexuality. Just as the mind and heart travel through the body to gain knowledge, the mind leaves knowledge in segments of felt reality.

Art, drama, body therapies, dance, developing new tradition, embracing old tradition, connecting to other women, connecting to political action — these are all part of the work of "re-member-ing" ourselves embodied.

Mental-health disciplines, particularly psychiatry, clinical psy-chology, and applied social work, have learned from women, from anti-oppression work, from the psychiatric-survivors' movement, the importance of linking cause and effect when understanding women's problems in living. Unfortunately, instead of being used to transform the work, this knowledge is altered or usurped by new, somewhat more complex re-creations of pathology, such as post-traumatic stress disorder, sexual dysfunction, self-defeating personality disorder, multiple personality disorder, and, most recently, false-memory syndrome. In the creation of false-memory syndrome, there is a concerted attempt to re-create silence and memory loss in women. This will not work. The arrogance and sense of entitlement to power reflected in this most recent venture are equalled only by the total ignorance and fear of women's strength. All of these constructs are harmful to women's lives, to women's ability to live in their bodies, their worlds.[9]

> *A woman speaks:*
> When you are away from the abuse you can go from one hell to another. Living in a world where people commit the same crimes over and over to friends, children, strangers; a place where my experiences as a ritual abuse survivor aren't believed, where people like me are seen as crazy; a world where women don't know who to trust; where it's not safe for me to walk alone in the streets at night. This culture, our systems continue to oppress me. I've changed but the world has not. The world would rather keep me quiet or dead. It is essential to find the strength I know I have and work from that place, to keep fighting to find others who are not afraid of the truth. I will not die.

To live in connection with other women, to see and be seen to understand and feel — this is both defence and growth. The same is true of feminist, anti-oppression–based counseling relationships (which must always be grounded in the "real" world, where food, shelter, clothing, refuge, human rights, child protection, and community are essential priorities), self-help and consciousness-raising groups, coalitions, political action, and loving friendships. Be particular and specific; always analyse the strands of oppression that bind; value difference in self and others; understand the accommodations made in strength, the accommodations made in fear or to maintain privilege. We must work on our own internalized misogynism, racism, and heterosexism, in order to work together. We need to hold the assailants (individuals and groups) accountable and make their assaults visible to all so women do not reabsorb responsibility. It is not more complicated than this: we do not need more theories about violence — it is brutal, it is simple, it works. We need the words, and minds, and pain and laughter, and sexuality and playfulness, and the huge fullness of embodied women — this need is insatiable.

✦

NOTES

1. Quotations titled "A woman speaks" are from survivors with whom the authors have worked. They have given their permission to be quoted here. This is the essence of the work we do — to speak, write, draw, learn together.

2. A recent Canadian study reported that one in five Canadian men living with a woman admitted to physically abusing her (Lupis *Canadian Social Trends* 1989).

3. Sistering Conference, Toronto, 1992.

4. Bart notes, rather cryptically, that men who are seen as being successful in attracting women are called "lady-killers."

5. Angela Davis speech on "Race and Rights" 1985.

6. These ideas are drawn, in part, from "self in relation" theories developed at the Stone Institute in Boston, in specific reference to the work of Janet Surrey. Margaret Powell and Patricia McGillicuddy developed a series of workshops for women in crisis, using these ideas and specifically relating them to sexual assault work with women.

7. Diane Ackerman, in *A Natural History of the Senses* (New York: Random House, 1990) richly details the power of the senses and the roaming of the mind through the nervous system.

8. This analogy with people in exile — particularly, poets in exile — is often drawn by Sandra Butler, who speaks and writes extensively on the subject of sexual abuse of women.

9. Maria Lagones (1990) writes about the need for women to travel to one another's worlds with love in order to love and to reveal plurality.

MAKING CONNECTIONS: FAMILY ALCOHOLISM AND THE DEVELOPMENT OF EATING PROBLEMS

Connie Coniglio

> Virtually all women in our culture are socialized to associate self worth with appearance. We learn to shave, paint, pluck, camouflage, colour, curl, trim, tuck, tighten, diet, and exercise before we begin to seek answers to other questions, like who we are and what we hope to do with our lives. These pressures to conform to society's standards of beauty and femininity cause us to become profoundly insecure about our bodies. Insecurity gives way to hate, as we come to realize how unattainable the ideals really are. (Rice 1988)

Weight and shape issues, eating problems, and eating disorders are undeniably connected to sociocultural issues and messages in Western culture. It has also become apparent, however, that for a great number of women, eating problems are linked to experiences of childhood trauma and victimization. Recent research indicates that 60 to 66 percent (Root and Fallon 1988) of women with bulimia have experienced some significant "abuse" in their backgrounds, including physical, emotional, or sexual abuse and/or witnessing woman abuse. The connections between growing up in an "unhealthy family" and the subsequent development of eating problems in adolescence or early adulthood are now being explored, and family dysfunction has received recognition as a complex phenomenon having tremendous impact on the development and adult functioning of both women and men.

One particular kind of unhealthy family currently being explored by researchers, clinicians, and writers is the "alcoholic home." An alcoholic home is essentially an environment where one or both parents are addicted to alcohol during the course of a child's development. The offspring of alcoholic parents have recently become the focus of extensive research efforts (Black, Bucky, and Wilder-Padilla 1986; El-Guebaly and Offord 1977; Wilson and Orford 1978), and are now recognized as a significant clinical population (Cermak and Rosenfeld 1987). Adult Children of Alcoholics (ACOAs) are receiving increasing attention in counseling circles today, and much energy has been devoted to exploring the early experiences, development, and adult adjustment of individuals from such homes.

UNDERSTANDING THE ALCOHOLIC FAMILY

The alcoholic home can best be described as chaotic, unpredictable, and inconsistent. At some time early in a child's life, one or both of her parents or her primary caregiver uses alcohol as a means for coping, as a way to face day-to-day stressors, or as a strategy for numbing out personal horrors such as childhood abuse or memories of life with his/her own alcoholic parent. The alcoholic parent is dependent, psychologically and physically, upon alcohol, and seeks it out in what could be described as a "compulsive" way. Relationships with primary others deteriorate as the alcoholic's communication style becomes increasingly marked by denial. "Denial" is a term used to characterize the alcoholic's strategy for dealing with the world, him/herself, and important others. The alcoholic does not recognize that he/she has a problem, nor will he/she take responsibility for any resultant behaviour. The alcoholic thus engages in a process of "distorting" his/her own views and those of persons in the immediate environment. Examples of denial can be found in the alcoholic's explanation of events, behaviours, and means for perceiving the world, him/herself, and everyone else. Brown (1987) very accurately describes the process of alcoholism and its effects upon children, focusing upon the principle of denial, combined with the presence of alcohol, as the facilitator of great distortions of reality within families. Denial is manifested in the following ways by the alcoholic: distorted logic, distorted perceptions of self and the world, illogical explanations for events, and enforcement of the rules "don't talk, don't trust, don't feel" (Black and Wilder-Padilla 1986). There is, of course, tremendous pressure to conform to the alcoholic parent's view of reality, and the family appears to orient itself around these principles. Honest communication, intimacy, and any sharing of thoughts and feelings disappear (if they existed at all) under these conditions. Children are blamed, criticized, abused, and forced to meet inappropriate demands.

Female children are particular targets in alcoholic families. While girls, as a group, are significantly less powerful, are most certainly devalued by the culture, and are socialized to be passive and to obey authority at any cost, in alcoholic families, these young women are additionally required to assume core beliefs that fit with those of the alcoholic; survival itself necessitates an acceptance of parental views of reality. In the face of these adverse conditions, a girl's sense of identity is underdeveloped, undermined, and repeatedly questioned; girls often come to believe that there is something wrong with them in order to cope with the distortions and a deepening sense of helplessness. No models for alternative, healthy reality are generally available, given the alcoholic family's relative isolation in the community.

Alcohol plays a core role in all essential interactions and relationships. Given that the alcoholic's needs come first, children exist only to preserve the parent's already shaky sense of self, and very often become an extension of the parent(s), not allowed to separate in terms of needs, thoughts, or feelings. Miller (as cited by Brown 1987) states that dependency precedes autonomy: children from alcoholic families lose the opportunity for dependence very early. While most children of their age receive nurturance, protection, and support from their parents, these children are required to assume "adult" roles in interactions with their own caregivers; they become the nurturers, the protectors, the supporters, the caregivers (to the degree that they are able) in order to meet the alcoholic's needs and demands. This is done automatically; survival requires the child to accommodate, to be a caregiver, and to be deprived of her own natural dependency needs. As a direct result, the childhood experience in an alcoholic family is marked by isolation, deprivation, emptiness, and a lack of emotional connectedness with parents. Children's needs are, of course, neither recognized nor acknowledged in a situation where adult caregivers are themselves too needy to give. All development, from the point at which alcohol begins to impact upon relationships among family members, is affected — cognitive, affective, and intellectual. This process has a progressive, cumulative effect upon children, as does alcohol upon the alcoholic.

Alcoholic families are noted extensively in the literature for the presence of the following adverse conditions.

• Parents are addicted to substances. Many adult women report extensive drug use, both prescription and illicit, on the part of parents, in concert with and sometimes separate from their alcohol use. Regardless of the substance, the outcomes are the same in terms of impact upon children.

• Addicted parents use denial extensively in their interactions with partners and children, thus reinforcing distortions in the perceptions and feelings of family members. The family rules — "don't talk, don't trust, don't feel" — are strongly reinforced.

• Abuses of power are perpetuated; emotionally, physically, and sexually, against women and children in the family. Rates

of physical, sexual, and emotional abuse, including witnessing woman abuse, are epidemic among women from alcoholic
families. Research is now being conducted to explore the
effects upon women's adult coping strategies.

- The emotional and physical needs of children are not attended
to consistently, or sometimes not at all. Women report a wide
spectrum of maltreatment including neglect, inconsistent caregiving, and being ignored and/or treated as invisible. Some
report, as adults, that even their most basic physical needs
(food, shelter, clothing, sleep) were not attended to.

- Parents and children exchange roles, such that children become
the responsible caregivers of the family. Adult women frequently report that they learned, very early, to care for their parents
and their siblings. Childhood chores often included cooking,
cleaning, putting others to bed, and attending to the physical
and emotional needs of family members.

- Members of the family have poor emotional/physical boundaries.
One adult woman reported that there was literally "no place"
in her home where she could go; no place where she had
personal space, her own, alone, where she would not be in-
truded upon and abused.

- Parents are inflexible about and intolerant of the individuality
of children: "Being different means being bad."

- Members of the family experience difficulty with change or conflict. Women repeatedly report that their families could not
tolerate difference, change, development, or the natural
conflicts that arise between family members. These
issues would typically be ignored, denied, downplayed or
considered "forbidden topics."

- Images and expectations of female family members are based
upon sociocultural norms and values of the larger culture.
The family believes in and promotes stereotypical images for
its members; for young women, an exaggerated focus is placed

upon weight control, traditional relationships, and compliance or passivity.

• Abuses perpetrated within the family (sexual, physical, emotional, and woman assault) are kept secret. Women report that, while everyone in their family may have had some knowledge of abuses occurring in the home, no one ever acknowledged or spoke of them.

THE EFFECTS OF GROWING UP
IN AN ALCOHOLIC HOME

Research indicates that children of alcoholic parents suffer serious effects well into adulthood. Adult Children of Alcoholics (ACOAs) are at high risk for self-defeating behaviour patterns in the course of adult life, including the development of alcoholism or other addictive behaviours (smoking, drug use), becoming a partner to an addicted person (Miller 1987), low self-esteem, compulsive achievement orientation, and/or serious difficulties in establishing and maintaining satisfying intimate relationships (Woititz 1983; Wegscheider 1981; Whitfield 1987). Clinicians reporting on the outcomes of group therapy cite restricted emotional spontaneity, denial of personal needs, unclear boundaries of interpersonal responsibility, difficulty trusting, and pervasive fears of abandonment as common reactions to growing up in an alcoholic home (Cermak and Brown 1982). In addition, ACOAs appear to display persistent concerns in the area of control, that is, a reaction to personal and intrapsychic complications of life characterized by increased efforts to control internal and external events (Cermak and Rosenfeld 1987). ACOAs are also noted for their use of "compulsive coping strategies" (driven to seemingly irresistible behaviours engaged in repeatedly in an attempt to ward off painful thoughts, feelings, or realities) in their attempts to deal with the debilitating effects of growing up in an alcoholic family and, of course, day-to-day life stressors (work, finances, relationships, etc) and adult difficulties.

THE MIND-BODY CONNECTION:
DAUGHTERS OF ALCOHOLIC PARENTS SPEAK

Daughters of alcoholic parents are affected by their early experiences in profound ways. With regard to the development of eating problems, women from alcoholic homes are considered a population at high risk. The relationship between eating disorders and alcohol has been explored empirically by Claydon (1987) who noted that ACOAs were twice as likely to report an eating disorder as were their peers from nonalcoholic homes. As well, students from alcoholic homes were more likely to report all forms of substance abuse — four times more likely to report a personal drinking problem and three times more likely to report a drug problem. Bulik (1987) also explored the drug and alcohol abuse patterns of bulimic women and their families, discovering that alcoholism occurred significantly more frequently in first- and second-degree relatives of bulimic women when compared with nonbulimic peers. Hudson, Pope, and Jonas (1983) examined the family histories of adult women self-referred or referred for outpatient treatment of eating disorders and found an incidence of substance-abuse disorders among the total number of relatives of bulimics at about 11 percent. Overall, researchers have found high prevalency rates of alcoholism among family members of women with eating disorders; 20 to 51 percent of individuals with bulimia have one or more first-degree relatives with chemical dependency (Herzog 1982a, 1982b; Hudson, Laffer, and Pope 1982; Leon et al. 1985; Pyle, Mitchell, and Eckert 1981).

JANET'S STORY: UNDERSTANDING
EATING PROBLEMS AS CREATIVE COPING STRATEGIES

Janet is 21, the youngest of three children. Her siblings, aged 29 and 30, left home when Janet was quite young, leaving her with two alcoholic parents. Both Rene and Stan (Janet's parents) abused alcohol as far back as Janet can remember. Rene and Stan separated when Janet was a teenager. Rene remarried, to another alcoholic, and died soon afterward.

Janet loves her mother, and notes that they are very much alike, both in appearance and manner. Janet believes that Rene was competent and creative in her career, and that she was a good and caring person at the core. Janet also believes that her mother's alcohol problems developed as a result of marrying the wrong man. Janet dislikes her father intensely, and has chosen not to maintain a relationship with him. She feels that Stan was the source of much emotional distress for Rene, contributing greatly to her abuse of alcohol.

Janet's family experience has been marked by chaos, inconsistency, violations of trust, contradictions, abuse, and neglect. Janet grew up watching Rene and Stan drink, party, and involve themselves in overt affairs, and at times has vivid memories of lying in bed at night counting their drinks, feeling terrified and out of control. Janet feels sure that Stan sexually abused her, but has no active memory yet to support this. She is sure that something happened, and cannot let him near her as an adult. In fact, Janet has very little memory of her childhood and feels that many things are blocked.

As Janet grew up, Rene's drinking worsened, and after separating from Stan, Rene became angry and abusive with Janet. Janet was forced to deal with Rene's radical mood swings on a daily basis, and experienced severe physical and emotional abuse over a number of years. Janet learned to predict Rene's pattern of drinking and the ways in which her behaviour changed with alcohol, and coped by staying away from home and keeping herself very busy. While staying away from home as a teen, Janet was sexually abused by a male teacher, someone she confided in and trusted as counsel during a period of severe depression.

Janet has experienced profound feelings of isolation and self-blame for her mother's drinking and for the sexual abuse that was perpetrated against her. The dynamics of her relationship with Rene necessitated that she not have any needs, that the focus be completely upon Rene at all times, and that she not express any feelings, particularly negative ones. At the time of her sexual victimization, Janet was unable to tell anyone, and was sure that Rene would blame her if she found out. Janet feels that a pattern of communication existed in her family such that since she was the youngest, no one bothered to listen or validate her. She continue to wrestle with the feeling that no one will ever listen to her and that she is really quite profoundly worthless. Janet feels she is a bad person, and that she deserves punishment, particularly when she is not doing what she perceives others as wishing her to do.

In therapy, Janet is dealing with body image and eating concerns. She calls herself a "compulsive eater," a coping strategy she developed to comfort herself when feeling very "bad." Janet sees herself as fat and unattractive. As well, she has used a variety of self-harming behaviours, since causing herself physical pain relieves her inner sense of being out of control, an intense feeling that she feels is related primarily to her relationship with Rene. Janet is working hard to identify and express her needs and wants, to show her feelings, and to set limits, all those things she was not afforded the luxury of doing as a child growing up in an alcoholic family.

An eating problem is paradoxically and simultaneously creative, confused, adaptive, nurturing, denying, beneficial, and harmful (Catrina Brown, personal communication). It is, for women from alcoholic families, a fundamental means for coping with unresolved and internalized experiences of neglect, abuse, and chaos during childhood and adolescence. It provides women with a way of functioning in the world that is essentially learned at home; a constant state based upon feeling chaotic and out of control, and utilizing compulsive coping strategies to avoid, cope with, or manage feelings, thoughts, and relationships. We all live what we learn, and women from alcoholic families develop a highly creative strategy based upon their early experience; a socially acceptable, even rewarded method of coping; focusing on food, weight, and shape obsessively, just as an alcoholic or addict focuses upon his/her substance. An eating problem can best be referred to as a "survival skill," assisting a woman at first to manage her life/family situation, but over time increasingly interfering, disrupting, or complicating her day-to-day functioning. Eating problems as a coping strategy ultimately create a "double bind" for women; they are essential to coping, but at the same time severely limit a woman's capacity to face and deal with the very issues creating such pain and difficulty in day-to-day living.

WHAT MAKES COPING STRATEGIES CREATIVE?

Women who struggle with eating problems report that their coping or survival strategies serve some vital purposes in their lives. First and foremost, as has been previously mentioned, developing difficulties with eating can be the absolutely most effective means for living in an impossible situation. This is particularly true for those women who have experienced sexual, physical, and/or emotional abuse. The eating problem can allow a woman to function, while taking her conscious focus off of memories and feelings related to abuse, pain, deprivation, and suffering. Woman repeatedly state that, when they are preoccupied with weight and shape issues, there is little time left for dealing with emotional issues and feeling states.

Eating problems additionally serve some other important functions in women's lives. For the woman who grows up in an alcoholic family, her eating behaviours and seemingly compulsive thinking style provide a sense of stability, predictability, focus, and pseudo-control in an environment that is chaotic, unpredictable, and ultimately out of control. She may feel that in controlling what she does or does not eat, her body size, or when and how she eats, she is exercising the only means of control available to her. Women also report that there is a sense of power, the only power they have access to, attached to control over eating or the manipulation of their body size to conform to desired societal standards and expectations.

Focusing upon weight, shape, and eating (or not eating) can offer some protection from painful realities. Women often utilize food as their sole source of emotional comfort or nurturance in an environment that is otherwise severely deprived of such connections. Eating behaviour can also contribute to the process of "dissociating" from negative experiences and feelings. Women often discuss how their eating behaviour allows them to numb out, to minimize the impact of life events and experiences, and to rationalize problems that occur with and around them. Blocking out, denying, and avoiding intense and disturbing feelings is essential when a woman cannot truly escape or come up with solutions or alternatives for dealing with her life. Eating and related problems thus create a venue for self-expression and a focus for living that is ultimately insular in nature.

Women express a variety of feelings through eating, and for those from alcoholic families these feelings may include anger, shame, destructiveness, a sense of badness; all of the natural, negative feelings that arise as a direct result of living in an unhealthy environment where there is no room for true, honest, healthy self-expression and development. Unfortunately, this process of internalizing feelings leads directly to their expression in a self-defeating and harmful way — through the body. As Steiner-Adair (1989, p. 151) has astutely noted, "symptoms have meaning and are a way of speaking when a woman cannot speak directly, for whatever reason." Eating problems are thus an essentially female form of expression.

A WORD ABOUT

EATING PROBLEMS AS AN ADDICTIVE PROCESS

A growing number of writers view eating problems as similar to "addictions," and discuss eating disorders and associated difficulties as essentially an addiction to food. Kay Sheppard, in her book *Food Addiction: The Body Knows* (1989), discusses the problem of "food addiction," maintaining that some foods can be as addictive as cocaine or alcohol or any of the other substances that are accepted and acknowledged as physiologically addictive. Based on the concept of physical abstinence from addictive "binge foods," Sheppard recommends a lifetime plan of eating that precludes the intake of those foods one is addicted to, just as Alcoholics Anonymous precludes the intake of alcohol, while allowing the use of other beverages such as water and milk.

The "addictions model of eating disorders," although interesting to therapists and women with eating problems, is fundamentally inadequate in its attempts to provide a useful explanation for understanding and treating eating disorders. The model assumes that an eating disorder is a purely individual problem, that certain foods have addictive properties for certain people, and that those who suffer from an eating disorder are "addicted to food." It advocates food restriction and abstinence as the solution — a strategy that, in reality, is responsible for getting women in trouble with food in the first place.

Sheppard's approach reflects that of a growing number of women, therapists and clients alike, who have come, very recently, to accept an "addictions" viewpoint regarding the development of eating problems in women's lives. Indeed, an eating disorder can resemble an addiction with regard to an individual's observable behaviour; being out of control in relation to food, hiding or stealing food, or abstaining from certain foods for periods of time only to slip back into old patterns of eating. In fact, a number of treatment facilities have sprung up in the United States that base their treatment approaches upon the idea that women with eating disorders are "addicted to food" and ultimately require special diets, restricted in nature, (no sugar, no flour, no starchy, sweet foods) in order to manage their disease.

While it is clear that addictions and eating problems are similar in that they can be described as compulsive coping strategies, they cannot be conceptualized as one and the same. The addictions model of eating disorders does not account for the obvious and overwhelming sociocultural issues that play such a tremendous role in women's lives, and on a more practical level, it fails to address the effects of starvation/deprivation, set-point theory, and the relationship that exists between restricting and bingeing. Additionally, an explanation of eating problems as an addiction fails to address the connection that exists for women between emotional deprivation, abuse experiences in childhood/adolescence, and a focus upon food as one of the few available methods for gaining a sense of control, getting needs met, and ultimately expressing oneself. Eating problems are, in reality, a means for relieving unbearable internal states. They are not an addiction, but rather a set of coping strategies reinforced over time by virtue of the absolute relief they provide; their compulsive quality should be viewed as a reflection of this reliable relief and the absence of alternatives in a woman's repertoire of self-soothing methods (Westerlund 1992).

THE THERAPEUTIC PROCESS

Janet continues to move along in her healing work. She is engaging painfully in the process of recovering memories of sexual, physical, and emotional abuse, and is reexamining and coming to a new understanding of her early life in an alcoholic family. She is slowly beginning to express identify and express feelings: anger, rage, sadness, disappointment, grief, loss, happiness, and joy. As she gains experience with self expression, she is formulating a true identity, and is coming to recognize her needs and wants for the first time. Janet is currently exploring ways to nurture, care for, and soothe herself, and her urge to eat "compulsively" has decreased drastically as she has become more in touch with herself and the options available for living her life. She is working hard, and recognizes that she is engaging in a process of change — one that may continue for a while to come.

In order to provide useful interventions for women with eating problems, it is vital to recognize that developing an eating problem can be the most effective means for coping with the traumas, abuses, deprivation, and conflicts of early life in an alcoholic family.

Creative coping strategies are essential, assisting a women to deal with and maintain a sense of pseudo-control in the face of unresolved trauma, victimization, and the resultant sense of powerlessness, helplessness, and internal chaos. At the same time, these strategies are constricting, preventing women from moving forward in their development. Women are thus held suspended in space; while the coping strategies are creative, allowing women to function in the world in a reasonable and manageable way, they also prevent progress, development, and ultimately resolution of the difficulties that led to their inception.

Coping strategies will, of course, assume a variety of forms, and vary along a continuum from adaptive and life-enhancing to maladaptive and self-defeating, or self-destructive. In addressing and understanding women's coping strategies, we are really asking a fundamental question: "How have you negotiated and survived your childhood and arrived at where you are in the world today?"

Women will naturally use whatever means are available to them, and eating disorders are, of course (given sociocultural imperatives), the strategy of choice. Women will also, however, criticize and punish themselves for utilizing these techniques for functioning in the world. A fundamental component of the therapeutic process involves honouring and congratulating each woman for her resourcefulness at surviving; it is the therapist's role to understand and support clients' successes in utilizing resources to negotiate early life and adulthood.

Feminist therapy involves facilitating a process allowing women to explore the purposes and symbolic meanings of their particular coping strategies, and to look carefully at how they have been so fundamentally important and useful but ultimately limited. The therapist's "job" is not to try to remove these strategies, but instead to work with women to replace them with more self-enhancing, less harmful ways of coping. Eliminating or pulling away well-developed coping or survival strategies will render a woman helpless and vulnerable in the face of her early trauma and victimization experience with no resources for managing her life.

Ultimately, the therapeutic work involves providing women with assistance in the process of differentiating between healthy and self-defeating aspects of thinking and feeling. As therapists, we need to work with women to celebrate strengths and to work towards lasting and successful changes in strategies and patterns of coping that are no longer viable.

PHILOSOPHY OF TREATMENT: SOME GUIDELINES

- As therapists, we need to assist our clients in developing an awareness of alcoholism as a societal problem and to focus on their traumatic and abusive early life experiences, to uncover the truth of their early lives, and to place responsibility for victimization and abuse upon the perpetrator(s).

- It is vitally important to help women to recognize their so-called personal pathologies as normal responses to and creative coping strategies for dealing with an early environment in which they have been oppressed, rendered powerless, and abused.

- The work of therapy must be conducted within a sociocultural context (particularly when working with eating problems), utilizing feminist, egalitarian philosophy/technique, and promoting healing and growth.

- Silence and isolation are the greatest barriers to recovery. Assisting clients to break the silence, form relationships, and communicate are fundamental to the healing process.

- Never get caught up with focusing upon and treating symptoms. Symptoms are metaphors — we need to work with clients to establish and understand their meaning and function.

- Remember that children have only basic, undeveloped means for dealing psychologically with their traumatic family experiences. It is thus necessary for the therapist to have a good understanding of developmental theory and the experience of the "child" when working with adult women in therapy.

- The therapeutic process will necessitate extensive work with the following "core" issues: *grief* and *loss*. Women from alcoholic families have literally lost their childhoods. Healing means accepting losses, giving up on urges to heal the family and focusing upon the self. Many women have to accept that they will never have the family/parents they want. This, of course, is the most difficult part of the work.

- The therapeutic process will include facilitating emotional expression and working with clients to uncover unconscious memories, thoughts, and feelings. Women often repress that which is too terrible, overwhelming, and traumatic to remember. They experience fear — of losing control and of the power of emotions — and rage.

SUMMARY

Daughters from alcoholic families are a population at high risk for eating problems in adolescence and adulthood. Their reactions to the traumas, victimizations, and abuses common to the alcoholic environment are most effectively conceptualized and treated as "creative coping strategies." Therapists need to familiarize themselves with both the sociocultural and the family issues of these women, and must provide interventions that address trauma and victimization accurately. It is vitally important to facilitate such women in an exploration of early-life experience and make vital connections to adult coping strategies within the context of the therapeutic relationship.

◆

THE POLITICS OF RECOVERY

Ellen Driscoll

In this essay, I will analyse and critique the recovery movement and its role in creating a context for women's resistance and empowerment. I argue here that the widespread proliferation of this social phenomenon warrants attention in that many women who are conflicted about their bodies and food also have histories of chemical dependency and/or sexual abuse and other relational trauma. Many are likely engaged with a 12-Step program in one of its various forms, or have been encouraged to do so. As will become apparent, my analysis is sympathetic to the goals and methods of AA and Al-Anon. However, the extension of the AA philosophy beyond "primary addictions" to "process addictions" is, I suggest, a disturbing trend. When I speak about "primary addictions," I refer to addiction to alcohol and other mood altering drugs; "process addictions" do not involve a chemical substance and may include, for example, codependency, workaholism, shopaholism. The issue is even more complex with respect to Overeaters Anonymous (OA): the question of addiction to food is problematic in that the compulsion to over- and undereat *is* psychologically compelling and, in the case of self-starvation, can certainly be life threatening. I am concerned, however, with the generalization of experience that occurs within OA; the dynamics of weight preoccupation are often considered without reference to what is particular about overeating, binge-eating, and self-starvation. More important, we need to be concerned about how the discourse of disease serves to pathologize the individual and neglects the cultural prejudices that motivate the current requirements to produce a thin, fit body. In other words, to say that women with body types and sizes that do not conform to the acceptable form are, in fact, suffering from a disease, is a reflection and a perpetuation of the fat prejudice that consumes our culture.

I examine the popularity and positive aspects of 12-Step recovery programs here, and provide a commentary in the form of a dissenting, critical voice so as to create a sense of "dialogue." The implications of the recovery movement for women's empowerment and healing, for our movement from retreat to resistance, from apology to protest, are also addressed. I question whether these communities are sites of transformation or of shame, and whether they actively support the radical altering of the oppressive conditions of women's lives. Finally, I briefly examine the contributions of feminist spirituality in offering alternative ways of envisioning women's empowerment. The comments that follow reflect some of the issues and concerns that have informed my life and my work as a therapist over the past ten years.

POWER, CONTROL, AND CONVERSION

There is little doubt that the conversion experience at the heart of AA, as articulated in the first three of the 12 Steps, has turned many away from the ravages of alcohol and drug addiction. For many, identity, meaning, and life have been radically reorganized.[1] A reevaluation of the meanings and functions of power and control in one's life is a central dynamic in this process.

According to Jo-Ann Krestan (1991, p. 183), a family therapist specializing in addiction and in gender-related issues, the notions of power and powerlessness are used very specifically within AA. She argues that the 1st Step ("we admitted we were powerless over alcohol — that our lives had become unmanageable"), and the serenity prayer ("God grant me the serenity to accept the things I cannot change, the courage to change the things I can, and the wisdom to know the difference") are requisite admissions if one is to begin a recovery process. She states (ibid.) that to admit one *does not* have "power over" a chemical is absolutely necessary and that the "misguided and exceedingly male attempts" to maintain "power over" are at the very heart of the addict's dilemma. We need, then, to reconceptualize power so that it is understood as "power to" and "power with"; in this reframing, power has to do with autonomy, responsibility, and choice. Following from this, how the notion of "higher power" is understood is related to one's sense of self. I agree with Krestan when she argues that the desire for "power over" and the refusal to accept one's limits have to do with the "flight from relatedness" (ibid.). For women and men, a profound paradox exists here: in order to experience the freeing power of choice, we have to give up the need for "power over," or, as Krestan says, the "project to be God" (ibid.).

I believe Krestan raises important issues for the addicted person regarding the danger of self-deception and illusory control, as well as the necessity of relinquishing false power so as to recognize one's "unexceptional ordinariness" (Kurtz 1983, p. 65). For those of the dominant group, i.e., white and male in Western cultures, accepting one's essential limitation may well be a necessary concomitant to becoming more human, to transcending self-centredness and self-deception. However, I would argue that it is from the position of "lack," of insufficiency and deficiency, of low self-esteem and a too-soluble sense of self that women more typically approach programs of the recovery movement. Many women entering a 12-Step group are burdened by the uniquely female "sin" of self-negation and of hiding (see Saiving 1979; Dunfee 1982). For example, when compared with men alcoholics and nonalcoholic women, women alcoholics have reported that they feel powerless and inadequate *before* drinking (see Beckman 1978; Gomberg and Lisansky 1984).[2] Also the anorexic, along with many women in Western cultures, learns to fear her deepest cravings, the "Yes" within herself (Lorde 1984, pp. 57–58). Her starvation represents a denial of what she knows about her body's vulnerability, its power, and its promise.

Women who starve, or binge and purge compulsively, agonize about their *lack* of control, and so organize rigid behaviours and complex rituals in their attempts to feel powerful and in control. We must remember that issues of power and control are understandably significant for women in a culture where myths of our influence are promoted, i.e, "the hand that rocks the cradle rules the world," while, simultaneously, access to societal resources and institutions is denied us (Chrisler 1991, p.140). It has been suggested that women use dependence and helplessness and other indirect, so-called manipulative strategies to exert power in the interpersonal sphere, a function perhaps of the inaccessibility of more conventional forms of power (ibid.). Assuming responsibility for how one deals with personal and political powerlessness in a culture that legitimizes and reinforces such "lack" is, I believe, a different process from that which occurs when one begins from a position of social power and is engaged in the "exceedingly male attempt" to hold on to "the project to be God" (Krestan 1991, p.183). In the AA and OA paradigm, as it is traditionally understood, women are advised/required to give up what they have never had.

Krestan refers to the "flight from relatedness" as a key element in the addict's attempt to maintain power over and control of that which is out of control in her life. Theorists and clinicians working in the area of women's psychological development are proposing a paradigm shift from a focus on the well-boundaried, autonomous "self" to a model that emphasizes a relational way of living. Carol Gilligan and her colleagues at Harvard are demonstrating that adolescent girls take themselves *out of* relationship, (by becoming less assertive, less knowing) as a way to *stay in* relationship. By moulding to the still-dominant model of femininity required of young girls and women, they are more assured of being acceptable and accepted, albeit in a limited and truncated manner.[3] In their research, Jean Baker Miller and her colleagues at the Stone Center for Developmental Services are writing about how relationships are central to women's growth and empowerment. They are arguing that women's movement towards connection is not neurotic or pathological, but rather "inherently healthy and life affirming" (Surrey and Kilbourne 1986–91). Janet Surrey says that women use and abuse substances in the service of "making and maintaining connections — to try to feel connected, energized and loved when that is not the whole truth of their experience" (ibid.). Women's use of substances — and women's preoccupation with weight and body issues — often represent an attempt to deal with the pain *in* our relationships, and our desire to create or maintain relational connections with others. For example, many women use and abuse substances in the hope of feeling joined and connected to their drug-abusing partners; they alter and transform themselves so as to adapt to the requirements of the relationships that are available to them. In a paradoxical twist on Krestan's notion, it may be, then, that the "flight from relatedness" is both warranted and necessary for women. Many women are living within relational contexts that are far from being mutually empathic and empowering. The truth of their lives, their actual lived experience, is too often that of disconnection and violation, of isolation and shaming; many women's lives *are* a "pilgrimage of survival" (Ettore 1989, p. 600). Eating-disordered and substance-abusing patterns may well be a profound mode of disclosure, albeit an ineffective and even dangerous one, of women's "liberatory urge" towards more personal integrity and meaningful connectedness (ibid.).

In the ideology of AA and OA the conversion process is based on the internalization of the belief that one must turn, or give, one's life over to a higher power, and that one is powerless over the alcohol, drugs, and/or food that have wrecked havoc with one's life. I am concerned both about the passive mode of acceptance that may be generated by such ideology, and by the transfer of it to, for example, "men-addicted women who love too much" (see Norwood 1985). Such concepts can reinforce women's socialization to negate self and to give of ourselves in yet another variation of the theme of "passive acceptance" and the "willingness to surrender" that have characterized treatment strategies for so-called "female illnesses" at least since the late nineteenth century (see Showalter 1985). For women who love too much, who eat too much or not enough, the giving over of oneself to a "higher" power is considered to be *the* "redemptive" moment — when, in fact, it can represent yet another moment of self-denial and sacrifice, of "letting go" of self-will and the passion required to demand change in one's circumstances. An example of this may be found in the mantra of the codependency movement the membership of which is 85 percent female. "Reclaiming the Inner Child" has too often meant that the central drama of recovery is that of wading into the "quagmires of childhood" so as to excavate the "buried injured child" only to find that one must adjust to what are, in fact, intolerable situations (Faludi 1991, pp. 351 and 353). I am concerned that the potential healing power of revisiting the crimes of one's childhood so as to integrate and transcend them may be tragically lost in this infantilizing strategy.

Bette Tallen (1990) makes an important critique of the recovery movement when she argues that the language of conversion, confession, redemption, and salvation are inherently Christian in ideology and thus are unfamiliar concepts to other religious traditions. I would add that turning one's life and will over to the care of God reinforces a hierarchical notion of self in relation to the "transcendent" and that in the 12-Step paradigm, God is conceptualized in anthropomorphic and patriarchal terms — *however* one understands *Him*. While 12-Step programs offer a way of exploring spirituality that is communal yet not confined within organized religion, I would argue that 12-Step spirituality does not go far enough in revisioning our images of God, power, and our relationships with the whole of the web of life. When women are open to doing so, I prefer to work with a notion of transformation that has to do with "power within," rather than the concept of relationship with a "higher power."

THE DISCOURSE OF DISEASE

The disease concept of chemical dependency has served to mitigate against the oppressive and undeserving moral stigma that was previously attached to addicts, and it has helped to reduce the profound feelings of guilt associated with being, or living with someone who is, out of control. The fact of addiction, that it is an issue in its own right, has been placed at the centre of recovery, which is an astounding reversal of traditional therapy wherein it (addiction) is merely symptomatic and adjunctive to the "real" issues. The program of AA describes alcohol and drug addiction as a disease, while promoting an understanding of health that includes the psychological and the spiritual. Furthermore, many women have learned in self-help groups like Al-Anon that they are not responsible for their partners' behaviours, and thus have been freed from the internalized blame and shame associated with their partners' addictions.

However, many women do not actively seek help because of the very real stigma still associated with women's addictive behaviour. Throughout history, women have been held to higher standards of behaviour than men, in keeping with women's status as the "moral guardians" of the culture (Van Den Burgh 1991, p.18). Women who abuse substances are often victimized many times over: they are considered to be very "unlady-like," to have little moral fortitude, and to be sexually out of control (ibid.). According to Janice Haaken (1990, p.403), the moral interpretation of addiction *does* persist in 12-Step programs: "Even though the alcoholic is not seen as morally responsible for the disease, alcoholism, like Original Sin, requires spiritual redemption and divine intervention. Just as the concept of Original Sin liberates the believer from personal responsibility for his/her 'fallen state' while at the same time making the 'sinner' responsible for seeking salvation, so too the AA disease model shifts the moral ground from alcoholism (a disease for which the alcoholic is not responsible) to the alcoholic's responsibility to seek recovery through a Twelve step program."

Haaken observes that there are some interesting parallels in how the "disease concept" in addictions, and the concept of the "devil" in fundamentalism, operate psychodynamically:

> The appeal of both fundamentalism and 12-Step programs is similar: the hope of connecting with a source of goodness and benevolent control amidst a world dominated by chaotic, destructive forces. Both belief systems permit a mystical transformation of bad feelings and experiences into good feelings of peace and well being. God comes to represent the longed for object of comfort and hope — the object that has failed the believer in reality but that she/he hopes to recover through faith and relinquishment of personal will. The complexity of experience is reduced to some basic unifying ideas, and anxiety is warded off by following a set of prescribed steps. (ibid.) [4]

I would suggest that continued uncritical use of the disease concept, when it is controversial at best, does little to reflect the integration within the research and clinical community of a more holistic understanding of addiction that takes into account physiological, psychological, sociocultural, and environmental phenomena. Also, it is "preemptive and callous" to extend the disease concept and the AA 12-Step philosophy beyond chemical dependency to the so-called process dependencies, i.e., codependency, and to activities and behaviours that are primarily white, middle-class, and gender-related problems, i.e., shopping addiction, work addiction. In order to label such behaviours "addictions," one must have privileged status in Western dominant culture (Lerner 1991, p. 16). Furthermore, there is a very real risk that the experiences of those women who have been too close to death may be trivialized when addiction is generalized to non–life threatening, albeit painful, behaviours (Brown 1990, p. 3). In the recovery-movement paradigm, the social and political sources of oppression are so obscured that the political is now personal, which is a dramatic reversal of the once-powerful feminist dictum (see ibid. and Tallen 1990). Tallen cautions us that "the reality of oppression is replaced with the metaphor of addiction," with the result that individual, personal solutions are applied to collective, political situations (Tallen 1990, p. 396). The metaphor of disease and addiction is not reflective of the fact that, for example, the "unmanageable" life of a fat woman can be the result of oppressive expectations generated by cultural requirements as to how women's bodies ought to look (Freeman 1989, p. 20). In the codependency framework, women's experiences of victimization are considered to be wrought by virtue of our pathology; it is a new, inventive way to "blame the victim," and carries with it the associated risk that neither she nor society is challenged to assume responsibility for her/its actions. Is it not less threatening for the dominant group culture to have "sick" women meeting in codependency groups, working on their recovery, than "angry" women meeting in feminist empowerment groups, working on social revolution? (See Brown 1990, p. 4). Lerner (1991, p. 15) points out that "the recovery movement ... is lulling us back into nurturing our weaknesses. It's also luring us back into other things: self blaming, parent blaming ..." More specifically, I would attest, it is a seduction back to wife, partner, and mother blaming, or more precisely, woman blaming, a process that both the codependency movement and aspects of the men's movement, i.e., as articulated by poet Robert Bly, are perpetuating.[5]

The codependency movement is so entrenched in our sexist and heterosexist views of the world that it provides a particular challenge to feminist practice. The concept of codependence originated in the alcoholism-treatment field to describe the characteristics and behaviours of spouses — usually women — of alcoholics. The question of gender-role socialization in the etiology of the so-called enabling behaviours has only recently been addressed, yet this movement has grown exponentially over the past decade and now includes the children, adult children, and grandchildren of chemically dependent people (for example, see Krestan and Bepko 1990). It is a movement that lacks clarity and precision in terms of definition and scope: there are as many definitions of codependency as there are authors in the field. It has been variously defined as:

a "primary disease" that "could lead to death."[6] It has been described as an "emotional, psychological, and behavioural condition" and a "family disease" that should be included in the *DSM-III-R* classifications of personality disorders.[7] The symptoms of codependency range from "no symptoms at all to headaches to suicide."[8] In Melody Beattie's (1987) list of 241 characteristics, organized into 14 categories of behaviours, being female and codependent are one and the same. Codependency can be, then, a "symbol of stigmatization," one that relies on the myth of the "normal," traditional, male-dominated nuclear family. We are learning that such families are often only "functional" for the men in them (see Tallen 1990, p.404; Kresten and Bepko 1990, p.224). The codependency movement labels women as "diseased" for doing what is expected of them within the patriarchal family; and women, recognizing themselves in these descriptors of people who focus almost exclusively on others, are embracing this identity, its language and its practices, thus pathologizing themselves.

SHAME, RELATEDNESS, AND COMMUNITY

Countless women — hitherto condemned to isolation and shame — have discovered healing communities and learned to "feel better" through their participation in 12-Step groups. The core movement of healing is a relational one; women and men are encouraged to move from their isolation to experience connection in the context of a mutually empowering community. This is especially significant, I believe, when we consider the impact of shame and its role in the problem of "lack" of self and power. I would argue that shame is a core issue in women's pervasive sense of personal inadequacy. The centrality of shame as a primary source of human discomfort is being demonstrated in the clinical literature and is certainly observed in therapeutic practice. For at least the past decade, it has been thought that shame plays a crucial role in the development and maintenance of abusive, addictive, and eating-disordered patterns. Along with its importance in terms of self-functioning, shame is central to the development of conscience, alerting us to transgression, and to insults to human dignity (Kaufman 1989, p.5). It is also critical to identity formation. It has been suggested that shame is the crucible from within which both our particular and universal sense of self is formed (ibid.). As such, it may be defined as "the affect of inferiority, ... the most poignant experience of the self by the self ... dividing us both from ourselves and others" (ibid. 1989, p.17). In other words, shame is "the affect of indignation, of defeat, of transgression, and of alienation ... shame is felt as an inner torment, a sickness of the soul" (Tomkins 1987, p.17). To feel shame is to see oneself and "to feel *seen* in a painfully diminished sense" (Kaufman 1989, p.22). I think this very dynamic marks a fundamental problem of patriarchal culture. Women are repeatedly seen through the gaze of men; it is the male prerogative to image and fashion women. Like the soul in ages past, the female body is an object of worship; women strive to attain the divine body demanded by the modern age. By virtue of the male activity of observing and assessing woman as "object," her sense of self is derived. "Mirrored in the eyes of men, women are spectral, not quite all there; paradoxically, at the same time, they are all too fearfully present in the flesh" (Kiceluk 1991, p. 216). Within this cultural configuration, woman as subject and as a self is repressed, thus allowing for the kind of oppression that is justified by her status as object. The pervasive effect of the male gaze — which is "always there" and "could be" but is "not necessarily" watching, is such that she participates in her oppression by her vigilence (Foucault 1979, p.202–3; see also Hunter 1992, p.7–26 where she examines surveillance of battered women). She internalizes the "normative gaze" to which she is subjected (Bartky 1988, p.80). I would argue that if the experience of oppression itself promotes shame, then shame must be borne by women in a very particular way. The meaning of shame then, must be considered in relation to both women's psychological and social situation (Bartky 1990, p.84). Both the shame of embodiment and the shame of personal inadequacy are pervasive and profoundly disempowering states of being for women — and both are assured us by virtue of our location in sexist society.

I agree with Bartky's assessment that this shame "is not so much a particular feeling or emotion (though it involves specific feelings and emotions) as a pervasive affective attunement to the social environment" (Bartky 1990, p. 85). Women's shame, then, is not just a consequence or effect of subordination. Rather, "within the larger universe of patriarchal social relations, [it is] a profound mode of disclosure both of self and situation" (ibid.). This, then, is the emotional tone of the well-documented observations that women are less assertive that men, have lower self-esteem, less confidence in themselves, and poorer self-concepts. It is within this universe that an alcoholic women desperately feels her powerlessness and inadequacy, and so drinks so as not to feel as much and so deeply; she turns to substances so as to take something for herself; it is an attempt, however doomed, to meet her own needs. This is the world the weight-preoccupied, starving woman inhabits as she both upholds the social order to be slender, and threatens the society with disorder. This is the world wherein all women are denied "autonomous choice of self, forbidden cultural expression, and condemned to the immanence of mere bodily being" (ibid., p. 31). All women, like Eve, through their desire for the forbidden fruit, face the following dilemma: "a choice between obedience and knowledge. Between renunciation and appetite. Between subordination and desire. Between security and risk. Between loyalty and self-development. Between submission and power. Between hunger as temptation and hunger as vision" (Chernin 1987, p. 182).

A feminist analysis of therapy and recovery work must question, then, whether "feeling better" is enough. Our counseling and therapeutic work certainly is oriented to help women move towards "more self" and towards more mutually enhancing relationships (Lerner 1991, p. 16). We must strive to keep this in balance with our belief that a focus on women's pain as an exclusively personal reality can be detrimental to and prohibitive of structural change. As long as women continue to be oppressed under the guise of being helped and healed, as long as the political is pathologized and interpersonal processes are favoured over external realities, then women *will* be lulled into perpetual recovery (Brown 1990, p.3). I would suggest that the current research on ethics in feminist psychotherapy contributes significantly to our understanding of the application of an analysis of women's oppression to the principles and practices of our therapeutic work (for example, see Lerman and Porter 1990).

A brief comment on the exclusiveness of this community of healing: while originally intended for men, AA has adapted to include women, lesbians, and gays, thus providing community based on shared experience and the desire for change. However, the sexism and heterosexism inherent in the organization of AA and Al-Anon and critical to their history continues. For example, Herman has (1988, p. 61) observed that lesbians often have to "fine-tune the 12-Step approach to their own personal philosophies" in order to remain in AA, which is, for Tallen (1990, p.401), a phenomenal contortion of themselves. Furthermore, I have observed that an all-women group does not necessarily mean that all women find it accessible.

WOMEN'S REALITIES AND
TRADITIONAL TREATMENT AGENDAS

It is important to recognize that, in 12-Step groups, women are learning skills that enable them to take better care of themselves; they are developing more self-enhancing ways of living in and outside of intimate relationships. Their private experiences of incest, sexual abuse, and addictions are validated and shared within a community that does not trivialize these realities.

However, while validation may be the experience of many women in 12-Step self-help programs, the treatment plan of many institutional programs organized around the medical model and the disease concept of addictions has traditionally required that a women deal with her "disease" — which is regarded as the *cause* of her substance abuse. According to this conceptualization, dealing with incest, sexual abuse, eating-disordered patterns, or physical violence is to "defocus," at least until one is well into recovery, i.e, after two years of sobriety. I would argue that the central therapeutic work with chemically dependent women is to support them in their movement towards abstinance, and that the work of therapy is largely ineffective until that is accomplished. However, we need to be able to work with our clients in sorting out the *meanings* around their return to self-starvation, compulsive over-eating, or, drug use if that occurs in the process of therapy. The realities of women's lives suggest that while the initial, immediate, and long-term goal in treatment for chemical dependency or anorexia is abstinence from mood-altering drugs and physical stabilization, respectively, the therapist cannot always ordain when memories will surface. Neither can we control when familiar coping strategies may become necessary for a woman in order to feel safe when she is feeling most vulnerable. There *is* a risk to sobriety, or to stabilized eating patterns, that accompanies confronting the horrors of one's life. However, it seems necessary for most of us to go to the sources, the roots, of our woundedness and our pain in order for radical healing to occur. Our treatment plans and programs need to reflect that it is impossible and unacceptable to "program" women according to traditional treatment agendas. A related issue is that of therapist accountability: we must have the skills to be able to effectively "be with" a woman where *she* is. Especially when working with women who live in areas with limited mental-health and therapeutic resources, this may mean, for example, respecting her decision to be engaged in a 12-Step program. When appropriate, the therapist can then support a woman in the reframing of her experiences in terms of oppression and power (Brown 1990, p. 4). As therapists, we also need to evaluate, in an ongoing and rigorous manner, how it is that we have not facilitated women's empowerment (ibid.). We need to question whether we have sought arduously enough for healing alternatives to offer women who, as yet, can only come "out from under" in the name of disease and recovery (Learner 1990,

p. 16). While admittedly the topic of another essay, I would briefly suggest that we need to be reflecting on the healing process as circular and complex rather than linear, hierarchial, and neatly compartmentalized. In such a process, therapist and client are engaged in a mutually transforming event. While the therapist is theoretically informed and skilled with respect to "what works," the stages of recovery, and the like, she and her client move together as in an improvised dance, open to the experience and responding in the moment to it. *Both* are changed in the encounter.

ACCESSIBILITY AND INTEGRITY

In 12-Step programs, criticism and judgement of one another is discouraged, and anonymity is observed; thus the much-needed safe environment within which one can reveal oneself is usually guaranteed. This is particularly true of AA and Al-Anon, where integrity is maintained through the observance of the Twelve Traditions (see Appendix), which are the governing principles of the organization. These principles assure that the organization is informally structured and member-led, that anonymity is insisted upon and no experts are endorsed (Tallen 1990, p. 402). Generally speaking, groups are structured so as to be autonomous, and are open to an ongoing process of self-critique and evolution. The community is nonhierarchical and decentralized; thus, consensus and continuity are assured. Twelve-Step programs have provided accessible and structured therapy and, in doing so, have provided a challenge to the hegemony and class bias that has so often resulted in therapy being a privilege of the middle and upper classes (Freeman 1989, p. 20). Treatment is based on the "collective efforts of ordinary people" (ibid.) rather than the costly alternatives of drugs, hospitalization, and expensive therapists. And contrary to some of its spinoffs in the recovery industry, AA in particular does not aggressively pursue big profits from its publications (Freeman 1989, p. 20). Furthermore, because there are now groups worldwide, one is never far from a meeting and a supportive group.

Unfortunately, these qualities that contribute to the strength of AA do not always exist within the rest of the recovery industry, and other 12-Step programs; too many contradict both the traditions of AA and the principles of feminism. For example, as Tallen (1990, p. 403) has pointed out, many in-hospital groups use the steps without the traditions, are therapist facilitated, and are not accessible to everyone; they do not share AA's insistence on anonymity, or its politics and practices about money. I would add that, even within AA, anonymity is an ideal often not met in practice, a problem especially prevalent in smaller communities and rural areas. Also, judgement *is* often made in "helpful" attempts to challenge a member to break through "denial" — an experience which can have devastating consequences for women whose sense of self is already seriously depleted. Many women with whom I have worked have found that some groups can be quite rigid and closed to any ongoing process of self-examination and critique.

SUMMARY AND CONCLUSION

I think it is tragic that many of us find it more acceptable to define ourselves as "recovering persons" than as feminists. A feminist analysis of the political, psychological, and spiritual underpinnings of the recovery movement suggests that it represents a "depoliticization of feminism" (Tallen 1990, p. 395). The recovery industry is based on a model of therapy that opposes the principles and goals of feminist therapy: self-empowerment and liberation from oppressive sociocultural conditions. It is a model that can drain us of our "vital strength and woman anger" (ibid., p. 406). Lerner (1991) writes eloquently of this when she says that we are returning "to the culturally ingrained belief that women who put their primary energy into their own growth are hurtful and destructive of others. Women tend to feel so guilty and anxious about any joyful assertion of self in the face of patriarchal injunctions that each small step out from under is invariably accompanied by some unconscious act of apology and penance ... it is an act of deep apology, especially to the dominant group culture, for women to move forward in the name of recovery, addiction and disease" (p.16). In the recovery paradigm, women's anger is focused on their disease rather than on the oppressive social conditions within which they live their lives. Existing power relations are maintained as women's rage and fear are subverted in the service of their recovery; in women's spending enormous amounts of time and energy "working their program," there is a danger that there is little passion left for the effort and commitment required to work towards social and structural change.

I believe this same dynamic is observed when discussing weight-preoccupation and eating-disordered patterns: just as women are engaged in multiple and varied normalizing strategies in producing and maintaining the youthful, slender and fit body, so too does our intense involvement in the practices of recovery suggest yet another strategy by which gender relations are maintained and reproduced. The practices of recovery provide a contemporary, dominating, and difficult-to-resist venue for the "disciplines of the self" and, more particularly, for the disciplinary technologies of women's bodies (see Foucault 1979, 1988). Women's desires — for food, sexuality, meaningful connection in relationship, power, — are appropriated by the dominant culture and construed to be inherently shameful, progressive, and fatal diseases. While I know in my life and work that the horrific struggle of addiction to alcohol and chemicals and the all-consuming passion to be thin is all *too* real, we need to be vigilant about how readily we apply the metaphor of addiction to struggles that are based on women's oppression within Western patriarchal society. We need to remember that the desire to connect with the "Yes within," and to be related to others in meaningful and mutually empowering ways is at the heart of our "disorders." We need to support one another so that these courageous attempts for "more self" and more life-giving relationships, are honoured for what they are — rather than pathologized as diseases and internalized by us as sick and shameful.

What, then, are our alternatives? Is it possible for us to "divine" new patterns of metanoia, of transformation (Keller 1986, p. 248)? I propose that we turn to contemporary feminist thought in religion and in psychology as we search for new mythologies that will be sources for different kinds of knowledge and power for women and for men. Many scholars in these disciplines are engaged in the work of creating new paradigms for seeing and acting in the world. I believe there is a conversation going on within these fields that is rooted in their concern for embodied human life. I think the commonalities and parallel themes between a relational psychology and a feminist spirituality provide a framework that can contribute to the recovery of feminine *jouissance* (pleasure),[9] and so displace the male ordering of desire. In creating new spaces for conversation between these disciplines, we can imagine and create a more "ensouled world" (Goldenberg 1990, p. 112). They can help us investigate the various meanings given to the body and to identify the implications of these meanings for our movement beyond patriarchal culture. For example, some feminist scholars in religion are suggesting that a return to the Goddess can support our attempts to resurrect and honour the body, not as object of control that is out of control, but as "personhood that is thoroughly enfleshed" (Keller 1986, p. 234). Others propose that claiming the erotic as sacred power helps us to encounter the wholeness of self and other (see, for example, Heyward 1989). Mary Daly enjoins us in the task of creating postpatriarchal space and time, a project that Catherine Keller (1986, p. 158) refers to as developing a "metaphysic of connection."

I propose that, if our work as therapists is to be truly transformative, we will be challenged to move from the denial of eros to living truthfully our erotic connection to all of life; from alienation in our relationships to an awareness of our interconnectedness; from inauthenticity in our communities to active responsibility for changing cultural oppressions. We need to rethink the place of the body in this culture so that at least some of the old chasms can be bridged: between desire and its object, self and other, appearance and reality, body and soul, material and spiritual, immanence and transcendence, power-over and power-with. We need to learn to speak for an ethos of eros and connection in our research and our therapies. Perhaps then the split in consciousness which is our religious and cultural heritage, born by women and inscribed on our bodies and in our lives, will eventually be healed.

◆

APPENDIX

AA'S TWELVE STEPS

STEP ONE
We admitted we were powerless over alcohol — that our lives had become unmanageable.

STEP TWO
Came to believe that a Power greater than ourselves could restore us to sanity.

STEP THREE
Made a decision to turn our will and our lives over to the care of God as we understood Him.

Step Four
Made a searching and fearless moral inventory of ourselves.

Step Five
Admitted to God, to ourselves, and to another human being, the exact nature of our wrongs.

Step Six
Were entirely ready to have God remove all these defects of character.

Step Seven
Humbly asked Him to remove our shortcomings.

Step Eight
Made a list of all persons we had harmed, and became willing to make amends to them all.

Step Nine
Made direct amends to such people wherever possible, except when to do so would injure them or others.

Step Ten
Continued to take personal inventory and when we were wrong promptly admitted it.

Step Eleven
Sought through prayer and meditation to improve our conscious contact with God as we understood Him, praying only for knowledge of His will for us and the power to carry that out.

Step Twelve
Having had a spiritual awakening as the result of these steps, we tried to carry this message to alcoholics, and to practice these principles in all our affairs.

AA'S TWELVE TRADITIONS

TRADITION ONE
Our common welfare should come first; personal recovery depends upon AA unity.

TRADTION TWO
For our group purpose there is but one ultimate authority — a loving God as He may express Himself in our group conscience. Our leaders are but trusted servants; they do not govern.

TRADITION THREE
The only requirement for AA membership is a desire to stop drinking.

TRADITION FOUR
Each group should be autonomous except in matters affecting other groups or AA as a whole.

TRADITION FIVE
Each group has but one primary purpose — to carry its message to the alcoholic who still suffers.

TRADITION SIX
An AA group ought never endorse, finance, or lend the AA name to any related facility or outside enterprise, lest problems of money, property and prestige divert us from our primary purpose.

TRADITION SEVEN
Every AA group ought to be fully self-supporting, declining outside contributions.

TRADITION EIGHT
Alcoholics Anonymous should remain forever nonprofessionl, but our service centers may employ special workers.

TRADITION NINE

AA, as such, ought never be organized; but we may create service boards or committees directly responsible to those they serve.

TRADITION TEN

Alcoholics Anonymous has no opinion on outside issues; hence the AA name ought never be drawn into public controversy.

TRADITION ELEVEN

Our public relations policy is based on attraction rather than promotion; we need always maintain personal anonymity at the level of press, radio, and films.

TRADITION TWELVE

Anonymity is the spiritual foundation of all our traditions, ever reminding us to place principles before personalities.

Reproduced from *Twelve Steps and Twelve Traditions* (Alcoholics Anonymous World Services, Inc., 1953, 1975).

NOTES

1. See Appendix for Alcoholics Anonymous's 12 Steps and 12 Traditions. Griel and Rudy, 1983, p. 6.

2. For an analysis of the soluable self, see Keller 1986, pp. 203–18.

3. See Brown and Gilligan 1992.

4. For a discussion of the similarities between self-help and charismatic groups, see Galanter 1990.

5. See Faludi 1991 for a description of how Bly, having awakened himself to the feminine principle in the 1960s, began to think himself to be consumed by it and only "superficially manly" by the early 1980s. He began running all-male workshops to "remedy this latest imbalance" and to "reintroduce men to the deep masculine."

6. Wegscheider 1981b and Schaef 1986, cited in Harper and Capdevila 1990, p. 285. See also Wegscheider Cruse 1985.

7. Friel, Subby, and Friel 1984, and Gorski and Miller 1984, cited in Harper and Capdevila 1990, p. 285. See also Cermak 1986a, 1986b.

8. Whitfield 1984, cited in Harper and Capdevila 1990, p. 285. See also Whitfield 1989.

9. I use *jouissance* in the way that it is understood by Julia Kristeva, namely, as the "totality of enjoyment ... total joy and ecstasy" (1980, pp. 15–16).

METAPHORS FOR HEALING
SELF-HARM BEHAVIOURS

Maxene Adler

Jan, a bright, attractive, 30-year-old female, is vividly describing the childhood traumas that led her to seek counseling. As she becomes more animated, she makes a wide gesture with her arm, revealing a series of scars on her wrist which were previously concealed by her long sleeves. When you mention her scars, she hesitantly rolls up her sleeves to unveil a line of consecutive scars extending up her inner arm, some superficial, others deeply gouged and barely healed. You attempt to control an immediate and involuntary response to recoil at the sight of exposed raw flesh. It is this one single observation that gives you immense insight into the depths of hurt, anger, and emotional pain experienced by your client.

Self-mutilation is one of the many forms of self-harm behaviours, ranging from self-effacement to self-starvation and possible death. Self-harm includes a continuum of behaviours, ranging from devaluative thoughts and statements to compulsive eating and/or exercising and dysfunctional behavioural patterns; and to more overt self-destructive behaviours, such as substance abuse, suicidal attempts, and severe, life-threatening anorexia.

Most self-harm behaviours appear on the surface to be an irrational, out-of-control response to a particular traumatic experience or series of traumatic experiences. However, on closer examination, they are, in fact, a very rational, response of the client to defend or protect herself from these experiences. In essence, self-harm behaviours represent ways of coping with highly unpleasant or life-threatening experience(s).

Within the course of therapy, a client begins to understand the purpose behind the self-harm behaviours. By identifying the specific purpose or purposes behind the behaviour, it no longer appears to be an irrational act, allowing the client to begin to take ownership of it and to develop some sense of control over it.

Self-harm behaviours result from a number of factors that can vary significantly from individual to individual. More commonly, they arise from one or a combination of the following: the desire to annihilate oneself, the need to disrupt or stop the emotional pain, feelings of intense self-dislike or hatred, and/or the need to punish oneself. Suicidality may lie at the deep unconscious levels of all acts of self-harm; however, generally death is not the conscious, desired outcome.

USE OF METAPHORS AS TREATMENT

Although a variety of treatment approaches can be employed in dealing with self-harm behaviours, metaphors have empowering qualities, which are the core of feminist therapy. Through the use of metaphors, the client maintains the locus of control through the therapeutic process.

Healing takes place within the context determined by the client; control over the process and the speed at which it occurs is similarly retained by the client. The therapist plays a supportive role and sets the backdrop for the metaphors to unfold, facilitating insight as required. Metaphors used within the context of feminist therapy also incorporate strong female characters and powerful feminine symbols or rituals, indicative of the inherent strength of the female gender. This symbolism is significant, for it uses women to help women, thereby avoiding many of the pitfalls of the traditionally male-focused therapies.

A wide range of therapeutic options exist, ranging from the more traditional therapies, such as psychotherapy and behaviour modification, to the more contemporary modalities, such as positive regression to exaggerated paradoxes. The effectiveness of these options varies, and is often dependant upon the skill of the therapist and the match of the therapy to the client.

Metaphors can be viewed as symbolic representations of a person's conflict that are used within the context of a therapeutic situation to facilitate insight and healing. Metaphors can be an effective medium in therapy because they provide a nonthreatening way to externalize one's reality (Durrant 1983). Through the process of externalizing, a client's reality is given substance and form, often challenging the internal assumptions and belief system at the root of the self-harm behaviours.

The metaphors that are employed have particular meaning and relevance in a person's life, and often reflect interests, cultural heritage, religious background, or personal preferences. This personalization of the metaphors is important because it helps the client to frame the problem according to her own situation and particular experiences. Similarly, for this reason, healing that takes place through the use of metaphors can be more readily incorporated into a client's life .

As part of the therapeutic process, metaphors require the use of techniques, such as creative visualization, guided or nonguided imagery, or symbolic representation. These techniques generally include the use of mental images to promote healing. (Some examples of metaphors and their strategic use in the journey towards healing are described later in this essay.) Establishing trust in the therapeutic relationship is essential before introducing the use of metaphors. Once established, clients are more receptive to the healing journey through metaphor.

Metaphors can be used as a single modality in therapy or as an adjunct to other methods. Metaphoric descriptions of a problem can assist clients, enabling them to actually visualize their problem. For example, a woman who was experiencing severe depression following an incident of self-inflicted harm was at a loss for words to describe the depth of her depression. She was, however, able to relate to the metaphor of having a wet blanket thrown over her, which evoked the tremendous effort required for her to make even the slightest move. As the depression lifted, the woman was able to use the metaphor to describe her desire to peek out from under the blanket.

While metaphors are a highly adaptive medium for healing self-harm behaviours, they are not suitable for everyone. For example, clients whose acute fear of loosing control makes relaxation and spontaneity impossible are generally not ready for treatment through metaphors. With a great deal of preparatory work, these clients may be more amenable to this kind of therapy; however, in these cases it is important that the therapist exercise caution, and not proceed too quickly.

For some clients, an inadvertent word may trigger flashbacks. For these clients, a more structured therapy would be indicated. Some clients may find it intimidating to use metaphors and should not be pushed. However, if clinical judgement is used wisely, metaphors can be used effectively in healing self-harm behaviours.

BEGINNING THE JOURNEY

The first, most important step in the healing process is assisting the client in honouring what she has done and is doing to survive (Bass and Davis 1988). By the time a client comes to see you, these behaviours have likely been labeled negatively by others, and by the client herself. Within the context of feminist therapy, it is essential to ensure that the dignity of all coping behaviours is restored, regardless of their severity or potential harm to the client. You do not ignore serious, life-threatening behaviours; but neither do you label them in a manner that will further traumatize the client and reinforce a negative self-image. In order to restore dignity to the self-harm behaviours, reframing is often necessary. Using such terms as "coping" or "survival" behaviours removes the stigma and provides purpose to what is seemingly an irrational act. By restoring dignity, you encourage the client to take ownership of the behaviour, free from the negative connotations she and others have bestowed upon it.

In traditional therapy, the coping mechanisms, of women in particular, are often given pejorative labels, such as hysterical, histrionic, or masochistic (Caplan 1985; Lerner 1989). These labels have the effect of placing the blame on the individual for her current problems, reinforcing an already poor self-concept, and promoting a distorted understanding of her current situation. Honouring the self-harm behaviours eliminates these harmful and counterproductive results. Reframing the self-harm behaviours will begin to allow the client an opportunity to gain conscious control over the behaviours and to identify their degree of usefulness in coping with the problem.

A 25-year-old woman with a history of childhood incest began eating compulsively during her adolescence and continued into her adulthood. By reframing the eating as a form of nurturance, which she was lacking in her childhood, and as a way of insulating herself from further male advances, she was able to reduce the frequency of her eating binges. Finding nurturance and insulation through eating was a way of surviving, and was one of the few avenues open to her at the time. The eating thus served a useful purpose. Giving dignity and seeing a clear purpose behind her compulsive eating allowed her to take responsibility for it and to exercise some control over it. As the therapy continued, she was able to find nondestructive behaviours to nurture herself. Reframing the compulsive-eating behaviour in this situation transformed a seemingly impossible-to-control behaviour into a palatable action. This small but significant change was the first step in restoring this client's self-esteem and continuing the long journey towards healing and wholeness.

While reframing can be an extremely valuable technique, it takes time to find the precise words that fit for the client. Until an accurate fit can be found, clients may not respond or may give only cursory acknowledgement to efforts at reframing. Timing is also important, since a client generally tends to hear reframing when she is ready.

CONTINUING THE JOURNEY

As a therapist, you may feel that you are constantly engaged in an uphill struggle of dealing with the trauma arising from past events in a client's life, by a system that further victimizes her, and by the client's own negative perception of herself, all of which reinforce the victimization. The strength of these interconnective bonds are difficult, but not impossible, to break. Reframing of the self-harm behaviour is usually sufficient to provide at least a hairline fracture in what seems to be an impenetrable armour.

Once the crack appears, however minute, it provides the opportunity to introduce another level of intervention, setting in motion a healing process that has the potential, if carried right through to final conclusion, to restore the wholeness of the person.

Metaphors can be introduced at this stage. They can be created by the therapist, but preferably will be of the client's choosing. The client will, in all likelihood, select a metaphor which will have the greatest symbolic meaning to her life. However, if the therapist is suggesting metaphors, several should be offered among which the client can choose.

Since working with metaphors should occur in a relaxed state; it is necessary to take the client through a process of relaxation. The following example of a relaxation exercise is one among variants:

Assume a comfortable position, either sitting or lying down. Relax your body. Begin to breath deeply, allowing the air to fill the full cavity of your chest. Count down slowly from 10 to 1, feeling the tension being released with each count. When completely relaxed, imagine a place where you feel safe and protected (or warm and nurtured). It may be a beach with warm sand heated by the rays of the sun or it may be a forest where the trees form a protective shelter around you. Stay there for a while. Feel the warmth of the sunshine on your body (or the protective glow from the trees).

The therapist should be aware that deep breathing is an essential part of this exercise. Shallow breathing tends to indicate lack of focus and blocked feelings (Hyde and Watson 1990). Should this occur, it is important to focus on the breathing again by describing the physical sensation of breath filling the entire chest cavity. If this is impossible for the client, you should reconsider her readiness for the relaxation exercise or discuss other factors that may be distracting her.

For some clients, relaxation represents a tremendous loss of control, particularly for women who have a history of childhood abuse that required a constant state of hypervigilance. In cases where control is a major issue, it may be necessary to focus initially on one aspect of the relaxation, for example, the breathing or the visualization of a safe place. If necessary, you can instruct the client to practise this at home over several weeks. Once she gains mastery over one aspect of the exercise, you can move on to the next step. In some cases it may be impossible for the client to allow herself to relax, despite your best efforts. If this happens, it's important to reframe it positively, for example, as a sign of being very alert or attentive; you can then switch to another therapeutic intervention that does not emphasize a relaxed state. The client will let you know if she wants to try the relaxation exercise again.

Successful completion of the relaxation stage is necessary before continuing with the metaphor, not only to relax the client, but also to put her in touch with her body. This reconnection of mind and body is essential, particularly in cases where there is a serious body-image distortion (Bass and Davis 1988). What often occurs in these cases is that the mind becomes out of touch with the body. In mainstream therapy, this is viewed as a defence mechanism, where, as a result of a traumatic experience, the mind disassociates from the body.

This splitting is common among people with backgrounds of emotional, physical, or sexual abuse. Reconnection of body and mind can be a difficult process, requiring a great deal of preparatory work before relaxation exercises are possible. This holds true for cases where body-image distortions are severe, particularly where serious sexual or physical abuse has taken place.

METAPHORS FOR THE JOURNEY

Metaphors, as the term is used here, are mental images that are symbolic of the person's past or present life. They may be drawn from fantasies, daydreams, stories, or myths, and are bound only by the imagination of the person. Generally, metaphors are not static; they progress with the healing process. New characters, places, or images may be introduced by either the client or the therapist as the healing process evolves. Changes that take place in the metaphors, as the journey towards wholeness occurs, can be used as a benchmark for measuring progress.

Since the client generally directs the metaphor through the healing process, she is able to speed up or slow down the process to allow her psyche a chance to absorb the new images. The therapist's role is often one of adviser/observer, ensuring the client does not overlook something that is critical to her healing. In this role the therapist provides vital feedback to the client, based on her observation of the process. Advice is given judiciously. Most often, the client is encouraged to rely on her own intuition. The therapist also protects the safety of the client and can, at any point, stop the process if it has become too threatening. In most cases, a client's own protective instincts will perform this function quite well.

Some metaphors are particularly powerful for many women. One is the healing circle, formed by women. Most ancient cultures, and particularly many of the aboriginal cultures in North America, make use of versions of this metaphor. The following case example demonstrates its use and therapeutic value. This particular metaphor was suggested by the therapist because of the client's Native ancestry. Kimberly was quick to pick up on the image of the healing circle, vaguely recalling her grandmother's stories of such a circle. The therapist assisted Kimberly in guiding the image, offering only words of encouragement and paraphrasing where necessary.

> Kimberly is in a relaxed state, breathing deeply, as she begins to envision a circle of women surrounding her. They are rythmically chanting something that she cannot distinguish at first. She recognizes some of the women: a life-long friend, a helpful neighbour, a colleague; others remain unknown. All are smiling at her, whispering words of encouragement between chants.
>
> She begins to experience warmth and protection from this circle of friendly faces. As she allows herself to relax a little more, one of the women approaches her and hands her a package, which she opens. It is a doll from her childhood, whose face has faded and whose clothes are slightly tattered. Kimberly notices that the doll's dress has torn at the seam because of her bulging tummy. She is somewhat distressed by the tear, and for a moment her breathing becomes shallow and rapid. One of the women notices Kimberly's distress and brings a needle and thread to quickly mend the seam. Kimberly holds the doll as the woman sews the dress. When completed, the tear is barely noticeable. The woman then wraps the doll in a warm, soft blanket and hands her back to Kimberly, who holds her lovingly. She is aware that all of the women are staring admiringly at the doll. On closer inspection, she sees that the women are actually staring at her. Their admiration is for her.

For Kimberly, this was a moving moment, for up to that point she had been acutely conscious of people staring at her for what she thought was an unsightly weight problem. She was unable to see beyond this image of herself, and maintained a poor self-image and underachieved, despite the fact she was extremely intelligent.

In the debriefing after the metaphor, Kimberly saw the doll as representing herself as a child and the tear as resulting from being heavy through childhood. Because she had avoided most social situations, she was both surprised and delighted that a woman in the circle had voluntarily sought to help her. Prior to that, she would resist any contact with people for fear they would be repelled by her figure. When the women first began to stare, she assumed that it was at the doll, never believing that people would gaze upon her with admiration.

This metaphor continued on the journey with her, as different women helped her at key juncture points in her healing. In fact, her own support network began to expand as she became more comfortable in the healing circle; she gained greater confidence and eventually exposed herself to more social encounters that provided her with positive feedback of who she was as a person, thus bringing her body image into a more realistic perspective.

The healing circle can be a powerful metaphor using women to help women. Particularly in cases of incest or sexual abuse by a male, an all women's circle is viewed as nonthreatening, with the power to nurture and heal. Also, women with different cultural and ethnic heritages frequently inject revelant cultural and/or ethnic symbols into the circle, such as spiritual chanting, ceremonial drums, costumes, and religious prayers.

Another effective metaphor can be rebirthing. This metaphor is particularly beneficial in completing the healing process. Metaphorically, it represents the act of creating life, which is specific to women and women alone. This power of creation has been worshipped, revered, and feared in cultures from time immemorial. Some historians even believe that the fear of such creative powers led males to systematically strip females of power (Morgan 1985).

Rebirthing also symbolizes transformation, renewal, and regeneration. If the healing process is complete, then one truly is transformed into a whole person, free of the anxieties, fears, and encumbrances of the former self, at harmony with past, present, and future. In the following case example, the metaphor of rebirthing was used as the final step in a long journey towards healing. Renata had originally presented in therapy as bulimic, caught in a serious binge/purge cycle that, in the course of therapy, was found to be related to severe physical and sexual abuse in her childhood.

Initially, when Renata began to use metaphors as a way of healing, she required the assistance of the therapist to guide her visual images. However, as she gained confidence and skill in unfolding the visual imagery, she assumed greater control over shaping her visualizations. This assumption of control over her metaphoric experiences was directly related to a reduction in her binge/purge cycle.

> After a long and arduous journey of healing wounds inflicted by severe physical and sexual abuse, Renata visualizes a long tunnel in which she is being swept along by a maelstrom. As she is whisked farther down the tunnel, the wind begins to subside and becomes a gentle breeze. She sees the devastation that the storm has wrecked; buildings demolished; trees and plants uprooted. Then she becomes aware of a small, glowing light. As she moves towards this light, it becomes brighter and brighter, so much so that she has to shield her eyes with her hand. At that moment, she becomes fearful and unsure of her footing as she is blinded by the light. Reassured that she should proceed slowly, testing the ground with each step, she moves farther into the light until it enveloped her. As the intense heat from the light warms her to the inner core, it begins to condense to a small ball that remains in the centre of Renata's chest. The tunnel then disappears, leaving the small, glowing ball as a lasting reminder and comforting companion.

Following this visualization, Renata had a sense that a major event had taken place, but was not precisely sure what. In the few subsequent remaining sessions, she described an inner peace with herself that she had never experienced. As well, she reported significant gains in further reducing her binge/purge cycle and in improving her relationships with men, including less approach/avoidance behaviour and better communication. Also, she began to make more positive statements about herself, which was something the therapy had focused on in the past but with little success.

In the two examples of use of metaphors given here, nonguided imagery was used, with the therapist playing a supportive role. The debriefing session following provided an opportunity for the clients to make the connections between the imagery and their present lives. In most cases, these connections are fairly obvious; however, if they are missed or unclear, the therapist can suggest a possible interpretation.

In the course of the imagery process, the therapist can encourage the client to identify the specific parts of the body that are affected by a particular feeling triggered by the images. For those with severe body-image distortions and disconnection between body and feelings, this may be a difficult task, requiring time and continual refocusing. In cases of sexual abuse, the reconnection of feelings and body may unleash previously suppressed memories of the assault(s). By slowing down the process, the therapist can allow the client an opportunity to incorporate these memories. For some clients, it may be necessary for the therapist to act as a guide through the imagery, particularly where the imaginative processes have been blunted through trauma or through total lack of confidence. As the journey towards healing progresses, spontaneity and imagination usually resurface and allow the client to assume direction of the mental imagery.

Several other metaphors have proved effective in healing self-harm behaviour, such as inner-body images of the womb, which represent a place of creation and nurturance. Almost every culture has a healing ritual, such as the healing circle described above, or the sweat lodge of the North American Native people, which can be adapted to the needs and background of the client. Other metaphors can be drawn from ancient rituals of cleansing and purification, and fertility rights (Meador 1990). Mythologies also offer a vast array of relevant stories, often with strong females deities as central characters (Buffalo 1990).

AFFIRMATIONS FOR THE JOURNEY

No process involving metaphors is complete without the use of positive affirmation. Affirmations are positive statements that are designed to promote self-worth (Picker 1978). In order to arrive at statements that are realistic and suitable for the client, the therapist usually explores with the client different statements that have particular meaning and can be incorporated into the client's repertoire. In essence, affirmations represent goals that, as the healing takes place, can progress with the therapy. For example, "My body is a source of important information," can be used as an intial affirmation. As the client gains greater confidence and self-assurance, the statement may become: "My body is beautiful."

Positive affirmations, often selected by the therapist, can be injected into the metaphor at strategic points or following the completion of the mental imagery. Clients are encouraged to practise their affirmations at home, for example, upon rising and looking at themselves in the mirror. Mastering the art of positive affirmations is more difficult than may first appear. People's first attempts generally tend to incorporate a negative-positive, such as "My body is not disgusting," rather than, "I am learning to accept parts of my body." With some gentle guidance and vigilance, the ability to make positive affirmations becomes easier.

Affirmations are essential in altering a person's negative self-image, which is always closely accompanied by a negative self-statement. At the core of all forms of self-harm behaviour is poor self-esteem. The self-harm behaviours are, therefore, in part, manifestations of the feelings of unworthiness. In conjunction with the use of metaphor, affirmations begin to alter the negative image and feelings of the self, and begin to promote self-acceptance.

Affirmations may cover a wide variety of topics related to the self. Examples of some affirmations are: "I can identify my feelings"; "I am capable of achieving positive things"; "I am a loyal friend"; and "I have strong survival skills."

THE BEGINNING AND END OF THE JOURNEY

With the completion of the journey towards healing and wholeness comes the beginning of a new journey, one filled with a sense of hope, love, and acceptance. Metaphors can be an effective tool in the healing process that will open the door to new vistas on life. When sufficient healing has occurred, self-harm behaviours should diminish and may disappear altogether. Most important, self-confirmation behaviours are practised to replace the dysfunctional self-harming ones.

The healing power unleashed by a metaphor has a tremendous capacity to free the individual from the nemesis lurking in her past and to set in motion a journey that allows her to become whole. As part of this journey, self-harm behaviours begin to disappear once the behaviours are no longer needed to maintain a fragile equilibrium. In their place behaviours emerge that reflect a newfound self-confidence and sense of inner control. With the completion of the journey towards healing and wholeness comes the beginning of a new journey — one filled with hope, self-love, and self-acceptance.

◆

Decoding The "Language of Fat": Placing Eating-Disorder Groups In A Feminist Framework

Sandy Friedman

The fabric of everyday life is composed of a multiplicity of events interwoven with feelings. Ask any woman about her day and she will most likely tell you it was "fine" and that "nothing much" happened. Our society teaches women to discount and trivialize their own personal experiences. But feelings do not occur in isolation. Rather, they are encapsulated by the situations to which they relate.

Now, ask a woman with an eating disorder to describe her day and she will most likely highlight those occasions when she "felt fat." Women with eating disorders learn to encode their feelings in the "language of fat." When women talk about "feeling fat" it is usually in response to something concrete — something for which they have no other means of expression or interpretation. "I feel fat" (or "ugly" or "stupid") becomes an alternative way of expressing anger, fear, insecurity, loneliness — and all of the other feelings in the human repertoire. "Feeling fat" (and its corollary: "needing to be thin") becomes a way of describing the myriad situations a woman encounters in life in which she feels she has little control or no context.

Without a historical context to provide them with a reference point and a societal context to validate the personal components of their lives, women discount or trivialize their own experiences as they have been taught to do, and encode them in the "language of fat."

THE FRAMEWORK

Women inhabit a world that is androcentric; that is, the male version of experience is assumed to represent all the human experiences. In trying to fit themselves into a norm designed for men, women come to see themselves as "other" — and as inferior.

Men and women grow into what are essentially two different cultures designed to prepare them for the differing functions that they are supposed to serve in society. Men are socialized to take their places in the work world, or in what we regard as the "public" sphere. They learn to function through a goal-oriented linear perspective that emphasizes separation and independence (Gilligan 1982, p. 30). From their childhood play with other boys, men learn a pattern of communication that is centred around contesting dominance in hierarchically structured groups (Minister 1991, p. 36). They learn to use talking as a way to obtain and maintain the attention of others, and therefore enhance their own independence and status. As a result, they seem most comfortable in large groups, with people that they don't know well (Tannen 1990, p. 77), and in speaking about tasks and power issues that reflect what they *do*.

While women do participate in the "public" sphere, they are socialized to take their place in the "private" one — in the realm of the home. Women learn to function through a perspective that is process-oriented, relational, contextual, and based upon intimacy and closeness (Gilligan 1982, p. 30). As a result, the processes through which women learn and integrate information are different from those of men (Belenky et al. 1986, p. 15). These differences are reflected in the ways that women express themselves and in the stories that they tell. For women, conversation is a way of establishing connections and negotiating relationships. In it, emphasis is placed on establishing equality and intimacy by displaying similarities and by matching experiences (Tannen 1990, p. 176). Women are more comfortable in relatively small and private groups, talking about issues that define *who they are.*

The societal assumption of male superiority forces women either to deny their own experiences or to reframe them in male-defined language. Reinforcing only the male perspective makes women feel that the very way that they speak is wrong and that the stories they tell are trivial. Expressing "female" stories in "male" language robs them of their context and of their point of reference. It creates a gap between the original meaning and what gets heard (Spender 1985, p. 35). Because our conception of education — our ideas of what counts as important knowledge and good teaching — has been designed by men, this too treats women as "other" and ignores their experience. The commonly accepted stereotype of women's thinking as emotional, intuitive, and personalized (rather than as rational and objective) contributes to the devaluation of women's intellects and belittles their obvious contributions.

The suppression of women's experience of the world renders them invisible. This systematically undermines women's confidence and self-esteem until women begin to doubt themselves and become susceptible to believing the myths of their inferiority (Spender 1982, p. 20).

Sexualization (which ranges from a heightened concern with physical appearance to episodes of incest and sexual abuse) teaches women to objectify and to disown their bodies. The requirement that women nurture others while learning to expect less nurturing for themselves means that they internalize a societal ethic of caring that is built on self-sacrifice and guilt. When the work that women do privately inside the home (without pay) is extended into the public workplace, it is poorly paid and undervalued. Work that is centred around "taking care of" or providing a service for others is often considered not to be socially important. This leaves women with few alternatives to economic dependency upon men or upon the state.

The systematic devaluation of women reinforces the sense of powerlessness that most women feel. It influences how they define themselves, how they interact with the world, and how they respond to the lack of choices offered to them. When women cannot criticize the society that victimizes them, they criticize themselves — turning their anger against themselves.

When women are able to express their feelings, and to provide a context for these feelings, they affirm their sense of self and create the opportunity for a connection with others. The "language of fat," however, is a dead end. By encoding their feelings and experiences in the "language of fat," women become alienated from themselves and become distanced from others. Speaking it means engaging with an obsession instead of with the individual herself. The more alienated they feel, the more they tend to minimize or negate their own experiences and rely on the "language of fat." Without a sense of self based on a cohesive history of personal experience to ground them, such women constantly look outside themselves for definition. Without a secure sense of self, they are vulnerable to those definitions most readily available. As a result they accommodate themselves to whatever role is defined for them by a male-dominated culture — reinforcing the sense of alienation they already feel.

Traditional therapy looks at what is wrong with the individual and at her failure to adapt to society. This view is extended into the traditional treatment of eating disorders. The labeling of eating disorders as a "disease" and focusing upon individual deficiencies or family dysfunction serves to pathologize both the behaviour and the individual. Treatment models which are based on a hierarchical relationship (i.e., between the professional and "patient") disempower women individually and collectively. The goal-oriented structure of these models is reinforced by a language which externalizes and generalizes women's experiences. Women are encouraged to speak about *their* "bulimia," *their* "anorexia," *their* "compulsive eating," or *their* "body image." This separates the preoccupation with food and weight (and the accompanying behaviours) from the realities of women's lives and dissociates them from their experiences. ("I have a bad body image" tells little about how the speaker feels about her body or of the context in which the sentiment is embedded.) This reinforces the alienation from their selves that most women feel.

A feminist approach to eating disorders weaves together personal and political issues as causes and potential solutions to women's preoccupation with food. Feminist counseling integrates three processes based on a feminist understanding of society: a healing process, an educational process, and a political process (Levine 1982, p. 202). An underlying assumption of feminist counseling is that women have the potential strength to forge changes in their lives, especially together with other women (ibid., p.203). The group setting provides women with an opportunity to examine their relationships with food and with weight within the framework of their own life experience, and to place these personal experiences within a societal context.

THE EXPERIENCE

Early on a rainy Wednesday evening, in a small suburb of a large Canadian city, women make their way through a familiar community building. Individually or sometimes in pairs they enter a room, which, for this evening, is theirs to share. Tonight is the weekly meeting of the Eating Disorder Support Group. Because it is structured as a drop-in group, its attendance varies. The women come in all sizes and all ages, and from all walks of life. Together they represent the whole continuum of eating-disorder behaviours — from anorexia to bulimia, to compulsive eating. Some women enter timidly, for this is their first time. Some come reluctantly, pressured by parents or spouses. For some, this is a moment of hope mixed with desperation — another attempt for a cure that might result in failure. For others it is a highly anticipated moment — they are the ones who have been here before. The women take their places in a circle inside the room.

The group format is a familiar one. It replicates the play groups and the type of interaction that women experienced as children — with the emphasis on mutual aid and the commonality of experience.

The two-hour group begins promptly at 7:00 p.m. The beginning of each group is highly structured. The facilitator always speaks first. She introduces herself and tells the group that she is a therapist and consultant in private practice. In describing how she works with her clients, she presents a feminist ideology that frames eating disorders as a response to women's experiences in a world that devalues them. She illustrates how these experiences become encoded in the "language of fat." She talks about her own struggle with weight and describes how this group setting provides opportunities to explore beneath the obsession with food and with weight; to acquire the skills and information with which to do so; and, most important, to learn from one another's experiences.

The facilitator helps the participants feel safe by establishing her knowledge in this area, and by sharing her own life experiences. Acknowledging that everyone (herself included) learns from the experiences shared by the group members, she establishes a format for the group that is relational and not goal-oriented. Each week she presents the same theoretical framework — one which situates the eating disorder and preoccupation with weight within the individual's own experience and places that experience in the context of a society whose institutions have a strong influence on shaping and directing the lives of women. She lets the group members know what to expect and what is expected of them. Whenever possible, she describes the process that is happening in that particular moment in order to increase the element of safety in the group and to help women name their own experience.

The basic philosophy of the group places eating disorders in a perspective that replaces shame with dignity, self-blame with curiosity, and self-criticism with tolerance and self-respect: "In order to change a behaviour (or a way of being in the world) you must be curious about its process. This means that you must find out as much as you can about it and what this means to you. Only when you have something to replace it with, and are ready to do so, will you give it up."

The facilitator tells the women that they will each have a turn to speak. She asks them to give their first name and to say something about themselves which includes both their eating behaviour and what is at present happening in their lives. She describes how women constantly compare themselves with others in an attempt to define what is "normal" for themselves, so that even in this group: "You look around the room and compare yourself with everyone else. This person is more profound, that person's story is better, this person is more articulate, that person is thinner ... and by the time you get to yourself, you're feeling like you're worthless."

She asks the women to be curious about these comparisons and to look for any clues that they might provide about their own insecurities. She talks about how hard it is to come to the group for the first time and then gives them all permission to just state their name and pass if they are not ready to talk. She is aware of how cautious women are and how fearful they are of making mistakes: "There is no way that you can fail this group. There is no right thing or wrong thing that you can say or do. Everyone's experiences are important. Sometimes people don't speak for many sessions — but they take a whole lot in."

She asks a member to begin. The group is now in session. After all of the members of the group have introduced themselves and the framework has been established, the focus turns to eliciting from the women the stories that are encoded by the language of fat.

There is no set agenda. Usually a theme evolves from the concerns that group members express. The group operates according to a specific format. Each member speaks without interruption. After she speaks, the facilitator responds to her. Then other group members may contribute their feedback. This is an important ritual. It provides the speaker with the experience of claiming time just for herself and encourages her to bear witness to her own stories. It allows the facilitator to validate that speaker, to address her specific needs, and, where appropriate, to provide her with a societal context for her individual experience.

Knowing that the facilitator will respond frees the other group members from the need to "take care of " the feelings expressed by the speaker and thus enhances their feelings of safety in the group. It also provides group members with the opportunity to practice setting boundaries between themselves and others. Women learn that they can provide encouragement and give feedback without taking on the burden of caring for the speaker. Because they are always part of the experience, this distance and objectivity provides the group members with a different perspective. It lets them see what happens if they don't respond right away. In learning to set boundaries between themselves and others, women learn that they can provide encouragement and give feedback without taking on the burden of caring for the speaker.

Those women who are ready to do so share an episode where they "felt fat" and tell the story behind it. On nights when there are many new participants, most of the session can be taken up just with describing and normalizing the eating disorder behaviours and the rituals around food:

> "I buy a dozen donuts and then tell the cashier that I am having company. How could you just buy one?"

> "My friend and I would go to McDonald's and order one of every breakfast and make up fictitious friends that we were buying them for."

> "Have you ever had ice-cream that reached its expiry date? Who ever heard of ice cream living long enough to get stale!"

Women learn from sharing the lives they have been taught to keep private. Their stories are different from men's — because the things that they talk about are personal. Their stories are sometimes painful, and the anxiety is intense. But by telling their stories, women create a context for their own experiences (Heilbrun 1988, p. 38). Stories encapsulate the feelings and provide them with a point of reference.

The women talk about bingeing and purging and about the miles and miles of cycling they do on stationary bicycles — exercising until they can hardly stand. They speak about how hard it is to diet and how equally hard it is to eat when you are anorexic. Their pain is evident when they talk about obsessing and of being out of control:

> "I used to lie in bed every night and go over every single thing that I had eaten that day. I would feel tense and anxious and guilty and promise myself that I would go on a diet. But the next day I would eat again and feel mad at myself."

> "I can't stand the fat. I have to know what all the ingredients are in everything that I eat."

> "I wash my food, to get out each drop of fat. Ugh!"

> "I know when I need to purge. I buy the right food. Some foods are easier to bring up than others."

The commonality of experience described in groups diffuses the shame that many women with eating disorders feel and normalizes both their appetites and their eating behaviours. Our society teaches women that eating is wrong — especially if they eat with enjoyment or eat all that they want. Eating is sometimes even seen as an act of aggression, in opposition to the passivity that is considered to be "feminine." As a result, it tends to be accompanied by guilt and self-blame. Because most bodily functions — especially vomiting and defecation — are considered repulsive, women who purge or use laxatives transform general societal attitudes into personal shame and self-loathing. And while anorexic control might be admired by some, anorexic rituals are usually viewed with bizarre fascination.

The facilitator addresses three components of eating disorders: the eating-disorder behaviour, the individual experience that triggers this behaviour, and the societal context in which both occur. She describes the psychological components of bingeing and purging, of the restriction of food through dieting and obsessive behaviour, and relates these behaviours to individual ways in which women learn to cope with a society that constantly devalues them. Most women have been taught to see eating disorders as a "disease" and "getting better" as controling the eating-disorder behaviours. The emphasis on "success" and "failure" usually succeeds in intensifying the obsession with food and with weight. By reframing eating disorders as a coping mechanism and by placing these behaviours in the context of real life, the facilitator normalizes them — they become one of many ways that people learn to cope with societal pressures and personal stress.

Members who are new to the group talk about the desperation that they feel and their fears that they will never get "better." They talk about their failures and talk about the experiences that have left them feeling unseen, unheard, and ashamed:

> "I got to the doctor's office and realized that I couldn't go in. She was going to weigh me. The first time that I saw her I hadn't been eating much and my weight was down. But now that I've been taking Prozac, I haven't been vomiting much, and she was going to see how much weight I've gained. She makes me take my clothes off. I never let myself see myself naked. Not even my boyfriend sees me naked."

> "My psychiatrist told me that the reason I was still bulimic was because I wasn't trying hard enough to get better."

> "No matter what's wrong with you — you can have an arrow sticking out of your back! — your doctor will tell you it's because you're too fat."

As the session progresses, one thing is clear — where there was once shame and secrecy, there is now the healing force of laughter: "He said I couldn't be anorexic. I wasn't thin enough."

Women decode the language of fat by telling their stories. They learn to bear witness to and validate their own experiences as they recount and react to them. Because feelings occur continuously, each day is a tapestry woven with many stories — which vary in length, intensity, and importance to the storyteller.

Mona is a 21-year-old bulimic student:

"I'm going to a formal this weekend and I'm scared that I won't fit into my dress. I rode my bike the 20 km to school and then went for a run at lunch time. I just need to fit into my dress. The guy that I'm going with has a girlfriend in Toronto and I'm not sure what his relationship with her is so I feel a little guilty — like I'm betraying her. Why is he asking me? And I don't know what to do if he comes on to me. I mean — I don't want to hurt his feelings. What if I say something to him and he says he wasn't coming on to me? Maybe I'm being too conceited and too full of myself. It's really hard. You don't want to come across as a slut, but at the same time you don't want to be seen as frigid."

Mona's story allows her to see how her focus on trying to anticipate what the "guy" thinks robs her of her own perceptions and feelings. This prevents her from acknowledging to herself that she is scared and insecure. Decoding Mona's fat enables her (and the group) to form the connection between her experience and her eating behaviour and obsessive exercise. It provides a concrete example of how these behaviours operate: not having a choice in their responses leaves many women feeling powerless and out of control. And the more out of control they feel, the more likely women are to turn to the illusion of control provided by dieting, anorexic rituals, and other eating-disorder behaviours.

This story generated a discussion about how much effort women expend trying to please other people, and about how afraid they are to say *no* even it it means having sex when they don't want to. The women talk about how they assume complete responsibility in their relationships with other people — they try to figure out how the other person would act, and then respond to their own assumptions. In trying not to hurt the other person, they suppress their own feelings and lose their sense of themselves — reinforcing the alienation that they feel:

"I've always written off what I *felt* as invalid — because I *should* be thinking, doing, feeling something else."

"If only I could do the right thing at the right time ... I wouldn't hurt them."

"I'm so afraid of hurting someone I can't even return a pair of shoes. Do you know how many pairs of shoes I have that I've never worn?"

"I can't housebreak my dog. I'm afraid that if I get mad at him, he won't love me."

Women constantly struggle against the powerful conditioning that makes it somewhat selfish and uncaring to worry about getting their own needs met. The intertwining of the labour component ("caring for") with the affective component ("caring about") creates an ethic of caring that is built around self-sacrifice and guilt (Baines, Evans, and Neysmith 1991, p. 15). When women can't do that labour, their love is called into question. Because caring is seen as the responsibility of women, dutiful daughters become sandwiched between the needs of their children and the needs of their aging parents. Many women encode the feelings that are generated by their caretaking roles in the "language of fat." An examination of the societal ideology of caring enables these women to recognize the forces which contribute to and reinforce their sense of inadequacy and guilt.

Ida is a 62-year-old widow. She is a compulsive eater who is finding it hard to diet:

"All my life I've taken care of people. I just told my 28-year-old son to move out — I'm so sick of doing his laundry! You young women have more choices. I spent my whole life taking care of my husband and children — and even though my husband was a good man, I'm so angry at him for never appreciating anything that I did."

Janice is married and has two children under five years of age. She works at home, doing childcare. She has been bulimic since her first child was born:

"Yesterday was a really bad day. I couldn't stop purging and I felt awful. My thighs were so gross. Both of my kids have been sick and they're whiney and demanding. I yell at them and then I feel guilty at yelling at them. I'm a bad mother. I don't have very much patience. So then I binge and purge and feel mad at myself. And then my husband Doug comes home and says: 'What have you been doing all day?' And of course the kids are fine now and so sweet, and he asks me: 'What's the big deal?' "

Marla is married and has a 10-year-old son. Her mother, who has lived with her for the past eight years, has developed Alzheimer's disease. Marla is a compulsive eater:

"My fattest day was on Monday. I'm thinking about putting my mother into a home and I feel really terrible about it. How can I do that to her? Then I tell myself that my son Kevin really needs me, and Mom won't know the difference. But I feel like such a bad person. On Monday, Kevin and I went to look at a place. He kept telling me how happy Grandma would be and I realized how hard her illness is on him and how squeezed I feel."

As individual women learn to decode the language of their fat, the stories that they tell reflect issues which concern most women.

Students speak about the alienation that they feel, because the presentation and evaluation of academic materials are in forms adapted specifically to the needs of men. Even when their courses raise isssues of importance to them, they feel concerned that anything they might contribute would be "wrong":

"Everyone seems so interested in their courses. I keep feeling that I'm missing out. And then I feel guilty because I think of all the people my age who can't afford to be students and wonder what right I have to complain."

"I've been thinking about going back to Weight Watchers. I've been feeling really depressed since the Christmas holidays and think that if I start another diet I'll feel more in control. How can I admit that I don't fit in here?

"I walk around campus and look at the other women — and all I can think of is how together they look, and how I must be the only one here who feels like such a phony."

Single mothers blame themselves for their poverty. They have been taught to view this as the result of their own inadequacy — rather than as the result of a labour market that consistently under-values their work, and a social-welfare system that defines them either as workers or homemakers but does not make it easy for them to do both (Evans 1991, p. 188):

"I'm getting welfare and I feel so ashamed. You'd think that at 30 I'd be more responsible — that I'd have my life more together. I lie awake at night and wonder how I'm ever going to get it together. I feel like such a failure. I can't seem to discipline myself. The dishes keep piling up. I keep making excuses so that I don't have to do my homework. That's really dumb, isn't it? I have to pass these courses so that I can get into nursing school and make something of myself. My daughter tries to help out when I'm at work, but she's only ten years old."

"I realize how I push away things that bother me. I took my daughter to the orthodontist yesterday. He said that her bite is really bad and that she needs $5000 worth of treatment. Can you imagine: $5000!! I went totally numb. All the way home I kept thinking about how fat I am. But I realize that's what I do when I get overwhelmed. And I felt really powerless in the ortho-dontist's office. Five thousand dollars might as well be a million! And now I feel like a bad mother because I can't provide for my kids."

Sharing these stories enables the women in the group to articu-late the incongruity between the societal conditioning that they receive as children and the personal feelings that they experience as adults. They come to see their eating behaviours as a kind of barometer — or "mood ring" — which signals to them that they are experiencing personal discomfort. This discomfort is connected to the unhealthy and unequal power structures in their lives. The more practised they become at naming their own experiences, the more adept they become at reclaiming their true selves.

Women's groups sometimes seem almost magical. They give rise to an exciting sense of possibility. There is an incredible energy that is generated by women who share and validate each other's experiences. When women begin to speak about their experiences, they individually gain the self-esteem and self-confidence necessary to make changes in their lives. And they collectively develop a public voice that can change the lives of others. Change is then seen as a circular process which moves from the personal to the political and back:

> "It's not about *never* being insecure again, or *never* having certain feelings or thoughts again — they'll *always* come up. It's about learning to cope, and allowing yourself to be true to what you feel and being honest with *you*."

> "My husband said, 'Janey, you're getting more and more uppity and it's all because of that damn group.' "

> "My mother told me," said Nancy, "that I only think about myself. And it's all because of that damn group."

> "Wow," remarked Michelle, "maybe we should just name it that way — you know, like tonight I'm going to *That Damn Group!*"

MECHANICS

The Format: The open-ended drop-in format of these groups means that women can attend as they choose. For many women, setting limits is so difficult that they will not attempt anything that requires them to make more than a one-time commitment. Here, they can come just once to check out the situation, knowing they don't have to come back. They can also take time out from attendance without feeling like they failed or hurt anyone's feelings. The continual mixing of experienced and new members is beneficial to the group process. Experienced members act as role models. They set the tone for discussion by introducing the wide range of issues that underlie the preoccupation with food and fat. Their active participation provides a breathing space for new members — who can wait until they become oriented to the process and feel ready to join in.

The Participants: The women most likely to attend feminist groups for women with eating disorders are those who see their disorders as "personal problems," even though some may have experienced hospitalization at some point. Most women with eating disorders are not likely to label themselves as "sick" unless and until they have an experience that teaches them to do so. Those closest to the institutional model may adhere to that model for quite some time.

Some women come because they are desperate, and there are very few services available for them. Some come thinking they will find a magic answer. Some women use the group as an adjunct to individual therapy, while others make changes directly as a result of their participation in this group alone. Whatever their motivation, many women are greatly affected by the group process and attend regularly. Women who are not yet ready for this process often return at a later time (sometimes as much as one or two years later).

Even though there may be a need for services for men, these groups should be segregated. Inclusion of a male participant shifts the dynamics of the group — everyone then focuses on the male and accommodates herself to him. The unique energy that is generated by women's groups — which is fundamental to the process of change — is either lost or diluted.

While a large percentage of women who come to these groups may have been sexually abused as children or experienced sexual assault as adults, the drop-in format of the group does not provide them enough safety to deal with this issue. A closed-format group would be more appropriate.

The Facilitator: The facilitator of this group must be a woman. The presence of a male changes the focus and type of interaction of the group. A sensitive skilled and sympathetic male co-facilitator might be of benefit in different ways to a woman's group. However, it would be inappropriate for a group that has as its goal the reclaiming of women's experiences and stories. It would inhibit the women in the group and provide a barrier to the level of interaction that is characteristic of women-only groups.

It is advisable for the facilitator to have had some personal experience with food and weight preoccupation and to have worked through her own issues. She must have a feminist perspective of eating disorders and must be comfortable working in the egalitarian counseling format.

The Location: Feminist groups for eating disorders are community based and as such should be located in a community facility with simple public access — preferably one that is accessible by public transportation. The room allocated to these groups should be private and relatively soundproof. Care should be taken that wide and comfortable chairs are provided for large women.

Childcare should be provided wherever possible, because many women who attend these groups are mothers. In cases where this is not possible, an attempt should be made to schedule these groups so that they accommodate the childcare needs of the women who attend.

FORMING YOUR OWN GROUP

Starting and maintaining a group for women with eating disorders means advertising consistently over a long period of time — so that the idea becomes familiar, and the group becomes identified as an established part of community services. It is sometimes also necessary to do outreach in the community in order to build a network for referrals. It takes time to establish full attendance, because many women are fearful of coming forward, and because many may come for only one "sample" session and then return later. Although there is a real need for many more such groups, their beginnings must be carefully nurtured — a great deal of patience is helpful until word of mouth stimulates attendance. And that it will, if the group is at all successful, because there is no better advertisement than enthusiastic regular participants.

There is something almost magical that happens when women get together and tell the truth about themselves. A sense of generosity and excitement occurs when they talk about things that are real, when they feel themselves to be seen and heard — and that doesn't happen often enough in any person's life — male or female. It is awesome and humbling to be a part of that process: it is truly a creative act — and an infectious one — and its energy can generate ripples of change from the individual women to the immediate community, and perhaps eventually the world.

◆

FEMINIST FAMILY THERAPY

Jan Lackstrom

In the literature on counseling women with anorexia nervosa and bulimia and their families, very little has been written that integrates feminist theory and family therapy. Given the similarity between the issues feminist theorists have identified as toxic to women and the accepted understanding that eating disorders are caused and perpetuated by a combination of individual, familial, and sociocultural factors (Garfinkel and Garner 1982; Garner and Garfinkel 1985), this lack is surprising. The past twenty years have witnessed an exponential growth in the understanding of eating disorders (Bruch 1973, 1978; Crisp 1980; Garfinkel and Garner 1982; Garner and Garfinkel 1985) and of effective treatements for them, including the use of systemic family therapy on its own and in conjunction with other forms of therapy (Selvini Palazzoli 1974; Selvini Palazzoli et al. 1978; Minuchin, Rosman and Baker 1978; Root, Fallon, and Friedrick 1986; Schwartz, Barrett, and Saba 1985; Sargent, Liebman, and Silver 1985; Vandereycken, Kog, and Vanderlinder 1989; Roberto 1987, 1991; and Woodside and Skekter-Wolfson 1991). A parallel growth has taken place in the exploration of women's life experience and the development of feminist approaches to the understanding and treatment of women's "problems" (Chesler 1972; Friedan 1963; Baker Miller 1986; Gilligan 1982; Jordan et al. 1991; and Chodorow 1978). The apparent failure to integrate theories and models may, in part, be a result of an ongoing debate between feminist theory and models of practice and those of systemic family therapy. Feminist theoreticians and researchers are critical of systemic therapy, including the notions of neutrality, circularity, and complimentarity, believing that it has failed to recognize the larger social context in which the family — and, subsequently, women — must function and, as such, that it ignores the realities of power differentials and the definition of normative behaviour, which, at best, deny and, at worst, support the psychological and environmental factors that constrain women (James and McIntyre 1983; Lerner 1988; Bograd 1988; Taggart 1985; and Avis 1988). Family models and therapies often fail to recognize just who the family is. The theory often rests in the idealized image of the intact, white, Anglo-Saxon middle class family. The issues of different families — those with unique constellations such as an older single adult living in the parental home, lesbian or homosexual couples, ethnic families, or single-parent, remarried, or impoverished families — are minimized or ignored.

This does not mean that large numbers of practitioners of family therapy and feminist therapy have abandoned the other; rather, they continue to struggle with both the theory and the practice of family therapy in order to integrate it with feminist theory and practice (Ault-Ritche 1986; Hare-Mustin 1978; Libow, Raskin, and Caust 1982; Schwartz and Barrett 1988; Goodrich et al. 1988).

In this essay, I present a model of family therapy that attempts a *rapprochement* between feminist concerns and the more traditional approaches to counseling families of eating-disordered women. As well, I briefly review the tenets of feminist family therapy and the family models associated with eating disorders, provide a concrete guide to family assessment, and finally describe a two-part model that addresses the dynamic of the family both as an isolated unit and as a member of a larger social community. This model can be adapted for use as a brief model, employing only the problem-focused stage, which is expected to reduce, if not eliminate, the eating symptoms and to help the family develop new ways of dealing with stressors, or as a longer-term model, building upon the problem-focused stage to address deeper issues from which attention was distracted by the eating disorder and which become more apparent with the elimination of the eating-disorder symptoms.

THE FEMINIST APPROACH TO FAMILY THERAPY

To integrate a feminist approach to family therapy, the clinician must begin by examining the values, beliefs, and knowledge that informs his or her practice. This does not mean abandoning specific models or techniques of family therapy or professional affiliations; rather, it means challenging, building upon, and shaping this knowledge base by incorporating new information about women's experience. Feminist therapy is an orientation, an approach, a philosophy in which one's practice is embedded. To this end, Ault-Ritche (1986) and Braverman (1988) have identified a number of theoretical underpinnings on which to shape a feminist approach to family therapy. The latter has itemized them as:

1) Understanding the impact of a patriarchal system on both men and women, and acknowledging that the social and political context ... as well as the family context have a significant influence on the problems of women.

2) Recognizing the limitations of traditional theories of psychological development based on a male model of maturity.

3) Familiarity with women's problem solving process which tends to focus on connection and relationships, rather than on logic, abstraction and rationality.

4) Understanding that the "personal is political" that is ... motherhood, child rearing and marriage are not simply life cycle events, but institutions that carry particular sociocultural legacies for women.

5) A sensitivity to the biological effect of the female life cycle ... on women's symptom presentation and interpersonal relationships.

6) Understanding women's sexuality and sexual responsiveness so that confused and mistaken notions ... are not perpetuated.

7) Valuing women's relationships with each other as a special source of support, different from their relationships with men. (Braverman 1988, pp. 8–9).

Clinicians are challenged to increase their knowledge of gender differences and the constraints that the larger environmental context places on both women and men. Therapists must be aware of their own gender issues and be careful not to replicate the specific dynamics that the presenting family are stuck in, or the larger patriarchal system in which the family and therapist are functioning. The process of therapy should allow for modeling of skill, competence, and collaboration. The clinician is a facilitator and partner, with recognized and respected skills, rather than a consultant or guru who is above the family by virtue of some well-guarded, mysterious knowledge and powerful techniques and tools to which the family must avail themselves for the cure (Libow, Raskin, and Caust 1982). The therapist is expected to treat the family as an equal partner who also brings valuable knowledge, skills, and competencies to the counseling process. The feminist approach rests on a genuine relationship, with mutual respect, that acknowledges a client's right to self-determination and the skills, knowledge base, and ethical principles the therapist brings to therapy. A feminist approach to practice must explore the impact of the social context on such issues as power, responsibility, and gender-role stereotyping within the family. A feminist approach values therapist shopping for an appropriate match, and views disclosure of personal values by the therapist as appropriate while allowing for a variety of direct, indirect, educational, and consciousness-raising techniques. Sexual contact between therapists and clients is clearly prohibited. The model provides for the use of a contract with clearly stated goals. The contracting process is aided by the recognition of the presenting problems as valid problems to be dealt with rather than as symptoms of some unconscious hidden problem. The meanings of problems are explored within the family and cultural context (Ault-Ritche 1986).

FAMILY MODELS

A number of people have been working over the past fifteen years to understand the families of eating-disordered adolescents and women. The development of theories of eating-disordered families closely parallels the evolution of family therapy itself as the theoreticians not only outlined family dynamics but also proposed models of practice to address those problems.

Salvador Minuchin and colleagues (1978) working primarily with anorexic families, identified five family characteristics found in psychosomatic families: enmeshment, overprotectiveness, rigidity, lack of conflict resolution, and involvement of the anorexic child in marital conflict. The anorexia serves a homeostatic function within a family that fears change. The structural model of family therapy was developed to address the dynamic within the family which perpetuates the symptom. The family therapist is directed to take an active stance to assist the anorexic daughter to surrender her symptoms and to help the family system restructure itself in an effort to meet its goals and tasks without the aid of any symptoms or distractions (Minuchin 1974, Sargent, Liebman, and Silver 1975; and Fishman 1979).

Selvini Palazzoli (1974) and colleagues (1978) developed a strategic model to treat anorexia at the same time as Minuchin was developing the structural model. The Milan group focused on the interactional pattern of a family, and identified four patterns: rejection or disqualification of messages; the lack of leadership and responsibility taking in the family, which in turn contributed to a lack of individual identity separate from "the family"; the use of secret and denied coalitions; and the valuing of self-sacrifice to the family. Individual moves towards difference or individuation were defended against by the family. The anorexic child is understood to be symbolically communicating the tremendous distress the entire family experiences. After formulating a systemic hypothesis, a strategic family therapist uses indirect methods to confirm or disconfirm the hypothesized function of the anorexic symptoms and to avoid the resistance the family presents (Selvini Palazzoli et al. 1978; Selvini Palazzoli 1974; Tomm 1984a, 1984b; Madanes 1981; and Haley 1976).

In the 1980s, Schwartz, Barret, and Saba (1985) and Root, Fallon, and Friedrick (1986) focused on bulimic families, attempting to differentiate them from anorexic families. Schwartz (Schwartz, Barret, and Saba 1985; Schwartz and Barret 1988; Barrett and Swartz 1987) confirmed the family characteristics identified by Minuchin and noted additional features in bulimic families, including social isolation, a hyperconsciousness of appearance, and the attachment of special meaning to food and eating. Incorporating structural and strategic techniques in their approach, Schwartz and colleagues included the use of concurrent individual and family therapy in an effort to help the family restructure itself to exclude the symptoms and accommodate change in a more functional way. The bulimic girl is understood to need individual and separate attention to help her take greater control of her own life.

Each of three stages of treatment — creating a context of change, challenging patterns, and expanding alternatives and consolidating change — have set goals and tasks (Schwartz, Barret 1985). Three bulimic family types were defined, based on how well the family adopted stereotypic American values. The "All American Family," "Ethnic Family," and "Mixed Family" are described as each having a unique constellation of dynamics and issues that predispose a young woman to bulimia. The bulimia was thought to be an expression of the individual's distress and need for individual expression in families that have rigid beliefs about propriety.

Using a systemic understanding of family, Root, Fallon, and Friedrick (1986) encouraged the use of structural, strategic, and Bowenian theories and techniques in their treatment model. For the first time, the addition of gender-sensitive issues and the recognition of sociocultural influences in the family are addressed specifically. The authors also present three bulimic family types, "The Perfect Family," "The Overprotective Family," and "The Chaotic Family," based on how the family copes with psychosocial demands. Issues of boundary, identity, expression of feeling, powerlessness, loss, and autonomy are examined in relation to each family type. The bulimic symptoms are thought to be an expression of the self and in particular express a need for individuation and autonomy. Symptoms may serve a self-soothing and affect-moderating function for those in chaotic families.

White (1983, 1987) and Roberto (1987) identified the issue of the multigenerational transmission of beliefs which predispose an individual to an eating disorder and are then activated by the sociocultural pressures to be thin. White identifies three transgenerational beliefs in anorexic families. These families value loyalty and family tradition at the expense of personal needs or wishes; hold traditional and rigid expectations of women, and in particular daughters, who are expected to sacrifice themselves to the care and support of others; and family problems are understood to be the result of personal inadequacy and disloyalty. Any girl who is unable to remain loyal, sensitive, and devoted to her family needs, despite poor parenting, triangulation, and intergenerational boundary violation, is thought of by others, and — more important — by herself "as bad." White suggests that cybernetic theories and strategic therapy are useful to explore and challenge the family structure and system of communicating, and to challenge the effect of the larger sociocultural system on the family.

Roberto (1987) assesses the family legacy of "covert themes, beliefs and world views supporting and perpetuating their interactional pattern ... in which the eating symptoms are deeply rooted"

(p. 2). If the family cannot modify their beliefs, relapse is thought to be inevitable.

Roberto identifies three characteristics of eating-disordered families, including intrafamilial loyalty, which creates obligation and mutual protection at the expense of individual development; a drive for success in the context of losses of earlier generations; and the prohibition of disagreement and conflict. Bulimic families placed tremendous importance on body image and general appearance.

Roberto uses a symbolic-experiential model of family therapy that employs structural, strategic, and cybernetic techniques in a three-stage process to identify and then challenge the existing family legacy and to construct an alternative legacy that frees the family and individuals from an organization that has contributed to the development of the symptomatic behaviour.

There has been a progressive broadening of the understanding of the role of families of eating-disordered women. There is an ever-growing list of factors affecting the individual and the family as a whole. With the integration of new knowledge about women as unique from men and the importance of this difference on such issues as identity formation, relationships, power, problem attribution and the definition of normalcy, the content of therapy continues to change.

Feminists have challenged the personal attribution of sickness, personality disorder, and general inadequacy that have frequently been placed upon women and families that do not conform to the traditional definitions of health and normalcy. Feminists have brought to attention the real impact of such issues as poverty and violence in the lives of women. A feminist approach to practice offers the opportunity to integrate the larger social context of the individual and their family into the treatment process. The recognition of the importance of the social context on the individual and their family broadens the information base the therapist can work with and provides the opportunity for a significantly more unique view of that individual and their family system. Feminist therapy, itself evolving, offers the hope of a therapeutic process that does not replicate the hierarchical and constraining aspect of the traditional social structure. The careful use of techniques such as modeling, contracting, self disclosure by the therapist, focusing on behavioural change, and accepting the problem as defined by the family and its members are just a few of the ways in which feminist family therapists are attempting to apply theory and knowledge to practice. The integration of feminist theories and models with those of family therapy will not be easy as each will need to be shaped by the other. Thankfully there are a number of clinicians actively working in this area. The following is an attempt to integrate feminist practice principles and techniques into the more traditional theories and models of family therapy when working with eating disordered families.

FAMILY ASSESSMENT

The purpose of the initial assessment is threefold: to engage the family in a collaborative process, to gather enough information to form a working hypothesis about the function of the eating disorder within the specific family, and to agree on a contract to work together. The family therapist is free to use any model of family assessment, but must incorporate additional areas of inquiry specific to eating disorders and a feminist approach to practice. Unlike the case of some family therapies, individual therapy for the anorexic or bulimic person is not an uncommon adjunct to the family work. Ideally, individual therapy will be done with the family therapist or with a like-minded colleague so that individual work, based on the feminist understanding of "self in relation" (Gilligan 1982) and focusing on identity formation, individual power, assertion, and boundary setting, will complement the family work.

ENGAGEMENT

To form a therapeutic alliance, the therapist must join with the family rather than work against the family. By accepting the family and individual definition of problems at face value and working with the family to fit those definitions into a systemic understanding, the opportunity to gather personal and unique data is intensified. The genuine recognition that family members have tried their best to understand and aid their daughter and sister is essential to the formulation of an empathic relationship with each family member. The use of techniques such as positive connotation and reframing work only if there is an accurate understanding of family rules. The therapist must work within the family rules and structures to be able to challenge those very rules and structures or be faced with a daunting task of managing resistance to the very process of being in therapy (Roberto 1987, 1991). The goodwill and trust developed during the engagement process provide the leverage the therapist will need to make demands for work in the future.

There is a danger of reinforcing power relationships within the family during engagement. By focusing on individual difference rather than on trying to uncover right or wrong answers to questions, the therapist can help to develop a culture which values individual perspective. By avoiding a search for "the truth," the therapist also avoids reinforcing the power of the person with that answer and has greater access to individual opinion and to the reasoning forming that opinion. The key to harvesting rich material from difference questions is to turn to the family to account for why people hold different beliefs or ideas. From this self-reported material the therapist can begin to detail the multitude of unique variables — past, present, intrafamilial, and extrafamilial — that influence the family. The content provides valuable information about what individuals think, about how certain beliefs and opinions are given greater value, and about the behavioural and interactional consequences of the differently held opinions. The process is a model for an individual and equitable style of relating to others. There are certain times when individuals may not feel free to speak up. The therapist can ask about this directly, more to let the entire family know that the therapist is aware of this problem than to get everyone to speak up immediately. The therapist must be on the look out for "leaked" information throughout therapy, and be prepared to address it directly. Equally, there needs to be some belief that over a number of sessions enough trust and relationship will be built within the therapy that all family members will feel free to identify increasingly risky information. For an adolescent girl, simply being in a room with three adults can be censuring. It is important to level the playing-field by relating to the young woman as respectfully and carefully as to her parents.

The Nesbitt family consisted of Mrs. Nesbitt, a "housewife"; Mr. Nesbitt, who owned and operated a successful car dealership; Samantha, 17 years old; and Laurie, 15 years old. Laurie had been experiencing restricted eating since 13 years of age and had recently been admitted to a General Hospital through emergency after fainting at school. She was diagnosed as having anorexia nervosa and treated on the Inpatient Unit for two months. The referral to family therapy was part of Laurie's discharge plans and was largely driven by Mrs. Nesbitt, who was afraid Laurie would relapse because everyone at home was getting on Laurie's nerves.

Mr. Nesbitt did not feel therapy was necessary but came at his wife's insistence. He described himself as a hard-working, self-made man who always supported his family. When others were asked about how they saw Mr. Nesbitt, his wife concurred he was a good provider, however also felt he had difficulty talking about his feelings and problems because his parents were unfeeling problem solvers who worked hard to put their only son through college. Samantha and Laurie both thought their father provided for the family well, but thought he was a "goof" who didn't know anything about what was going on in their lives. Laurie did not believe her mother when she was told her father cried the night she was admitted to the hospital.

Mrs. Nesbitt described herself as a "typical housewife" who was happy to stay at home. She described a traditional role for herself, including taking Laurie to early-morning swimming lessons before and after classes so that she could pursue her interest in competitive swimming. Mrs. Nesbitt also described debilitating headaches that meant she has to "take to her bed" for days at a time.

Mr. Nesbitt complained bitterly about his wife's commitment to running the "show," saying she never had any time for their relationship or herself. He thought this drive for the perfect family came from a need to protect herself from her family of origin who were very critical and demanding of perfection and gossiped about those family members who were "not doing so well." Again Samantha and Laurie saw their mother similarly. They both described her as an "old bag" who was interested only in making sure they did what they were supposed to do. Samantha had some ability to feel sorry for her mother however thought she was "totally faking" her headaches. Laurie described her mother as out of touch with anything "real." The two often had terrible arguments, and Laurie would threaten to kill herself if her mother didn't stop making demands.

In the case of the Nesbitt family, Laurie and Samantha were initially reluctant to talk about their own thoughts, although they would talk about their feelings. The "push" in the family was to solve Laurie's problem fast and to get back to normal. By taking time with both Laurie and Samantha, asking them direct questions and asking family members of comment on the "I don't know" responses, the therapist was able to include them more fully in the conversation. Each young woman responded directly to another family member's opinion about her behaviour. With some effort they were able to identify their fears of hurting their mother with their thoughts and getting in "trouble" because they knew it was going against "the rules" to be critical. They feared Mrs. Nesbitt would get a headache and that Mr. Nesbitt would work even more if they began to really say what they thought.

The next few weeks of family therapy with the Nesbitts was spent exploring the influences of the extended family and how intergenerational demands were understood differently. After asking their mother about her experiences with her own mother,

Samantha and Laurie began to have a greater appreciation of the reasons why Mrs. Nesbitt placed so many demands on them. Although resolving loyalty and identity issues were to be the work of ongoing therapy, in two sessions Samantha and Laurie had a greater appreciation for the seriousness with which Mrs. Nesbitt took her job. By understanding the different contexts and factors, the girls were not so quick to fight with their mother, and Laurie was able to promise she would stop threatening to kill herself. A similar exploration of Mr. Nesbitt's life experience led to a greater intellectual understanding of their father. The girls continued to see him as having limited capacity to form a relationship. The therapist reframed his lack of social skill as a training issue, not a personality issue, based on how Mr. Nesbitt's family of origin was described. This reframing made it much easier for the girls to accept his social struggles and provided the basis for a much later task of teaching him how to be a father to two teenage girls. By focusing on parental limitations and constraints, the focus came off of Samantha, in particular, and pointed to the fact that all family members, not just Samantha, had problems to deal with that effected the whole family.

Context of the Referral

The therapist must be cognizant of the referral route when treating eating-disorder families. Typically, the family is referred by one or two people who are pushing for change. The family physician, individual therapist, or even a family member may be referring because of anxiety or frustration with the individual or treatment process. The referral process should be addressed directly with each family member to assess why they are seeking help now and what their goals and hopes for treatment are. It is not atypical to discover that family members will hold divergent goals; for example, an anorexic woman may wish to give up vomiting and reduce tension within the family, while her physician wants her to gain weight, and her family wants her to be happier. A direct approach will prevent scapegoating the eating-disordered individual; help her develop ownership of her eating; identify boundaries, alliances, and power issues; and model a mutual and respectful approach to relationships. The family therapist is typically trained to assess within the family system; however, it is incumbent upon the therapist to assess the larger sociocultural forces at play. This is an area where traditional family therapists can easily incorporate a feminist approach. What groups of institutions — for example, educational, child welfare, or religious — might be invested in the family seeking treatment or changing their behaviour in a prescribed way? What roles do the extended family or friends play in this referral? This information will be used, as appropriate, later in therapy, as it may, on the one hand, hinder family efforts to change, and, on the other, be a valuable support for the family.

Collaboration with Other Professionals

The anorexic or bulimic woman may be seeing no other person for help or have a large treatment team working with her. The family therapist is encouraged to develop an open and collaborative relationship with key professionals, and in particular with the family physician. The individual and family need to be aware that an open and frequent exchange of information will take place throughout treatment to facilitate the provision of high-quality and coordinated care. It is not atypical to find a woman with an eating disorder telling different helpers different stories. This pattern is understood to rest in a need to protect or defend against painful issues. This interpersonal pattern can lead to fighting among the various professionals, each of whom feels he or she is the recipient of the truth or holds the key to recovery.

The family physician is responsible for addressing the physical well-being of the individual. A joint meeting with the family therapist, family physician, and family, including the individual with the eating disorder, is worthwhile. The family physician, family therapist, and eating-disordered individual must have a clear understanding of the minimum weight and health requirements and the use of hospitalization as part of the treatment contract. This meeting could incorporate the initial assessment or be held separately. A joint meeting should involve contracting a clearly stated approach to collaborative treatment and the specific responsibilities of all concerned. It is easy for the various helpers to abuse the powerful positions they hold, given the knowledge base and service they control. To model a truly collaborative and conjoint approach to practice, the helpers must be prepared to listen to what the anorexic or bulimic woman has to say about her own care and to value this as being as vital as their own "professional" opinions. Including the "patient" as a vital member of the treatment team is an essential tenet of feminist family therapy. The family therapist, although not expected to be expert, is well advised to develop a familiarity with the medical issues and complications of anorexia and bulimia (Kaplan and Woodside 1987).

Shame

Individuals and their families generally experience a great deal of shame about the eating disorder. They may hide the extensiveness of the symptoms or minimize additional problems in an effort to preserve some sense of integrity. The family therapist must prepare an accepting, tolerant, and empathic approach to the problem, while at the same time not colluding with the anorexic or bulimic woman about the seriousness of the symptoms and subsequent problems. A thorough assessment of symptoms is important so that the family therapist can be aware of the woman's health. Symptoms can also be understood as metaphoric or nonverbal language, which the family therapist should have access to. The anorexic or bulimic woman's health does effect her ability to think clearly and participate fully in therapy. If the individual is to be a full partner in the therapy, the family therapist must keep an eye on her physical well-being, although constant checking on symptom levels should not be the primary focus of treatment. The use of specific close-ended questions generally ensures a more complete answer from the individual with the eating disorder. The use of a symptom checklist is not altogether inappropriate as it ensures a thorough assessment of the symptoms; however, it should be used in combination with more open-ended questions that facilitate discussion and explanation. Because the individual may not speak forthrightly in front of her family, an individual assessment of eating behaviours is recommended. An individual appointment also begins the process of boundary definition and responsibility taking. By meeting with the individual alone, the therapist is able to begin the work of realigning who is responsible for the actual eating symptoms. The mother or father are not asked to report on symptoms; rather, the woman herself is trusted to do so. This intervention speaks to many levels of issues: first, it gives the message that the "sick" person deserves respect and trust; second, it begins a much longer process of differentiation which allows the anorexic or bulimic woman and members of her family to be both individuals and members of the family at the same time.

Blame

Family members frequently feel they are to blame and, in fact, often are blamed for the eating disorder. The issue of blame must be dealt with directly at the beginning of treatment, as if it is not, it will likely present an insurmountable barrier. Both the popularization of therapy and beliefs that "psychopathology" rests in the parent/child, in particular the mother/child, relationship have served to reinforce the defences of many parents who already blame themselves for their daughters' eating disorder. It is important to assess for the larger sociocultural content in which these parents are feeling their blame. Assessing if anyone has actually blamed parents and siblings for the eating disorder and, second, whether they have absorbed the belief that they are responsible, are ways of joining with the family. The issue of blame is embedded in the family communication and is readily identifiable. An empathic approach allows the family therapist to reassure the parents that they are not to blame, while at the same time recognizing how their efforts to parent their children well and stop the eating disorder may have inadvertently contributed to or perpetuated it. The nonblaming approach is not appropriate, however, when there are issues of abuse and violence. In most jurisdictions, some sort of official reporting procedures are required when the victim is considered in need of child-welfare protection. If the victim is adult, the therapist must be clear and direct that violence of any kind is intolerable and must stop. This is not to say that, by defining abusive behaviour as unacceptable and demanding, it will stop. By defining behaviour as abusive and inappropriate, the therapist throws the balance of power out of alignment. This has implications for the family at all levels. This realignment of power must be explored over time, and always with safety as a priority. It may take a long time to understand the abuse and its impact on the family. Therapists need to prepare themselves for the stress of working in a context of possible danger until it stops, or the woman gathers enough strength to leave. The function of the eating disorder should be included in the assessment of the abuse. Feminist theory and practice are clear in these situations. Abusive situations are not to be formulated within a systems context and are to be understood as unacceptable. Traditional family therapists will understand that no change will occur if someone is in danger, as the context significantly skews the balance of power and energy in the family.

The feminist approach to practice provides one of the key elements for dealing with both blame and shame, as the exploration of the larger social expectations and pressures on both mother and father can help free the family from paralysing guilt.

> Mrs. Ross, a single mother, brought her 17-year-old daughter, Lisa; her 19-year-old-son; and her 14-year-old daughter to family therapy. Lisa's anorexia began four years earlier when Mrs. Ross and her husband separated. Mrs. Ross's family warned her not to separate because the poverty and hard times of being a single parent were far worse than living with a man who had the occasional drinking binge. Mrs. Ross worked as a secretary and took on additional work as a sales clerk part time to ensure her children were well cared for. As predicted, the child-support payments were sporadic, at best. In family therapy, Mrs. Ross spoke openly

about her sense of guilt that she had not been there to take care of Lisa when she needed her the most. Mrs. Ross's own parents added to her guilt when they told her none of this would have happened if she had stayed in her marriage in the first place.

Patrick burst into tears when asked what he thought had contributed to his sister's developing anorexia. Patrick thought he had caused the anorexia, because when his parents separated, he fought a lot with Lisa. He reported being jealous that school always seemed easy for her and that she seemed to be more popular than he. Patrick tried to put Lisa "down" by calling her names like "fat pig and ugly" and if she did not do what he said he would physically punch her until she said "uncle."

Time was taken initially, and later in the context of ongoing therapy, to explore the impact of individual behaviours and events and of the sense of blame and responsibility on the family relationships. This exploration of beliefs — where they stemmed from, what reinforced them, and how they effected interpersonal behaviour — helped to develop an understanding of the behaviours within the context of time and place, and helped the family think about change rather than remaining paralysed by their sense of guilt and shame.

INFORMATION GATHERING

The information necessary for developing an understanding of family functioning and a working hypothesis is standard. Rather than outlining a specific model here, attention will be given to those issues that are unique to eating disorders, including the family's understanding of the eating disorders; the role and importance of food, appearance, and exercise; and the impact of the larger sociocultural values and beliefs on the family. A three-generational genogram and family history are helpful in the collection of information and, in particular, will trace any issues that may cross a number of generations. A complete assessment generally includes individual and family developmental history and issues of attachment and loss, power and control, victimization, problem solving and conflict resolution, roles, communication styles, boundaries, values and belief systems, and earlier experiences with counseling.

The Family's Understanding of the Eating Disorder

Each family member is asked how he or she found out about the eating disorder. This question should elicit information about what made each family member become suspicious, when that occurred, and how they came to talk openly about the eating disorder. The content of the answers, as well as the way the information is processed by the family, will give the therapist an opportunity to hear about and observe the family communication pattern, boundaries, roles, and beliefs.

A second set of questions addresses what the family knows about the present level of symptoms. Based on information the therapist has already gathered, from the anorexic or bulimic individual, the accuracy of the information each family member has is noted as it contributes to information about secrecy, denial, alliances, and power in the family. The way the family speaks of the symptoms — with shame, disgust, indifference, concern — also gives the sense of their feeling about what their daughter or sister is doing. Family members are asked how they feel about their daughter or sister's eating disorder and the accompanying symptoms. Family members, like the person with the eating disorder, are often greatly relieved to be asked to speak about their feelings directly. These moments of disclosure are very important for the therapist as they offer an opportunity to join with each member of the family at a feeling level and to connect with those family members, including the anorexic or bulimic woman, who appear ambivalent or indifferent. Often lying just below the surface of indifference is the fear, frustration, or self-criticism of someone feeling inadequate to help a family member. Frequently, those expressing indifference have retreated to protect themselves.

Mr. Thomas, a 50-year-old banker, had a 30-year-old daughter with a 13-year history of bulimia. He faithfully attended a number of attempts at family counseling, but left the talking to his wife. By asking directly, the therapist discovered that rather than feeling indifferent to his daughter, as the entire family had reported, he had a number of strong feelings; however, they were contrary to his wife's feelings. Mr. Thomas wanted his daughter to move home so that the family could take care of her. He was very worried she was not able to take care of herself and she would end up chronically ill, or dead. Mrs. Thomas wanted her daughter to have her own apartment but did agree the family should help out financially. When Mr. Thomas could not "win" with his wife, who had been supported by an earlier therapist, he began to withdraw and generally became busier at work. Mr. Thomas spoke about his absence initially in the context of his busy job and stating that his wife "knew best." With some encouragement from the therapist, he began to describe his fears for his daughter — for her physical well-being and for her future. He wondered if she would ever have the things he had hoped she would — a career, marriage and children, and a general sense of well-being and happiness. She seemed so unhappy to him. Mr. Thomas spoke of his responsibility as a father to provide and care for his daughter, and his sense of failure that he must have done something wrong to cause the eating disorder. Mrs. Thomas, on the other hand, showed impatience with her husband and reported she always had to take things in hand.

The couple had work to do to balance their individual responses to the eating disorder and each other. By focusing on Mr. Thomas's fearfulness, he was able to develop, with his daughter rather than his wife, ways he could help that they could each appreciate. He came to the sixth session reporting that he had given his daughter a gift of a tool box since she had decided that she had to live on her own. He offered to teach her how to repair the things that broke in her apartment.

Mr. Thomas was thought to be indifferent to his daughter's health problems when, in fact, he was very concerned but distant in reaction to three issues: his fearfulness about his daughter's health, an accompanying sense of shame that he had not cared properly for her, and anger with his wife about unresolved control issues that dated back to the beginning of their marriage. Given the opportunity to speak directly and within the context of helping his daughter he was able to challenge family beliefs about him and much later began to deal with the longstanding control issues.

The family is also asked what they think has caused the eating disorder. This question is designed to provide detailed information about each family member's belief system. The answers to this question frequently provide the point of entry into the family system. It is important to identify individual beliefs, as they shape and drive behaviours and feelings, which, in turn, are observed and reacted to within the family relationships.

Questions about what the family has done to try to help, what they have found successful, and what has failed contribute information about the family's problem-solving abilities, boundaries, parenting skills, roles, and power and control. The anorexic or bulimic woman must be involved in this line of questioning. What does she find helpful and what has made it more difficult to eat normally? Has the family already asked her this question, or are the answers new information to them? If the family has asked for feedback but ignored it, and continued to do unhelpful things, why didn't they stop? Do they trust that she will answer their questions honestly, or is she lying to get them to leave her alone? Again, this line of questioning gives the therapist, and ultimately the entire family, access to information about how individual members are feeling and how their behaviours interact and influence one another and reflects such issues as power, control, trust, and roles. Such questions recognize the collaborative approach that will be taken with the family. The therapist can take the opportunity to acknowledge that the family has not been passive or uninvolved in this process, and that they can contribute significantly to the treatment process by jointly thinking about, trying, and evaluating new solutions.

The family is asked how the eating disorder has affected the family in a good way and in a bad way. These two questions are designed to test the family's ability to observe themselves, and to begin to test their ability to understand and tolerate alternative ways of viewing the anorexia or bulimia and the role the disorder plays in the family.

Role of Food and Importance of Appearance and Exercise

Assessing the role of food is important because anorexia and bulimia are such powerful metaphors. Exploring the meaning and rituals of food and eating is a means for determining what is being so rigidly resisted and symbolically expressed. Questions about mealtime rituals — who buys, prepares, and serves the food; how and where the family eat; what the tone of meals is like; who joins the family and who does not; what food preferences people have; what health problems, if any, require special diets; what other family members, if any, have an eating disorder or a tendency to diet or eat carefully; and how the family manages the anorexia or bulimia at mealtime — give the therapist information about both the meaning of food and family functioning. Issues of appearance and exercise are important, given the drive for thinness and body-image disturbance associated with anorexia and bulimia (Chernin 1981; Garner and Garfinkel 1980; Steiner-Adair 1986). The therapist is assessing for family beliefs that reinforce the importance of both physical appearance and the appearance of success. Each member is asked to comment on others' weight, shape, style of dress, grooming, and exercise pattern. What initially may seem like a painful or insensitive set of questions is, in fact, an invitation to speak about a "taboo" subject. If the family is not already commenting on this issue openly, it is important to know what they are saying to each other and how they treat each other, and to discover the thoughts they are keeping to themselves but showing in a nonverbal or masked way. Making explicit those thoughts and feelings that are implicit in nonverbal behaviours often brings a tremendous sense of relief to family members who were afraid to comment. In situations where anger, shame, hurt, or sadness is expressed, an opportunity emerges to discuss the feelings directly, with the hope of some resolution over time. For those families that comment indirectly, an opportunity is offered to do some consciousness raising and to explore the purpose of indirect communication in the family. The family is also asked about what they think is an ideal weight for their daughter or sister, which is a basis on which to assess their ability to judge "normal" weights. Any family members who also idealize a superthin or anorexic shape might sabotage the recovery process, as would anyone who wanted the anorexic or bulimic person to "control" her weight at an artificial level, using means other than normalized eating and healthy activity. It should be noted that younger sisters may idealize their older sisters, and want to follow in their footsteps. Other family members may idealize the anorexic shape for a variety of reasons. Equally, they are asked about the importance of exercise and what it is used for; for example, is exercise related to health concerns, body shape, weight control, or recreation and leisure? It is important for the therapist to explore and challenge weight and shape issues that might compromise the individual's efforts at normalizing her eating.

The Frank family discovered Christine had bulimia when Mrs. Frank was called by the Emergency Department of a downtown hospital. Two of Christine's friends had taken her there when she fainted at a party. Mrs. Frank reported being suspicious for some time as food was missing and the bathroom smelled of vomit. She reported her concern to husband two years earlier; however, he said it was nothing. Mr. Frank was proud of his daughter since she had become a lovely young woman. Since turning 16, she lost her "baby fat" and taken great pride in her appearance, grooming herself in a sophisticated fashion. Mr. Frank enjoyed taking his daughter to lunch and introducing her to his business associates.

Mrs. Frank thought the eating disorder was caused by Christine's boyfriend who is always commenting on how he likes his girlfriends to be thin. She thought her own dieting might have influenced her daughter somewhat. She thought Christine could stand to lose five pounds or so, but that vomiting was stupid and sick. Mr. Frank thought his daughter was sick and crazy.

He was clear that it was an emergency and that his wife had better do something right away before it got worse and the rest of the family had to be told.

The Frank family had clear issues with weight and shape that they spoke about openly and directly. Although the issues of weight and shape were powerful in themselves, they also became a metaphor for more profound issues of power, family loyalty, identity, and marital distress. Discussion of the family weight-and-shape issues provided an entry into the more profound issues, as body image was a far less threatening place to begin. The Cheung family presents a different picture.

Lilly worked as an X-ray technician at a small city hospital and took extra shifts to save money and keep busy. It was clear there was something wrong with Lilly: she had become very thin and picky about what she would eat. However, the family did not speak openly about Lilly's problem. Lilly's older sister had tried to speak to her several times, but Lilly had been angry and abusive to her sister, who then stopped expressing her concerns. Mr. and Mrs. Cheung tried to help their daughter by preparing food that Lilly liked and taking her to her favourite restaurants. The Cheungs invited friends and extended family for dinner, but declined invitations to eat at friends' homes because they did not wish to leave Lilly alone. She refused to accompany her parents, because she could not be sure of the menu, and they would not leave her alone for fear she would spend the entire evening doing exercises. Mrs. Cheung bought larger wool clothes at Lilly's request. Only later did Lilly tell her mother that she hated the clothes but wore them because they hid her emaciated shape and helped to keep her warm.

When Lilly began making mistakes at work, her supervisor sent her to the employee health department. Lilly told her mother about her problem because she was sent home early and required a note from her family physician to be able to return to work. Mrs. Cheung accompanied Lilly to the doctor's office and insisted on counseling for Lilly and their family. The family found great relief in being asked about Lilly's anorexia, weight, shape, and dress.

The Cheung family placed value on family peacefulness and harmony. Lilly's angry outbursts and moodiness were a result of starvation and were a defence against the shame she felt she was bringing to the family. Mr. Cheung had had a minor heart attack earlier in the year, an event that had frightened the family and served to push stress and tension underground for fear of triggering a more severe recurrence. The family's feelings began to be expressed in nonverbal ways that everyone could readily understand, but also ignore. The family, although initially hesitant, leapt at the invitation to speak openly about their fears and concerns for both Lilly's and Mr. Cheung's health.

Impact of Larger Sociocultural Beliefs and Values on the Family
The therapist should be assessing for the impact of the larger culture on the family, including specific expectations from the social-support system of the family, as well as the more subtle influences of the patriarchal hierarchical culture that demarcate the roles, responsibilities, and expectations of men, women, and children in the family. Equally important to assess is the process of censuring any family or family member who dares to challenge the rules. Assessment of cultural influences will help guard the systemic therapist from guiding the family to a new level of functioning that either accommodates or tolerates many of the factors that are readily identified as contributing to and perpetuating the eating disorder. Systemic therapy that does not include the influence of culture, ignores the reality of the constraints of poverty and powerlessness, or misunderstands the importance of biology and the value of relatedness to women will serve only to reinforce the family structure and process that contribute to the anorexia and bulimia.

It is important to recognize that there is no single culture; rather, each family has a unique culture of its own that is influenced by a multitude of variables. Just as it is a mistake to ignore the role of the larger social system or community in which the family lives, it is also a mistake to make assumptions about some sort of static monolithic culture that victimizes and controls helpless families and individuals. The therapist must assess the interaction between the family and larger community. It is important to explore issues of membership, loyalty, boundary, and censuring that occur between family and community. The therapist must be mindful of a gentle balance when working in this area — no blame must be placed on them for behaviour resulting from constraints and expectations placed upon them by cultural standards of normalcy, yet it should be made clear that they are responsible for their individual decisions. It is useful to explore with the client which beliefs, feelings, and behaviours directed their choices.

The Frank family (see above) illustrates the impact of cultural beliefs on the family and how those beliefs then reverberate within the family itself. The Frank family is father-directed and -controlled, as is evident in Mrs. Frank's need to "report" to her husband, and Mr. Frank's power to label his wife's concern and Christine's behaviour as "nothing" and, as such, to control the subsequent action taken by his wife. Mrs. Frank's own lack of power and self-esteem is reflected in her need to take direction from her husband. Her role and responsibilities rest in the home and in feeling issues; however, even these responsibilities can be overruled by Mr. Frank.

Both Mr. and Mrs. Frank described real concerns with appearances. Each believed their status and esteem was reflected in how well they presented as a family unit. Mrs. Frank always took great care over her appearance. She groomed herself carefully and strove to remain thin. Her husband gave her a generous allowance to buy fashionable clothes. Mrs. Frank dieted throughout her life, and thought Christine could stand to loose a few pounds. She was very upset at the prospect of aging, and spoke continuously to her children about the importance of taking care of themselves so they would look young as long as possible. She believed her best years were behind her. North American culture, which values beauty and youthfulness, has little room for women once they reach middle age. Mr. Frank began to take his daughter to lunch, not to treat her or enjoy her company, but to use her as a reflection of his own importance and esteem. He "appeared" to be lunching in the company of a much younger and beautiful woman; in fact, these scenes had incestuous overtones. Christine participated in lunches because she seldom saw her father otherwise, was afraid to say no, and thought she might as well get a free lunch. Mr. Frank did not know Christine would excuse herself from the table after lunch to vomit in the restaurant washroom.

Both parents insisted that the family always convey a good image in public. Mr. Frank reported that, among his peers, he was considered a "softy" who gave his children far too much. Mr. Frank was insistent that the bingeing and purging stop before he had to tell his family. He was fearful of what his parents would think, and joined with Christine in demanding that "this thing" be kept a family secret. Mrs. Frank insisted on help only when Christine had a health crisis. When asked about the delay in seeking help she reported not wanting to upset her husband. Her role in the family was to ensure the children were well cared for and ready to proudly represent the family in public, and not to distract her husband from his job of earning money for the family. She was equally embarrassed and appalled at Christine's behaviour and very upset that she would be looked upon as a bad mother by those who might find out about the eating disorder. Mr. Frank believed his wife had not taken a strong enough hand with Christine. Mr. Frank firmly believed in control and punishment as a method of teaching and socializing his children to the correct adult roles and responsibilities. By the time of the assessment, Mrs. Frank had taken to policing Christine, following her around the house, controlling the food in the house, and accompanying her on as many outings as possible. Mrs. Frank developed this plan on the advice of her mother who, like Mr. Frank, believed a "strong hand was needed to take care of the situation." Mrs. Frank had doubts about the stern approach proposed by her mother and husband. She did not challenge their plan because she had long ago learned to comply with them as a response to the constant devaluation and ridicule of her ideas that has occurred over the years. What she did do was never quite implement the plan completely. Christine was very unhappy with her mother's efforts "to help." Initially she asked her mother to stop. When Mrs. Frank did not stop, Christine attempted to push her mother away by initiating aggressive arguments. When asked about her behaviour Christine reported being deeply ashamed by it and added that her mother's policing reminded her of what a "loser" she really was.

Families easily answer questions about how they feel the larger culture has impacted on them. Such questions as: what role do you think the larger culture has played in your daughter developing an eating disorder? are frequently answered with insight and sincerity. Families seem to be aware of the cultural focus on thinness, appearance, and the accumulation of the products of success. The family can generally be engaged in talk about how they fit into and how they differ from the predominant culture. Some family members may struggle to answer questions about the influence of the culture on their role, identity, and parental disciplining or censuring behaviours. Families are very aware of being "politically correct" and can be afraid of being labeled bad or afraid of being forced to change by one of those "women's libbers" who will tell them what is right and wrong. It is critical that the therapist ask questions and work with the family in a nonjudgemental way. Again, this nonjudgemental approach is not to be taken when abuse (including emotional abuse) and violence are occurring in the home. These questions must be embedded in curiosity and positive recognition of the work the family has done to be unique and to fit in to their larger culture. Questions that are hypothetical or make-believe, such as "If you could change any family traditions without any concern for what people think of you, which ones would you likely change?" should also be explored, along with questions concerning the "cost of such change." Equally, a family should be asked about which traditions and influences of the predominant and family culture they would like to keep and why.

Maria's family believed her bulimia was a way to get back at her parents. Maria binged and at times left vomit to be found by her mother when she went to clean Maria's room. When her parents were asked how they thought their culture affected Maria and themselves, they reported that Maria is embarrassed by her Italian heritage and ashamed of them, and that she wants to pretend that she is a Canadian girl. Her older two sisters had married Italian men and were raising good families. Mrs. Pelloso had begun to work part time and was seeing more of her friends after her second daughter married. Mrs. Pelloso was also taking English as a Second Language classes and doing well. Mr. Pelloso did not like what his wife was doing. Although she kept up her house work, he thought all money should be put into the family pot, not kept separately. Although the subject was not spoken of at home, Mr. Pelloso also objected to his wife taking English lessons. None of his friends' wives spoke good English, and they managed. Since Maria's vomiting was discovered, Mrs. Pelloso had stopped seeing her friends as much and was only sporadically attending a drop-in English class.

From her culture's standpoint, Mrs. Pelloso became a deviant in her efforts to develop an identity and life more independent from the family. Not unlike her daughter, Mrs. Pelloso was not doing what a "good Italian wife and mother" should do, according to the standards of Mr. Pelloso, his peer group, and his extended family. When asked what initially attracted the couple to each other, Mr. Pelloso said he found his wife attractive, liked her commitment to her family, and found her interesting. Further questioning revealed that Mrs. Pelloso did some untraditional things as a young woman; for example, she traveled throughout Europe on her own as a teenager, and in defiance of her father she paid her mother rent, even though her father thought he should support her completely until she married.

Maria was angry with her mother, whom she felt was upsetting her father with the result that he, in his role as family leader, became more controlling at home and made Maria's life miserable by lecturing her, comparing her with her sisters, and threatening to not let her see her friends any more. Maria felt her mother had her chances earlier on, and now she should sacrifice for the family. The Pelloso family used a variety of means — guilt induction, demands for behavioural change, and conformity and shaming — to force Mrs. Pelloso to return to their expectations of "normal" behaviour within their family and social context. Maria's bingeing and vomiting speaks of the family's belief that "children should be seen and not heard" and that family loyalty is paramount. Speaking out of turn indicated disrespect to parents and was thought to be the harbinger of worse chaos and change for the family. Efforts to be individual or to separate from the family flew in the face of family and cultural norms and were guarded against by all family members to a greater or lesser extent. Therapy with the Pelloso family centred not on traditional hierarchies, but on difference and bravery. Mr. Pelloso was initially attracted to his wife because she was untraditional. Therapy focused on how they had lost the energy to be different and unique. Much centred on the couple's immigration to Canada and a retreating to old but safe roles, as well as the limited choices they had because of their positions as unskilled immigrants who spoke poor English. The couple reviewed their adventure in coming to Canada and the decisions made along the way. They were able to recognize the great amount of energy, bravery, and risk that they took to begin a new life. Over a number of months of therapy, they reviewed what they wished to keep of the old ways and what they wished to discard. Maria and Mrs. Pelloso began to see similarities in their lives, which joined them rather than divided them. Maria began to develop a more individual identity that was not dependent on her parents' approval. Her Canadian boyfriend was welcomed into the family. Mr. Pelloso was very concerned about what his friends would think about the "disrespect" his daughter was showing from time to time. His wife and oldest daughter spoke with him about his need for external validation from his friends. In the last family meeting, Mr. Pelloso reported a friend had approached him about problems the friend was having with his son. This request for help reinforced for Mr. Pelloso that he had to be less concerned with what others thought and do what he and his family thought was important for themselves.

CONTRACTING

Negotiating the contract is the final stage of the assessment process. A feminist approach to contracting is extremely valuable in working with eating-disordered families. The contract is a useful as a direct and practical tool; however, it can also be effective as an indirect technique and intervention to begin to challenge the power and process within the family. The contract makes mutual responsibilities clear. A written contract is particularly useful for a family that initially appears to be chaotic and may have trouble working within the rules of therapy. The contract makes clear the business part of therapy: the when and where of appointments; what the fees, if any, are; how extra therapy contact and confidentiality will be dealt with. Education and exchange about what the family can expect from the therapist and what the therapist can expect from the family are important elements.

Mutual and realistic goals are negotiated rather than set down by the "expert" therapist, as are measures of accomplishment of the identified goals. It is essential that every member of the family be part of the contracting process and goal setting. The therapist must find common ground on which to proceed.

Family members often present with different goals and degrees of power, which can affect the contracting process. Power issues can be addressed directly, especially if they are affecting contracting. The therapist should be assessing the currency that contributes to power in each family and how that power is used. For example, if a father claims power, based on the money he earns, the mother's contributions to the family need to be explored and validated. So too, the contributions of each child should be validated as contributing to family functioning in an important way. Mothers are often disqualified if their primary role is parenting, and they are blamed for causing, or at least not stopping, their daughters' anorexia or bulimia. The father may step in and take charge of setting the goals and objectives for the family therapy if the mother is seen as failing to do her job.

Therapists can deal with power and alliances by shifting their own alliances in keeping with the goals of treatment. This does not mean the therapist must always agree with what the individual says but rather that the therapist ally with all family members through a variety of means — content issues, feelings, personality similarities, views, and attitudes. (Hare-Mustin 1978).

Heather, an 18-year-old high school student, was referred, with her family, for treatment of her anorexia by Mrs. Hamilton's life-long friend, who was also a colleague of the family therapist. The Hamiltons were seen quickly as a professional courtesy and because of the degree of reported distress. A contract for counseling could not be made with the Hamiltons. Heather had some desire to stop vomiting and to feel better, but would not gain weight or normalize her eating. Mrs. Hamilton, a newly graduated lawyer, could not make time for regular family sessions. Mrs. Hamilton was upset and stressed with her own father, who blamed her for Heather's problems. The grandfather thought that mothers have a responsibility to raise their children and not fuss about careers. Mr. Hamilton wanted family counseling because he was tired of having to take care of everything. Stephan, Heather's 14-year-old brother, was not interested in counseling. He thought that she was "stupid" and doing this for attention. He might come for one session if it didn't interfere with football and it would get Heather's friends off his case about her health. The referring physician/friend was tired of hearing about family stress and upset from his friend. He had hoped that, if they got help, the friendship would return to normal. Mrs. Hamilton was also worried about the friendship.

No one in the Hamilton family or their support system was really prepared to accept a different way of understanding the eating disorder or to invest in therapy of any kind. Often fear of the consequences of anorexia or bulimia pushes a family to seek help and, with the therapist, they can begin to identify problems and make changes, but this was not the case with the Hamiltons. Because no clear point of entry could be found it was impossible to establish a therapeutic contract and proceed with family therapy at that moment. Heather was referred for individual counseling and followup with her family physician. The family were welcomed to return should they feel family therapy would be useful in the future. The family therapist heard at a later date that Mr. and Mrs. Hamilton had separated and that Mrs. Hamilton was accompanying Heather to therapy sessions with her individual therapist.

INTERVENTION

Intervention can be brief or longer term, depending upon the working contract. The first, or problem-focused stage has a life unto itself or can be the introduction and preparation for further family work. The problem-focused stage is designed to be brief and solution oriented. The goal is to significantly reduce, if not eliminate, eating symptoms; to help the family support the person with the eating disorder in more helpful ways; and to generate new responses to family stressors.

Stage I : Problem Focus

Families come to treatment looking for a "cure" for the anorexia or bulimia. The problem-focused stage is designed to provide concrete suggestions about the management of the eating-disorder symptoms by the person with the symptoms and by the family. Depending upon their knowledge base, the family may find a session devoted to education valuable. In the format of presentation and questions and answers, information about such topics as defining anorexia, bulimia, nutrition, fitness, relapse, medical emergencies, and treatment can be a useful way to check false hopes, while also encouraging those that feel anxious or hopeless. Sharing information and helping to educate the family contribute to the demystification of therapy and help make the family an equal partner in the process.

The purpose of the problem-focused stage is to work with the family and the person with the eating disorder to design new ways of managing the eating-disordered symptoms and to help the family develop a new way of relating that does not include the constant presence of some kind of symptom. By the time most families seek help, they have usually exhausted their own solutions and gone way beyond the bounds of "normal" helping behaviours. Their efforts to help are likely contributing to the perpetuation of the anorexia or bulimia, and have likely skewed all levels of family functioning, creating a preoccupation with the eating disorder at the expense of most everything else.

Initially, family members try to help by talking to the anorexic or bulimic person. If being verbally supportive and encouraging does not work, the parents typically become angry, frustrated, and frightened. They begin to use more punitive measures, such as "grounding," restricting use of the telephone, making money contingent on eating properly, and subjecting the individual to more serious discussions/lectures. These tactics, although well intended, are doomed to failure as the eating disorder may now become secretive and at the same time more powerful. It should be noted that, during this time, the anorexic or bulimic individual is generally trying equally hard to bring her eating into some kind of control. In addition to the frustration, fear, and anger that the family feels, she is likely experiencing shame and self-loathing at her inability to take care of herself. Next, some family members may begin to separate or distance themselves because of their fears and frustrations, while others escalate their involvement. Typically, although not always, fathers tend to take a distancing or punitive stance, and mothers, embracing the more traditional role as nurturer, escalate their involvement.

In attempting to be more helpful, mothers may consult with their daughters. However, often they do not, particularly when policing their daughter's behaviours. Mothers cook separate meals for their eating-disordered daughters, keep only nonbinge (or appealing) food in the house, and reserve specific bathrooms for her use. Mothers ask siblings to place their requests and needs on hold because of their "sick" sister. When even these efforts fail to stop the person from bingeing, restricting, or purging, mothers escalate their involvement out of a sense of responsibility to care for their child and to try to appease other family members who demand some sort of change. Mothers may hide food; put locks on the refrigerator and freezer; complete daily food inventories; search their daughters' bedroom and the bathrooms for evidence of ongoing bingeing and purging; join their daughter at all meals; offer unending opportunities to talk; and offer up numerous reasons to teachers, employers, and shopkeepers to excuse their daughters' behaviour. Although all family members are well intended, after some time and much failure the process of helping can take the family far off the course of "normal" development; distract from other serious problems; and contribute to increasing levels of fear, resentment, anger, and frustration.

The anorexic or bulimic person is encouraged to recapture control of her eating symptoms. The remainder of the family are encouraged to let go of control of the eating disorder and to become reinvested in their family relationships, free of responsibility for the symptoms. This can be easy for some families and very difficult for others. Behavioural change in the form of a symptom separation (Schwartz, Barrett, and Saba 1985) is introduced. A symptom separation is simply examining with the family who is responsible for what behaviours. Ownership and responsibility for oneself is addressed in a practical way that encourages families to experiment with new ways of relating to each other. The family has the right to evaluate and stop an experiment at any time. When the reality of what the family can actually do is explored, family members quickly accept that they cannot make their daughter or sister eat normally if she does not want to. They are left with their fear of her possible death or a chronically limited lifestyle. Parents are encouraged to take control of parenting and their marriage in a new way. The immediacy of the eating disorder will likely have distracted parents from their long-term goals for their children. The parents, with their children, can be encouraged to return to a more longitudinal view of parenting and family development, including the need for adolescents to develop their own identities and for young adults to become more independent of their families.

The reaction of the family members to the new behaviours produces a rich cache of information at a more abstract and systemic level, and as such should be closely monitored and stored for future use. Although desperate for relief, families also have tremendous ambivalence about change. This ambivalence rests in many levels of fearfulness and often drives a strong resistance to change. The family therapist is well advised to develop an understanding of the use of the technique and art of restraint and advocacy for change. Making suggestions for change in a manner that emphasizes the difficulties individuals may experience while changing their behaviour, the cost of change for the family as a whole and to individual members, while also instilling hope is important; misused, it can sap the energy of therapy and turn it into a punitive, abusive experience for the family. It is essential to have a respect and an ear for the message embedded in resistance.

Guided by the therapist, the anorexic or bulimic person and her family begin to negotiate new rules about the eating disorder. A number of commonly negotiated methods of symptom separation are described below. It is important to remember that these are not directives issued by the therapist, but are mutually negotiated plans. The more a behaviour change is unique to the family, the greater the likelihood the family will be able to embrace the change and make it their own.

Parents are asked to stop monitoring eating and purging, which means no more listening at bathroom doors for vomiting; searching dresser drawers for laxatives; or buying, storing, preparing, and serving food to "help" the eating-disordered person. These suggestions serve to challenge enmeshment and to stop frustration and resentment, as family members can return to eating what they like and look forward to spending time together or individually, doing things they enjoy.

The anorexic or bulimic person is asked to take control of her own eating, to make her own selection of choices and quantity of food with the freedom to supplement family meals, if need be. Equally, she is expected to return the bathroom and kitchen to previous levels of cleanliness should she purge or binge. Binge food should be replaced by the bulimic person.

Some families will make excuses for the "sick" individual and will need to let her take responsibility for her own mistakes and choices by refusing to make or accept excuses about tardiness, absences, illness, and unlawful activity such as shoplifting. This does not mean parents cannot support their daughter at school, in court, or at work; rather, they must stop protecting her from the natural consequences of her behaviour.

While their daughter is taking increasing control of her eating — and, metaphorically, of her life — the family is asked to assess realistic consequences for all family members who break the rules. The use of the notion of natural consequences is easily embraced by families; however, they will likely struggle with extreme consequences, like telling their daughter she has to leave home. Families may need help recognizing and negotiating rules that are no longer age appropriate or simply do not work. They may need help making explicit rules that, until now, were implicit and remained unspoken.

Parents are also directed to take time to plan what they will do with their time individually, as a couple, and as a family, now that they are helping their daughter in a different way. These ideas should be brought back to therapy and discussed with the children in an age-appropriate manner. The family may initially use the therapy time for such discussion, but later may be able to do it in meetings at home.

While the family has been problem solving to discover ways to let go of the eating disorder, they have also been learning to communicate with one another in a much more direct and clear manner. For the family to be able to negotiate the practical issues of symptom management, they must also address the relationship issues embedded in them. Feminist family therapy can guide the family therapy. A feminist approach supports both direct and indirect techniques, but does require that the therapist collaborate with the family. The entire family is directly included in planning the methods by which the individual will retake control of her eating disorder and the family will redefine their responsibilities. The therapist is also responsible for helping the family review the indirect changes that they have made so that they can develop awareness by learning from their experiences now, and in the future.

Once the family has established new ways of relating about the eating disorder, they will be surprised and reflect back on the consequences of change. Although family members are still anxious, generally the tension levels are greatly reduced, and issues of control and power are more evident. Issues that the illness masked or distracted attention from are more clearly identifiable by family members who, once confident about the stability of their daughter or sister, will introduce other stressful situations to be dealt with. Issues such as abuse, battery, alcoholism, and martial unhappiness can now be accessed more directly, if the family contracts to do so.

The family may choose to end therapy at this point, confident that they have now developed new skills and have been released from the rigid responses made out of fear for their daughter or sister. Other families will want to continue with more family therapy to address more underlying concerns. The decision to continue therapy will usher the family into longer-term treatment.

Mrs. Lamb had devoted herself to the care of her 20-year-old daughter, Freeda, and 18-year-old son, Misha, since the unexpected death of her husband three years earlier. Within a year of Mr. Lamb's death, Freeda developed bulimia. Mrs. Lamb was a well-respected and highly valued vice-president of a drug company. The company initially provided her with tremendous support at the time of her husband's death and upon her daughter's illness; however, Mrs. Lamb was feeling tremendous pressure to return to work, which included conducting several evening meetings and working weekends. To help Freeda, she kept all binge food out of the house, including food Misha liked. He felt growing resentment that he could eat ice cream, chips, and cookies only outside of the home. Dinner was prepared by Mrs. Lamb, who threw all leftovers out. She joined Freeda for dinner every night and, although she did not stop Freeda from going to the bathroom, she did invite her to have a leisurely coffee in the living room with her every evening, right after dinner. Mrs. Lamb also "overlooked" the money missing from her purse on a regular basis. Freeda was moody, so both Mrs. Lamb and Misha were walking on eggs. Mrs. Lamb curtailed her social life completely, working at home or spending the evenings with Freeda, who had largely isolated herself from her friends, if she did go out, she returned upset, saying that no one liked her because she was so fat and boring.

After symptom management was returned to Freeda, Misha reported tremendous relief. Mrs. Lamb and Freeda had an initial period of heightened anxiety and tension, especially when Mrs. Lamb closed her purse and insisted Freeda not binge in the home. Over a six-month period, Mrs Lamb returned to work full time. As she set limits with her daughter, she was able to do so at work as well, insisting that her weekends were for family exclusively. She and her children developed more age-appropriate activities. Misha became more involved with the family; Mrs. Lamb cultivated her own social circle; and although Freeda remained isolated and anxious among peers, she now used her therapist for this work rather than her mother.

Brief therapy focused on grief and realigning control in the Lamb family. Everyone's thoughts and feelings about the help he or she was providing were explored. Everyone was afraid of the eating disorder. Misha had enjoyed doing "things" (bike riding, talking, and hanging out) with his sister. Now, he felt he couldn't do anything right, resented the attention Freeda got, and exclaimed: "After all, I lost my father too!" Misha felt all he could do was withdraw. Mrs. Lamb felt she had to give Freeda more, that if she could only give her enough love and attention, Freeda would not be so insecure and would feel better about herself and be able to eat normally. Freeda felt her mother cared, and knew that Misha was mad at her; however, she also felt that their efforts to help did not work, except when her mother listened to her problems after social events. Freeda did not trust her mother's supportive comments, believing Mrs. Lamb was just telling her she looked fine or had done well to make her feel good. The therapist positively framed what everyone was trying to do and invited the family, first, to explore intellectually what the stages of "normal" family and individual development were, and how they compared with the theory. Misha felt he was only beginning to get to know who he was. Freeda said she was totally confused about who she was, but felt she was good at taking care of "things" and could be responsible if she had to. Mrs. Lamb was also confused about her identity since the death of her husband. She was unhappy to see Freeda so ill, but also glad that she still had her role as a mother since she was no longer a wife. She was frightened by what the future held for her and thought there would be a void until she became a grandmother. She began to recognize that she needed to attend to rebuilding her own life as a woman.

Meaning and Metaphor

The decision to engage in longer-term therapy rests in the family's readiness to make more change and endure the anxiety associated with fears about the consequences of change in the family. As the family enters longer-term therapy, the focus shifts from the management of the eating disorder to family problems. The eating disorder may reappear at time of systemic stress, and can be used by the therapist and family as a barometer of stress levels and resistance to systemic intervention. It is a mistake to return to a day-today approach to symptom management at this point. Management should be in the hands of the individual, her physician, and individual therapist, and not the family therapist.

The therapist should be prepared to explore with the family systemic and individual dynamics within the family itself and between the family and their extended family, their personal support system, and the culture at large. It may be necessary to work with subsystems and individuals as the meanings of reactions to change are explored. Depending upon one's theoretical orientation and the wishes of the family, the therapist may see all constellations or refer family members to and collaborate with individual or marital therapists, as appropriate.

Themes identified and partially worked on during the problem-focused stage are explored in more depth with the goal that the issue of eating disorder will be resolved and the family will develop a new way of relating that is free of both the eating disorder and the issues it both masked and highlighted. The list of content issues that frequently emerge includes:

1. Loss — separation, attachment, longing
2. Victimization — abuse, shame, safety
3. Multigenerational legacy — loyalty, self-sacrifice, differentiation, secrets
4. Identity formation — self-image, self-esteem and confidence, individuation, separation, autonomy, relatedness
5. Power and control — decision making, conflict management, equality
6. Boundaries — ownership, responsibility, safety, independence
7. Expression of feelings — anger, grief, anxiety, protest, self-regulation
8. Gender issues — personal support system, larger system, family, individual
9. Marital relationship — as it impacts the family system
10. Shame and blame

Through examining such content issues, the therapist and family together can identify and refine issues that keep the family stuck in a style of relating that no longer functions well for them. Content can be addressed directly in an accepting, enquiring way, encouraging family members to explore their own beliefs, behaviours, and feelings, and to begin to track their interaction with those of other family members. The use of difference questions — How do you see your role as a daughter differently from your mother? How does your father's need to provide you with good training to be an adult differ between you and your brother? How do you account for the difference between your mother and father on the issue of dating? How do you think your sister will be different when she gives up her bulimia? Difference questions avoid the right/wrong, good/bad dynamic that engenders the blame and shame that families are sensitive to. Content and process need to be tracked. How the family censures and encourages information and behaviour is as important as the collected content.

The therapist and family together form a hypothesis about how historical events and present circumstances have come together to influence the family's functioning. The joint hypothesis forms the focus of work in therapy, to be worked and reworked as therapy progresses. The role of the eating disorder is positively connoted as helpful, given what the family has had to contend with. The eating disorder is seen to be a tool or coping mechanism for the entire family, and one that freely taken up can be freely given up when the circumstances are right.

At this point the therapist must move away from content issues to process issues. Content is the story of what goes on, and process is how the story comes to be. This is not to say that content is not important, but that it is less so than process. Being focused on detailed content is a sign of some sort of resistance to change, as is the reappearance of anorexic or bulimic symptoms. Resistance is often understood to be a bad thing. Families that "don't do as they are told to do" are trying to say something to the therapist. What they are saying is not always clear; however, what is clear is that whatever the plan was, it didn't work for the family. The therapist must work with the family to understand the meaning of the "resistance." While advocating for and supporting change, the therapist must also help the family explore the high cost of change for its individual members and for the family as a whole. By focusing on timing and the pace of change, the family can find a pace at which they can accommodate to new ways of relating without a sense of having to keep up to some time line established by the therapist.

Mr. Benvenuto emigrated to Canada after 10 years of taking care of his mother's farm in Italy. He took on this responsibility at age 12, when his father died. He returned to Italy at age 30 to find a wife. He met his wife, an old friend's younger sister, and married her within a week. Being the youngest, she had stayed home to help her parents, but at age 20 was eager to get married and have a child of her own. Her father begged her, first, not to marry, and then, not to leave, promising he would die if she left. Mrs. Benvenuto did leave, and within two months of her arrival in Canada her father died. Mrs. Benvenuto was filled with guilt and did not return for the funeral. The couple worked hard for two years to prepare for a family. When Mrs. Benvenuto became pregnant, she left work and has raised her three children.

The family has had a number of successes and losses. Mr. Benvenuto has worked hard to give his family a comfortable living and has also gone to school to become an engineer. Mrs. Benvenuto was able to bring her mother from Italy, and she now lives with the family. Unfortunately, the family also suffered the loss of the family home in a fire, and Mr. Benvenuto has had a break with two of his brothers over money they owed him. Although they have many friends, the larger family, with the exception of Mrs. Benvenuto's mother, are very critical of and competitive with each other.

Bonita, the 15-year-old daughter, developed bulimia six months after she failed her school year. Her entire family were upset by the failure, and even more upset when they found out how she threw up the food bought with Mr. Benvenuto's hard-earned cash and lovingly prepared by her mother and grand-mother.

The Benvenuto family, as might be expected, worked hard in therapy, were prompt, did their homework, and so on. At the outset, the family presented as looking for expert advice from the therapist. They had a difficult time grasping the notion that they had the solutions to the problems already and that the role of the therapist was to help them recognize those solutions. They managed the symptom separation well, developing unique ways to let go of the symptoms and allowing Bonita to manage her own eating. Mrs. Benvenuto had the greatest difficulty because of her role as caretaker. It was recognized that feeding the family was her responsibility and that much of her self-esteem rested in preparing high-quality meals. She and her mother spent much of the day either shopping for or growing food to prepare for family meals. Mr. Benvenuto, who was largely absent, was able to support his wife when he understood she needed his help. He was not a naturally demonstrative man; however, when his wife became upset about her daughter and her own abilities as a mother, he would acknowledge and remind her of all the things she had done for the family over the years. He helped remind her that by doing less she was doing more for Bonita. When the family entered into longer-term treatment, Bonita had only occasional bouts of bulimia. Themes that pervaded treatment were those of loss and family loyalty. The children led discussion about the struggles between the old and the new ways. The entire family explored their beliefs and expectations about family roles. The bulimia was seen as a wish for greater independence on the part of Bonita, and as a metaphor for a family who, because of losses and emigration, were unclear about how they wanted to keep the old traditions while also adopting their new culture. The greatest fear of change came from concerns about whether they could manage in a new country. The old ways were retained more as a life preserver than as something the family really wanted. Once each parent dealt with "leaving home," all family members, securely and jointly, were able to redefine themselves and their relationships with one another. Mr. Benvenuto found it particularly difficult to give up his role as head of the household and all that this entailed, for example, the right and power to make family decisions and to have the unconditional respect of his children. Mr. Benvenuto initially became angry at the lack of respect, verbally abusing those within shouting distance; when this tactic did not work, he became quite despondent. Mrs. Benvenuto almost returned to the old ways when her husband became despondent; however, with the help of her son Peter, 20 years of age, and discussion of this urge to go back to taking care of everything in the therapy sessions, she was able to stop acting as a go-between for her husband and children. She was aware that she could stay out of the fray when he was angry, but she wanted to rescue him when he became despondent and protect him from having such a hard time with his children. Her son was able to help her hold off acting, and in therapy the entire family discussed the role of women as "natural" helpers and caretakers. This is not to say the family lives happily ever after; they continue to struggle and fight, however they no longer need to have a symptom to distract or speak for them.

ENDING

Therapy is recognized as coming to a close when the family come to sessions, reporting what they have done, rather than seeking answers. Ending therapy may be a time of heightened anxiety for the family, who may fear managing alone or who have loss issues in their lives. It is a time to jointly reflect back on work done and changes made. A relapse of symptoms is understood within the context of the stress of termination and is met with cautious but optimistic prediction of a return to normal eating. Therapy may be tapered off, with a final check-in session six months after active treatment is completed, or therapy may be brought to an end within the context of the normal schedule of sessions, based on what is negotiated between therapist and the family. It is important to include issues of relapse and the possibility of returning to family therapy for brief booster sessions as part of the ending process.

◆

WORKING WITH EATING-DISORDER CLIENTS IN INSTITUTIONS

Niva Piran

My experiences of working in hospitals with women with eating disorders has left me with two daunting questions that seemed to cast a dark shadow on years of effortful work: Can we, as counselors in institutions, help women heal in a way that transcends the restrictive institutional mileau in terms of gender and power, sexist values, limited awareness and sensitivity? And, what are the costs for client and counselor in working within such a context?

When one conceives of the symptoms of eating disorders as reflecting trauma to the body, either through sexual or physical abuse or other forms of abuse and alienation-inducing conditions, such as the media's abusive, aggressive, and deprecating portrayal of a woman's body, and the objectification of the woman's body by our culture, then one cannot but wonder about the potential effect of a setting where the body is controlled by the treating team, or the effect of having a physical exam being conducted by the physician who later assumes the role of the therapist. When one conceives of the symptoms as also reflecting a disturbed sense of self with associated experiences of powerlessness, helpelessness, self-devaluation, and a lack of acceptance of authentic aspects of the self (related to one's experiences within a particular familial, social, and political context), then one could wonder about the potential effect of devaluing and invalidating women's experiences, devaluing or abusing women staff, or disrupting a sense of human connection through creating a barrier between counselor and client.

My focus on institutions reflects the importance I ascribe to the context within which the counseling dyad or group takes place. The counseling relationship does not occur in a vacuum. It has been my observation that a working context which contradicts major aspects of the counseling paradigm — in this case, the feminist counseling paradigm — erodes the relationship in different ways. It disallows the important occurrence of continuity between what happens inside and outside the counseling sessions, resulting in confusion, invalidation, and frustation. It erodes the counselor's confidence, awareness, values, and beliefs through the selective dispersion of punishments and rewards to the counselor. Since the client is typically fully aware of the counselor's negotiated role within the system, as well as of the counselor's internal relations with dominant institutional values towards women, the client can detect "harmful adaptation" (Ballou and Gabalac 1985) in the counselor. Erosion in the counselor is a scary and devastating experience for the client. Such erosion is so subtle and "adaptive" in terms of inherent rewards and power structure that the counselor may not be aware of it. I have followed several colleagues whose services have been enlisted by powerful male-dominated institutions, and have been struck by the power of this process of erosion and by its often unconscious nature. No one can be immune from such a process, which requires ongoing monitoring.

Three components in a healing feminist context I value highly in my work with eating-disorder clients: a woman-centred experience involving the valuing and cherishing of womanhood and empowering women; connection from an empathic, nonhierarchial position without the "we"-"them" barrier; and the reversal of a destructive internalizing process through feminist ideology and contextual formulations. The interaction of a woman counselor's stance in relation to these dimensions with the institutional stance on these three dimensions would affect the woman counselor's experience at work, as well as the experiences of the clients.

In order to ground these observations in women counselors' experience, I decided to include in this essay a short description of women counselors' experiences of working with eating-disorder clients in four different settings. These women have all agreed to have the particular description included as part of this essay. Each counselor's story is divided into three parts: localizing the setting, the woman counselor's experience, and the counselor's impression of clients' experiences. The clients' own accounts, clearly lacking in this format, would have been invaluable for our learning.

A COUNSELING EXPERIENCE IN AN EDUCATIONAL SETTING

LOCATION

Women compose the majority of this counseling centre, which is also directed by a woman. Most counselors hold doctoral-level nonmedical degrees, and conduct demanding professional work in terms of counseling, supervision, teaching, research, and community work. These counselors as a group subscribe to feminist ideology, both in the understanding of women's issues and in the application of feminist principles within the counseling paradigm. In this setting, the continuity between the counseling office and commuity activism is particularly stressed. The health services centre, headed by a man and staffed by physicians of various specialties, provides counseling as well, through the psychiatry department. However, both the understanding of women's issues and the paradigm of counseling as practised at the health centre contrast sharply with the feminist approach of the counseling centre.

WOMAN COUNSELOR'S EXPERIENCE

The woman counselor and her colleagues have been under attack by the medical services at a personal and professional level. The attacks have been devaluing, humiliating, and at times threatening.

The counselors' competence and personal integrity have been questioned. These attacks have been made publicly and had been conveyed to clients using both services, for the purpose of discrediting the counselors. These attacks have introduced disruptions in the alliance with clients and required repair at both the personal and the ideological levels. There have been efforts to silence the counselors, for example, by silencing complaints about client experiences in the medical service (including sexual harassment) or by impeding plans for public engagements by feminist counselors.

There are important components in the setting that allow for continued noncompromising work for women's issues in a way that is ecologically safe for the counselors. The woman director of service, holding strong solid feminist beliefs, mediates the experience for the other staff. There is also an explicit ongoing discussion of the political issues leading to the character and professional assassination. This political clarity works against the destructive internalization of external pressures. The counselor said, "It makes me feel that it doesn't mean anything. I understand it means something about the power struggle. This way of undermining feminist services is a backlash against feminism at a personal level." There is a reinforcement and support between counselors. In countertransference groups, these issues are discussed, as well as in individual supervision.

COUNSELOR'S IMPRESSION OF CLIENTS' EXPERIENCES

Clients need ideological continuity whenever other services are needed, as is often the case with individuals with eating disorders who require medical monitoring. However, such continuity is hard to find. Instead, at times, clients end up subjected to revictimization or to diagnostic labeling. These experiences are destructive to the clients.

Another issue for clients is the challenge of forming and keeping the alliance with counselors; as a result of medical practitioners' stigmatization and deprecation of the service, "clients are confused, their loyalties questioned." A reported effect on the client's sense of herself when experiencing the deprecation of her women counselor is that "they question whether they can trust the women counselors" (and themselves). One could also question the effect on the client of the counselor's lack of political power, for example, in cases of client harassment or in the silencing of her voice.

A COUNSELING EXPERIENCE IN A HOSPITAL SETTING

LOCATION

The eating-disorder service is located within a psychiatry department, composed mainly of, and directed by, male physicians. In terms of the understanding, treatment, and conceptualization of the counseling relationship, the setting is antithetical to feminist principles: eating disorder is seen as a disease and the practitioner-client relationship is highly hierarchical; clinical formulations are intrapsychic and not anchored in social-political context and experience; and respected, adopted, and guiding professional knowledge is not based on women's experiences.

WOMAN COUNSELOR'S EXPERIENCE

Women counselors of various mental-health disciplines found the power structure to be abusive in many different ways; for example, their contributions and work were presented as the male psychiatrists', their powers were construed and labeled negatively, their services were devalued, their needs as women were not respected, and their voices were silenced. Barriers were erected between providers and clients, between clients, and between women counselors. Women counselors felt isolated, devalued, and angry.

COUNSELOR'S IMPRESSION OF CLIENTS' EXPERIENCES

A lot of clients' experiences had to accrue without validation before clients' histories regarding sexual abuse were listened to and addressed in treatment. Clients' internalizations of their difficulties were reinforced. Their bodies were still controlled from the outside, and they were not connected to one another in a common sense of womanhood. Rather, their interrelationships were replete with comparisons and competition.

One theme that comes through strongly in such an oppressive environment is that there is a considerable parallel in counselors' and clients' experiences. In such an environment, unless women counselors are able to unite as a group and find a way to deal with their oppression, counseling work may involve particular losses to both counselors and clients, including the restriction of important personal development and transformation.

A COUNSELING EXPERIENCE IN A WOMEN'S HEALTH CLINIC

LOCATION

The clinic, staffed, managed, and directed by women, focuses on health issues of women. The eating-disorder section had strong feminist ideology, especially regarding the oppression of women.

WOMAN COUNSELOR'S EXPERIENCE

The counselor felt that there was a particular challenge in translating feminist ideology to practice, and in training women staff. However, training was beneficial, and women physicians, as well as women from other mental-health disciplines, were ready to work closely with counselors, especially in cases of medical concerns, so as to avoid hospitalization whenever possible. The centre seemed to be particularly successful in offering consistent ideology to clients as far as dieting, weight, and control were concerned.

However, there was an irreconcilable difference in the centre between those who viewed eating disorders according to a disease model, erecting a barrier between "them" and "us," and those who supported the continuum view of eating disorders. Women who supported the continuum hypothesis were encouraging of anti-dieting groups, peer counseling and other grass-roots approaches, and were respectful of the expert viewpoint of women with eating disorders. Other women were "worried and scared" about the process of allowing greater room and power, both for clients' own voices and for counselors who held lower academic degrees but were highly competent and successful. This worry about women's grass-roots wisdom and power led to major administrative revisions, which altered and limited the service. The counselors' experience was that of loss, depression, personal isolation. Power was taken away, but not before misconstruing the counselors' competence and success negatively.

COUNSELOR'S IMPRESSION OF CLIENTS' EXPERIENCES

As did the counselors, clients felt hurt, devalued, powerless, and angry when peer counseling was not approved.

A COUNSELING EXPERIENCE IN A CRISIS SHELTER FOR WOMEN

LOCATION

A time-limited shelter for women in crisis.

WOMAN COUNSELOR'S EXPERIENCE

There was little training regarding the approach to eating disorders, and little support to staff in dealing with their own struggles around weightism and fat phobia. As a result, staff were at a loss as far as management of eating disorders was concerned, with the result that they were more controlling and punitive with women with eating disorders. There was also a greater sense of threat from the physical consequence of eating disorders than from other forms of self-harm related to the lack of familiarity, training, and support.

COUNSELOR'S IMPRESSION OF CLIENTS' EXPERIENCES

There was a risk of staff being punitive towards disordered eating, and thus a staff collusion with a past pattern of victimization.

COMMON THEMES

POWER

All counselors were accomplished in their work and had important impact within their setting. Their agency and power did not follow the hierarchy of power upheld by their institution: by being women, nonmedical, and/or nondoctoral mental-health professionals. It is therefore important to note that a process of misconstruction of their power, strength, ambition, and competence was invariably present. Backlash aimed at their power and ideology was an invariable part of their experience and occurred in political administrative, and personal venues. Susie Orbach's description (1992) of the effect of a political defeat appear relevant to the counselors' experience. Orbach described the feelings of anger, anxiety, despair, and bereavement related to the disappointed hope of political change, representation, or expression. In all counselors, one could find the hope for change and the investment in the cause aimed at women clients' well-being and the quality of their experience. All counselors, however, found ways to express their commitment and their creativity in the same or other settings.

KNOWLEDGE

For both counselors and clients, the issue of which knowledge was respected and amplified and which invalidated and silenced seemed to be an important one. Voices that were silenced were clients' voices as experts in regards to their own situation; women counselors' voices grounded in their lived experience of being women in this culture or their voices of protest regarding possible client harrassment or victimization; and theoretical knowledge derived from women-centred experience, such as the understanding of eating disorder as related to trauma (Herman 1992), oppression (Jack 1991; Steiner-Adair 1986), and suppression (Surrey 1991). In that process, women lose their authority (Young-Eisendrath and Wiedemann 1987), their confidence in their knowledge (Spender 1982). Moreover, as mentioned earlier, the women counselors did not hold the academic degrees that came with the highest power in their organization, and that was further used to question their expertise. Two of the counselors, therefore, pursued further degrees in order to deal with this political challenge, even though these degrees may add little to their relevant body of knowledge.

SELF-CARE

Working within institutions may posit particular challenges to counselors' self-care. Institutions work towards the perpetuation of their own existence, and the dissemination and transmutation of limiting images of subgroups lower in the existing power structure, such as women, is one aspect of such perpetuation (Ballou and Gabalac 1985). In addition to destructive values and beliefs, noncompliance with existing power structure is responded to by a variety of penalizing mechanisms which have both personal and economic consequences. For women counselors in institutions, any consequent compromises related to connection with and respect for their own and other women's voices and the sense of agency and power are detrimental. Psychological distress, negative self-evaluations, denial of self-identity, and arrest in the ongoing process of personal development are all possible consequences of this struggle. Just as internalized destructive images may adversely affect a woman counselor–woman client counseling process (Bernardez 1987), destructive internalized images of women may adversely affect women counselors' positions in women-governed organizations as well.

A woman counselor in institutions has to use her perceptual and intellectual abilities and her creativity to become as aware as she can of the institutionalized and upheld image and treatment of women. Many sources of information will converge to yield this type of information; for example, her own sense of well-being and self-worth while working, institutional reactions to refusal to comply with an inferior or subservient status or reaction to her power, experiences of other women in the setting and of previous employees. The greater the clarity, the easier it is to work against the internalization process, to anticipate penalizing mechanisms and possibly employ resources that could buffer these operations. It is a taxing and difficult process with no assurances of success. Maintaining this clarity and monitoring one's own reaction to the system may help prevent unconscious collusion with institutional destructive treatment of women in order to secure rewards or avoid punishment.

A woman counselor may want to use all forms of expression and creativity, private and public, to deal with her reactions to the system within which she works. She can use her agency to elicit all constructive input she can get, and make informed choices conducive to her ongoing process of personal development, including the decision to stay or leave the setting. The most important recourse is to organize or join a group of women in which the woman counselor's experience will be of connection, validation, support, self-worth, greater awareness, understanding, and a sense of collective wisdom, power, and agency.

◆

GAPS BETWEEN FEMINIST UNDERSTANDINGS OF EATING DISORDERS AND PERSONAL EXPERIENCE

Éva A. Székely and Patricia DeFazio

The important point is that *woman in contemporary patriarchal society is fundamentally identified with her body. Her body is her power.* Men are their brains; women are their bodies. Man is culture; woman is nature. Woman is Woman as Body. (Greenspan 1983, p. 164.)

The theme that runs through almost all contemporary feminist writings is women's oppression in and through our bodies. For a woman, her body has long been considered her "only real asset" and also her "greatest liability" (Greenspan 1983, p. 165). The contemporary phenomena of weight preoccupation and "eating disorders" may be the best illustrations of what a double-edged sword a woman's body has been. In this essay we describe, from our own experience and those of other women, some of the difficulties in trying to overcome the fundamental identification of ourselves as bodies. We point out a few gaps and contradictions, both within feminist analyses of eating disorders and weight preoccupation and between feminist understanding and personal experiences in struggling with or against the tyranny of slenderness.

In a graduate class one of us recently taught on gender relations, the students, ten women ranging in age from their twenties
to fifties, were asked to describe a situation in which what they
looked like really mattered. The women were also asked to describe
a situation in which they felt that their knowledge, rather than
their looks, was important. The question was phrased in such a way
that either pleasant or unpleasant incidents could have been
recounted. When they described situations in which their "looks"
really mattered, most women wrote about feelings of shame, rejection, hurt, exclusion, and painful struggle. One woman remarked
that she could not come up with a single situation, because she
always worried about how she looked. Women described comparing themselves with others they knew, or with some ideal image,
and invariably, finding that they did not measure up. Their clothes,
their hair, the shape or the size of their bodies were somehow
wrong. Compared with the culturally defined ideal of feminine
beauty, they felt inferior in relation to their appearance and insecure about themselves. As they described these incidents, the
women noted that, despite all they had learned and done in their
lives, they could not fully overcome their conditioning in today's
society .

When it came to describing situations in which they felt that
their knowledge was really important, most women said that they
had a hard time finding examples. And even in the examples they
provided for when knowledge was really important, women often
made references to their looks. They worried about whether they
looked the part they were to play, and they prepared their appearance extra-carefully. Many of them wrote about being fearful,
uncertain, and anxious about demonstrating what they knew. But
some of the women also noted feeling excited, exhilarated, proud,
and competent. They felt that they were of value, they had something to contribute and could make a difference. In striking contrast to some of the good feelings associated with situations in
which what they knew really mattered, the feelings associated with
their looks were mostly negative. Even though they knew what is

outside is not what counts, they were still gripped by the tyranny of looks.

How can the accounts of these ten highly educated feminist women be explained? Are they an anomaly among feminists? We think not. In our experience, despite our critical analyses and understanding, we are all vulnerable to the tyranny of looks. It is not unusual for feminists interested in eating disorders to refer to their own experiences of anorexia nervosa and bulimia. The references, however, point to past, rather than current, concerns and struggles, and the descriptions are often very brief. Probyn's article "The Anorexic Body" (1987) is a good example of such brief descriptions. In this article, Probyn argues that we need to return to the "everyday body," the body as we live it, yet she uses only four words — "and I became anorexic" — to refer to her own experiences (p. 112). Some of us would have liked to know more about Probyn's own experiences when she was anorexic as well as postanorexic with regard to the body. Feminists typically argue for placing the eating disorders on a continuum (cf. Squire 1984), but the sense of the continuum is lost, at times, in some of the writings. The conceptual and language schemes employed may quickly move the anorexic into the "sick" category, which severs the connections, typically brought out early in the writing, between the eating disorders and women's socioculturally constituted situations.

Feminist accounts of anorexia nervosa have suggested that, in relation to the relentless pursuit of thinness, there are two groups of women: those who fight for "feminine power" and those who "retreat from it" (Chernin 1981, p. 99). Presumably those who fight for feminine power do not become (or are no longer) anorexic, and those who retreat from it are (or may become) anorexic. This either/or dichotomy, however, does not correspond to reality. Feminists also care about their appearance. In our experience, even feminist therapists can be distressed by weight gain. There are times when a feminist may have more invested in and feel prouder of her success in losing weight than she does in regards to any of her other accomplishments. But the pride she feels may be kept private or

admitted to only the closest of friends. When feminists make reference to their recent weight gain or attempted weight loss, it is often
with a sense of embarrassment, shame, or even guilt. Many of us
are conflicted, because we are concerned with our appearance yet
view this concern as inconsistent with our feminist political consciousness.

Feminist authors discussing female development in relation to
the onset of eating disorders have noted that "a sizable number of
our young women — poor and privileged alike — regard their
body as the best vehicle for making a statement about their identity
and personal dreams" (Brumberg 1989, p. 271). Or, as Susie
Orbach (1985) put it, the adolescent girl "speaks with her body"
(p. 90). Brumberg and Orbach both suggest that there is too much
emphasis on the appearance of the body in adolescence, at the
expense of other concerns and interests. Brumberg even talks about
a "brain drain" of female intelligence and creativity that results
from excessive attention to the body (p. 275). We agree that there
have been severe repercussions for women of overfocusing on our
appearance. The point is, though, that we all "speak" with our bodies; we all use our bodies to make statements about our identities.
After all, the human body is a "communicative body" through
which the bond between self and society is created (O'Neill 1985).

The body is the most immediate means of communication we
have. "What we see, hear, and feel of other persons is the first basis
for our interaction with them," wrote O'Neill (1985, p. 22). It is
our body that others see first, and they make an initial judgement
about us based, inevitably, on our appearance. We use our bodies to
communicate to others our identities, but our bodies also become
the objects of social and individual projections about our characteristics, including our health status. Psychologists have found that we
attribute socially acceptable or unacceptable characteristics to people based on their body size. For example, when children as young
as six years of age were presented with silhouettes of overweight and
"normal"-weight people, they attributed more socially unacceptable
characteristics (such as lazy, mean, dirty, stupid, ugly) to the over-

weight than to the "normal"-weight silhouettes (Staffieri 1967). Reviewing the literature on the stigmatization of fat people in our society, Ciliska (1990) noted numerous other studies with similar findings. Fat children and adults, especially women, have been evaluated less favourably than their nonfat peers. The research results are consistent with our everyday experiences: "overweight" people, especially women, are seen as being less healthy in general and as having more psychological problems than their "normal" weight counterparts (Székely 1987, 1989).

FEMINIST VIEWS ON EATING DISORDERS

Feminists have been most concerned about anorexia nervosa because it is "almost exclusively a distress symptom associated with girls and women" and because there has been a dramatic increase in the incidence of the disorder since the 1960s (Orbach 1985, p. 83). Researchers disagree about the historical continuity of anorexia nervosa, however. Some view it as a "modern disease," a contemporary "sociocultural epidemic," or a "stylistic breakdown" resulting from recent cultural pressures for women to be thinner (Bruch 1978; Garner 1883; Levenkron 1982) and, as such, a qualitatively different phenomenon from earlier reports of the disorder. Others suggest that today's anorexics are engaged in similar struggles for autonomy and liberation from a patriarchal family and society as medieval female saints (Bell 1985). Yet another view is that the "new disease" of anorexia nervosa emerged from the economic and social transformation that took place at the end of the last century (Brumberg 1989).

Although there is no consensus with regard to the issue of historical continuity, almost everyone in the field agrees that the anorexic population has a "highly specific social address" (Brumberg 1989, p. 13). It occurs predominantly in countries or among the strata of society where food is plentiful. Anorexia nervosa is more common among populations with the highest standard of living. Furthermore, the wealthier an individual woman,

the less likely she is to be fat. Reviewing 144 published studies of
the relationship between socioeconomic status (SES) and "obesity,"
Sobal and Stunkard (1989) found that, among women in developed societies, "obesity" was least common among the higher SES.
In developing societies, obesity was rare, but its prevalence
increased with rising wealth. These observations, along with the
growing incidence of anorexia nervosa among young white women
since the 1960s, have been the bases of sociocultural and feminist
analyses in the last two decades. In formulating answers to the
question of why it is overwhelmingly women who become anorexic
and bulimic, feminists have pointed to women's devalued position,
sexism, the objectification of women's bodies in our consumer-ori-
ented society, and the perceived hostility towards everything associated with femininity (Chernin 1981; Friedman 1985; Woodman
1985). Several authors have discussed in detail Western societies'
harsh treatment of fat women (Millman 1980; Orbach 1980;
Székely 1988a, 1988b; Wooley and Wooley 1979). Issues of power
and space have been addressed as central to our understanding of
women's concerns with our weight and size. For example, Laura
Brown (1985) has suggested that women strive for a small and thin
body because it occupies a minimum amount of space. A small
woman is less visible, hence less threatening, and considered by
men as more attractive than a large-bodied woman.

Several authors have concentrated on analysing women's changing roles and women's bodies as the arena in which the conflicts are
played out and are attempted to be resolved (Boskind-White and
White 1983; Orbach 1986). Women receive conflicting messages:
to be feminine in the traditional ways and to be masculine in so far
as it is a requirement for success in roles that have been previously
closed to us. By the time women receive this double message, they
have already been made to feel insecure about their bodies. They
are dissatisfied with their appearance, which they have learned is
currency in the male realm. It has been argued that what makes
women particularly vulnerable is that they have not been taught to

recognize and identify their own needs (Orbach 1986). Utterly confused about how to become everything her mother was and wished to be, and everything that, presumably, a modern woman could and should be, she turns her attention to her body, the one aspect of her existence over which she thinks she has control. As her attention shifts towards her weight, she may become anorexic or bulimic, or a chronic dieter.

We do not yet have any well-worked-out feminist theories of the body. Nor do we have one common approach with at least a core of agreed-upon assumptions regarding the development of eating disorders. Research on adolescent female development has only recently begun (cf. Gilligan, Lyons, and Hanmer 1990). Still, feminists have made many claims about the development of eating disorders. These claims have not been critically examined, and even the most obvious gaps and contradictions have been glossed over. In the remainder of this essay we describe some of the gaps and contradictions in this body of writings.

BODY SIZE

One major issue is that of body size. Some feminist authors suggest that any size is a "good size," and the whole range of women's shapes and sizes should be portrayed in the popular media as acceptable. Some of the writings inspire us to celebrate large women in particular. We are encouraged to allow our bodies to become whatever shape and size they were "meant" to be. It is acknowledged that, for most women, the loss of the dream of her thin body is a painful experience, but it is one that she must undergo in order to liberate herself from the tyranny of slenderness and from patriarchy. In other feminist writings, we come across the notion that fat provides women with a certain kind of power, the power of safety. Fat is a shell and an armour to keep out the world by essentially desexualizing women. However, as Orbach's early accounts suggest, both for her and for the women in her compulsive eaters' groups, thin remained the privileged form; the "real self" (the "real you") was assumed to be contained in one's thin body (Diamond 1985).

According to a third view, it is desirable to be thin for health reasons. We should diet (reasonably) and work out (reasonably) to improve our physical health and our psychological well-being. As we feel leaner and more muscular, presumably, we will be stronger both in body and in mind. Our self-concept will become increasingly positive, and we will like ourselves better. Although this latter view has been clearly challenged by many feminists, it is by no means dead (cf. Székely 1987). "Even *Ms.*, which eschewed preoccupations with appearance, was conquered by this ideology. While it was one of the few magazines to defend the overweight and to argue that fat could be fit, it nonetheless endorsed the health ethic's precepts of proper diet and exercise," noted Seid (1989, p. 246). There are, of course, many nuances within each position, and variations containing elements from two or all three views. The point we want to make here is that there is not a single feminist perspective regarding acceptable, desirable, or healthy body size.

In our experience, women in particular are keenly aware of discrimination against overweight individuals. Many women tell themselves that the size of the person should not matter and we should look beyond appearance because, after all, "it's what's inside that counts." Yet, a number of women have remarked to us that they cannot help feeling compassion for a person of size. Many women have clearly dealt with their own fat phobia and prejudice, but there are others who continue to think, almost automatically, that overweight individuals would be so much happier and healthier if they lost some weight. As we have seen, the attributions that are made to overweight people are largely negative. In contrast, thinner individuals are perceived to be more attractive, energetic, and possessing the qualities that are needed to be successful.

When dining with an "overweight" person, some women continue to feel uncomfortable. They may want to give advice on how to improve her eating habits but resist the temptation to do so. Some women may avoid discussing with her their own concerns about weight for fear of hurting her feelings or for fear of being seen as prejudiced. They somehow feel she needs to be protected. Consequently, topics such as dieting, food, and the women's own insecurities regarding weight are considered by thinner individuals to be off limits. Why should women feel this way if they truly believe that the size of the person does not matter? One may say to oneself, it shouldn't matter, but it has been most women's experience that it does. When many women see a thin and fit woman they are envious and wish that they could look more like her. The woman who says to herself "If only I could lose weight and exercise more, I could have a perfect body" may even know that, for many people, being thin is not so easy. Not all bodies can be exercised and dieted down to "the perfect body." Still, the ideals and role models that have been presented to most of us in this society are thin and attractive women. They are the ones to emulate. In the 1960s and 1970s women dieted to approximate Twiggy's shape. Since the mid-1980s many women have tried to eat "sensibly" and exercise to the videos of Jane Fonda and other celebrities. There are even feminists who see "nothing wrong" with the fitness and health consciousness propagated over the last few years. They do not see the connections between fitness and health consciousness and the oppression of women in our society.

Some women argue that they strive by dieting and exercise to achieve what they perceive to be the perfect body not primarily, or not at all even, to attract men. They say, they "feel better" when they are thinner and fitter, and many claim that it has nothing to do with societal pressure. They view their weight loss as "a private, personal choice." They presumably do it all strictly for themselves (Donald 1986). Results of recent research suggest that women actually want to become thinner than men prefer them to be (Zellner, Harner, and Adler 1989). The notion that women diet and exercise simply to please themselves can be challenged easily, however. None of us grew up in a vacuum; we all learned to like or dislike ourselves through our interactions with other people. And it is through the body that one communicates one's identity. Theroux

(1982), among others, has suggested that being thinner is a way of achieving physical perfection and self-satisfaction. But it may also be a way of attempting to gain advantage in a work force where women now have to compete with one another for jobs that were previously closed to us. And women can be just as competitive, judgemental, and critical of other women as any man can be of us.

We asked women we knew personally who were previously fat and maintained weight loss for several years what life was like for them before they lost weight. The responses varied, but a few women said that their corpulence prevented them from being involved in many physical activities. They tired more quickly than their thinner counterparts. They felt very self-conscious about engaging in sports, for example, even if they were physically capable of doing so. They felt embarrassed at the thought that people might be staring at them or making fun. For these women, shopping for clothing was most frustrating and nearly impossible. They had trouble finding clothing stores that catered to the larger woman, and the stores that did cater to the large figure were extremely expensive. They thought that losing weight would liberate them from a host of physical limitations and emotional constraints they experienced. They wanted to stop feeling ashamed, humiliated, left out, and "miserable."

These women reported that, once they lost weight, they began to feel more self-confident, could now enjoy physical activities, and claimed that their sense of worth and self-esteem improved. Whether it was truly the weight loss or the compliments they received from others for "looking great" is difficult to say, but for the first time they were being noticed, complimented, and somehow the self-consciousness that had plagued them for so many years dissipated significantly. Most of the compliments these previously obese women received were from other women, which is of little surprise since women in this society cannot help but internalize the message that "thinner is better." Interestingly, when men complimented them, they did not immediately attribute the change in appearance to weight loss. Rather, they noted the woman's new hairstyle or new clothes. In contrast, women immediately attributed this change to weight loss, which is consistent with women's socially conditioned heightened awareness of our body size. The women who were previously fat felt that life was not merely easier but truly better following weight loss.

The changes women have described who maintained weight loss read like an advertisement for weight-loss programs. Our intent is certainly not to advocate such programs but to give voice to some of the women who have struggled with the tremendous social pressure to be thin and the only way they had to feel better was to lose weight. In our society there continues to be very little support for women to feel accepted, respected, confident, competent, and in control of our lives, regardless of what the scales show when we step on them. It is therefore very important that counsellors validate as real the difficulties women face when they strive to accept their bodies at whatever shape or size they happen to be.

The fat oppression so characteristic of our society today has driven many overweight women to go on diets that are not safe, to exercise until they drop, and to adopt other drastic measures of weight control that are potentially life threatening. They may alternate between restricting their food intake and eating copious amounts of food, which they then purge. Vomiting and ingestion of laxatives and diuretics can cause potassium deficiency. One woman who engaged in these purging practices and was treated for severe potassium deficiency illustrated her fear of obesity by relating an experience she had while in the hospital. A nurse that had been caring for her told of her own personal struggle with bulimia. She spoke of having undergone treatment herself in another facility. Following treatment, this nurse gained more than 100 pounds. Listening to this nurse's tale of years of unsuccessful dieting, which eventually led to an eating disorder, the patient was horrified at the thought that, if she complied with the staff's recommendations and treatment program, she too would be doomed to a life of being overweight. She told herself over and over again that she would not allow this to happen to her. The idea of becoming fat terrified her to the point that she thought she would rather be dead than become like her nurse. Even though the nurse's intention was to help, the mere fact that she had gained 100 pounds following treatment, of course terrified the patient. She admonished herself to resist all attempts to restore weight to a point that the staff deemed "healthy." The patient felt torn between wanting to stop the destructive cycle of bingeing and purging and wanting to remain thin. After hearing the nurse's story, she believed that she could not comply with the hospital's treatment without becoming fat. This fear remained with her for years, and the destructive cycle of bingeing and purging continued. Through many years of therapy and strong support from close friends and family she was finally able to come to terms with the fact that restoring weight to a level that was deemed healthy did not necessarily mean gaining 100 pounds. Slowly, she began introducing foods in her diet that had previously been absolutely forbidden. Slowly, she gained weight to a point where she was no longer emaciated and now able to come to terms with the fact that, even though she felt fat, in reality she was now at an "ideal weight" (i.e., according to health insurance charts) for her frame and height. This example illustrates that, although we know we should accept people of all shapes and sizes, and size should not matter, it might very well matter when we fear our own body may one day become fat.

Although an increasing number of men seem to be concerned about their weight and are dissatisfied with their body size, weight preoccupation continues to be more prevalent among women than men. There is a propensity to judge a woman's weight more harshly than a man's (cf. Orbach 1980; Wooley, Wooley, and Dyrenforth 1979). We are deluding ourselves, however, if we think that obese women are the only targets of discrimination. As far as some people are concerned, fat is fat, whether it is on a woman's body or a man's. There are some studies that found no difference in the severity of discrimination against obese individuals of either sex (Harris, Harris, and Bochner 1982). The results of a survey indicate that the income of male executives drops by approximately $1000 a year for every pound of "excess" weight (Ciliska and Rice 1989, p. 14). Still, the fact remains that, in our society, the overwhelming majority of people who become weight preoccupied, anorexic, or bulimic are women. This is not surprising given that the day-to-day and long-term social consequences of being fat are much more severe for women than for men.

When a therapist is working with a population that is either fat or suffering from an eating disorder, the size of the therapist may also become an issue. As Ciliska suggested in her book, *Beyond Dieting* (1990), it may be advantageous to have a fat group leader when the group is designed for women who have been fat and have found dieting to be unsuccessful. The presence of an "obese" facilitator could provide these women with a role model and help them accept that dieting may not be the answer for them. In the minds of some women, however, this attempt at providing a role model of size may be seen as a justification on the therapist's part to be fat. In contrast, having a fat therapist lead a group or work individually with anorexic or bulimic clients (of normal weight) may be problematic. These clients may adamantly refuse the therapist's interventions for fear of becoming like her. They may also be concerned that any expression of their dread and hatred of fat may offend the therapist. They may censor themselves and not discuss issues that are crucial to their well-being. If the therapist is thin and works with obese people, this client population might feel threatened and think that their struggles with weight will not be understood by someone who has not been overweight and who has never had to diet. Therapists who are thin know all too well that their clients wonder how they became and manage to remain thin.

Clearly, there is not an "ideal" weight and size for therapists working with anorexic, bulimic, or obese clients. The point is that the therapist's weight is relevant to the therapeutic process and, at least initially, the therapist's credibility may hinge on her size. The therapist's weight and size, however, are only one factor. If the therapist demonstrates openness and understanding of the client's feelings and thoughts regarding the therapist's body size, in the context

of a supportive relationship and with encouragement from the
therapist, the client will probably be able to state her thoughts and
feelings regarding this issue.

THEORY AND THERAPY

Another set of issues pertains to how feminists have explained the
development of eating disorders. As with body size, we encounter
major differences. The medical-model view of eating disorders has
been criticized for being individualizing, pathologizing, insensitive
to women's issues, and even dangerous, but a coherent feminist
alternative has not yet emerged. Parenthetically, many women writers in the humanities and social sciences also individualize, pathologize, use derogatory language, and even blame the victim. Caskey
(1986), for example, refers to the anorexic woman's "peculiar over-
sensitivity" (p.179), "visual distortion" (p.181), "cognitive retarda-
tion" (p.183), and "literal mindedness" (p.184). (For a review of
this literature, see Székely 1988a and 1988b.) Numerous explanations of anorexia nervosa borrow unexamined notions from established psychological theories and combine these with analyses of
female socialization or with essentialistic postulates about a feminine nature or self (Caskey 1986; Friedman 1985). Ultimately,
these accounts fall into either psychological or sociological reduc-
tionism. In some of the writings, the elusive concept of patriarchy
is offered as the final explanation for eating disorders (Brown
1985). The realities of living in a capitalist social system are rarely
considered in their concreteness and immediacy.

In feminist accounts that have borrowed from self-psychologi-
cal, object relations, and Jungian theories, the social character of
our existence means little more than the psychodynamics of family
relations. Instead of mapping out connections among social relations and the concrete events in the lives of anorexic or bulimic
women, family dynamics are subjected to speculation at an abstract
level. Influenced by semiotics, several authors have discussed "the
meaning" of particular behaviours associated with anorexia nervosa

and bulimia. The "hunger strike" of the anorexic is one example of this point (cf. Orbach 1986). In her book bearing the same title, Orbach writes: "A woman who overrides her hunger and systematically refuses to eat is in effect on a hunger strike .... Like the hunger striker, she is in protest of her conditions .... Like the suffragettes at the turn of the century in the United Kingdom or the political prisoners of the contemporary world, she is giving urgent voice to her protest" (pp.101–2).

In our view, it is questionable that the anorexic is purposefully refusing to eat to make a political statement. There is no doubt that her behaviour expresses something, that it is meaningful, but we doubt that a universal meaning can be associated with her food refusal. Similarly, behaviours characteristic of bulimia, such as laxative abuse or vomiting, do not reveal a single common meaning. Meaning is a product of learning and association that is coconstituted between self and others in a social world, and not a matter of *a priori* categorization. Although there are shared features of our world, we do not all live in the same environment. Furthermore, we do not simply receive and internalize meaning; we also create and externalize what something means to each of us. The same behaviour can mean a host of different things to different people, and even to the same person a particular behaviour can have different meanings at different times. We therefore reject the view that anorexia and bulimia have universal meanings.

Finally, a number of studies have reported a high incidence of sexual abuse among women with eating disorders. We must be careful, however, not to make claims that sexual abuse "causes" eating disorders. The existence of a relationship between sexual abuse and eating disorders does not indicate causality. To our knowledge, there has been no controlled research (not even critical reviews of the literature) to investigate the etiology of eating disorders from a feminist perspective.

A corollary of the lack of adequate theorizing about the etiology of eating disorders is that we cannot explain why a particular woman becomes anorexic or bulimic. How do we account for the fact that most women, even in our society, have not become anorexic or bulimic? How is it that, despite our presumably pervasive socialization into femininity, most women do not act or experience ourselves in "typically feminine" ways all the time, or even most of the time? If we all live under patriarchy, why have not the majority of women developed a severe eating disorder? From a feminist perspective, what explanation can we offer for why some "recover" from anorexia nervosa or bulimia and others do not? As therapists, we come up against these and similar questions routinely, and we each try to answer them, based on our individual and collective knowledge, but in the absence of systematic research focused specifically on these questions.

The gaps and contradictions in feminist writings about eating disorders have obvious and serious implications for what we do when we work with an anorexic or bulimic client. They want to know: "Why me?" "Why now?" "What do I do to get better?" Not surprisingly, two therapists, both calling themselves feminist, may, in fact, give entirely different messages to the client. And the client is not always female. A minority of them — that may actually be larger than thus far estimated — are men. Feminist analyses have been silent on why some men become anorexic or bulimic. What do we tell them? Or is that not our concern because they are men? Finally, we must ask, how is what we actually do in therapy different from other approaches that do not call themselves feminist? We all use a variety of theoretical notions and techniques, and we do not have a common set of values, assumptions, and practices that describe us uniquely and exclusively. There has been little dialogue, and even less self-criticism in feminist theorizing about eating disorders. We think both are long overdue.

CONCLUSION

We have felt uncomfortable about the gaps and silences in the feminist literature regarding our own and other feminist women's weight and shape consciousness in our everyday lives. That, in different ways and forms, feminists are also concerned about how they look is obvious. Even the clients are concerned about the therapist's body shape and size. With eating-disordered clients, the therapist's own weight can be an issue in therapy. The client's concerns with the therapist's shape and size can have both positive and negative implications for treatment. For example, a fat therapist can be a role model for thin clients, and a fat client may initially find it difficult to trust a thin therapist. And, similarly to everyone else, feminists cannot help but form our initial impression of others based on their appearance, including their shape and size.

Our views as feminists on the importance of appearance and everything associated with it are quite varied. As with other issues, we have a wide range of feminist analyses of eating disorders. The divergent feminist interpretations often complement and sometimes contradict one another. Paradoxically, when it comes to our own bodies, feminist therapists may be having even more difficulty than women who do not profess to be feminists because the former are not supposed to be conflicted and concerned. So feminists may whisper, deny to others or even to themselves that not all is well, that we are not entirely comfortable with our own bodies, and that we do worry about how others see us. As women who do therapy we must address our own unease regarding body size and weight.

We all know that therapy can be successful only if the goals we set are realistic. To encourage a client to become the size she was "meant" to be is a very difficult undertaking because of the pervasive fat prejudice and discrimination in our society. The example of the woman who was hospitalized with severe potassium deficiency illustrates this point clearly. Most women in this society dread the possibility of becoming fat. We feel that therapists must acknowledge and continuously keep in view the importance of social perceptions and the stigma attached to being obese. Therapists have to take very seriously the client's fear of becoming fat. With clients who have been chronically fat, therapists have to work through the loss of the dream of one day becoming thin. Loss is the most painful of therapeutic issues for client and therapist alike. In some sense, the work is always unfinished. The only real ray of hope in helping chronically corpulent clients accept their bodies and themselves is feminist psychoeducational work, both inside and outside of therapists' offices. Feminist therapists need to challenge the myths and prejudices regarding fat through public education, media watch, and other activities at the social level. Numerous opportunities exist in everyday interactions as well to challenge the tyranny of slenderness. Women need to learn to support one another in not losing weight. Rates of successful therapy outcome with chronically fat clients are likely to be low until the social perceptions change towards acceptance of all shapes and sizes, and both women and men have thoroughly internalized these changed perceptions. Feminist therapists and educators have an important role in initiating and working towards these changes.

◆

·III·

COMMUNITY
EDUCATION
AND
POLITICAL
ACTION

INTRODUCTION

CHANGING THE CONTEXT

Karin Jasper

A distinguishing characteristic of the feminist approach is its recognition of the social, political, and economic forces that constitute the context in which eating problems among women are prevalent. Helping individual women resolve their problems with food and weight is important, but equally important are addressing and changing the broader social context. This section includes essays describing the efforts of women in diverse regions of Canada to have an impact on systemic forces that act to perpetrate the pressure to be thin.

One of the subtler ways the focus on being thin has been supported is through the *absence* of non-dieting programs for large women. Two of a growing number of such programs are described here. Donna Ciliska writes about "Beyond Dieting," a group program she originated in Toronto which is designed to assist large women in getting off the diet track. Suzanne Bell describes "Fitness for Large Women," a program based in Vancouver that provides the opportunity for large women to develop fitness without focusing on weight loss.

It is critical that women who are looking for help in resolving eating problems have a choice about the approach that is taken to assist them. In Canada, the health-care system provides services at no charge, but these services do not usually represent the full range available. Catrina Brown and Robyn Zimberg describe the work of the Women's Health Clinic in Winnipeg. Its "Getting Beyond Weight" program, as well as other services, have offered women a feminist, non–medical model approach, covered by medicare, since 1985. Their approach depathologized eating disorders by placing them on a continuum of eating problems, including "normal dieting." Providing such "alternative" services under the medicare plan usually means fighting ongoing political battles.

Merryl Bear and Alisa Gayle describe another government-supported and feminist-oriented program, this time in Ontario — namely the National Eating Disorder Information Centre. Through public-awareness campaigns and public speaking, the centre's staff make links between societal oppression, women's life experiences, and food and weight concerns. Through their information and resource service, they link those looking for services with appropriate service providers. Operating within a hospital setting holds challenges a new management structure has been designed to meet.

The pressure women feel to be thin is carried by the media, and often supported by trusted professionals. Challenging their messages publicly is an important step in raising consciousness at a social level. Karin Jasper describes the work of a small group of women in Toronto who, for five years, have worked under the name "Hersize" to do just that. Speaking to groups large and small, on television and radio, Hersize members have taken a feminist approach to weight preoccupation and made information and ideas available to a wide audience.

Work is currently being done to develop systematic prevention programs from a feminist perspective. Such programs are badly needed. We look forward to the time when they can be implemented.

BEYOND DIETING

Donna Ciliska

Most women experience some degree of body dissatisfaction. A program called "Beyond Dieting" was designed for women whose weights are above the culturally prescribed norm. In most cases, these women have a long history of "yo-yo" dieting. The purpose of the program is to improve self-esteem, normalize eating, and reduce body dissatisfaction and weight and shape obsession. There is no good term to describe the weight of the women in this group. Body shape has been medicalized, but there is no universally accepted standard for what constitutes "overweight" or "obesity." The social pressure to be thin affects all women, but is most severe for women who are the farthest from the "norm." They experience the stigmatization and discrimination more acutely than women who are closer to the ideal. The medical term is "obese," and while this term will appear in this essay when I discuss the literature, "fat" and "overweight" will also be used. "Fat" is not used in the negative sense of the usual stereotype, but as a descriptive term for one who has body fat. "Overweight" is used to convey that a woman may be considered, medically, to be at an unhealthy weight, but be at a normal weight for her.

THE PROGRAM

"Beyond Dieting" began in 1985 in response to two experiences: work with women who wanted to be thinner, had tried several times to be thinner, succeeded in being thinner for a short time and, despite continuing to follow the weight-loss program, were unsuccessful in maintaining their weight loss; and a review of the literature in which it was discovered that the experience described above was the overwhelming norm rather than the exception.

In their intensive review of the literature on dieting and weight control, Susan and Wayne Wooley (1984) called into question many assumptions that have determined approaches to weight loss. They documented that treatment for weight loss is unsuccessful, primarily because of the biological control over weight. The biological factors include the genetic determination of adult weight, and the reduction in metabolic rate that results from calorie restriction. Second, they concluded that there is a lack of evidence that fatness alone is a significant health risk factor. Third, they found that the stringent cultural standards of thinness for women have been accompanied by a steadily increasing incidence of severe eating disorders. They conclude that "it is very hard to construct a case for treating any but massive, life-endangering obesity [sic]. What is needed is to vigorously treat weight obsession and its manifestations: poor self and body image, disordered lifestyles, often marked by excessive or inadequate exercise, and disordered eating patterns, metabolic depression and inadequate nutrition caused by dieting" (p.191).

"Beyond Dieting" was developed to provide an affirming *alternative* to dieting for "overweight" women. It is *not* a weight-loss program. The purpose is threefold: to improve self-esteem and body image, to reestablish normal eating, and to learn to deal with size discrimination.

The women who attend vary in age (17 to 68 years), race, cultural background, socioeconomic status, sexual orientation, education, interests, and size and shape. However, they share preoccupation with weight, shape, and food. They have tried for years to attain the cultural ideal through "yo-yo" dieting. The cycle of loss/regain has led to feelings of body betrayal ("I keep following the diet but cannot lose any more weight"), low self-esteem ("If others can do it, why can't I? I must be a worthless person"), and chaotic eating. There are two typical eating patterns. Many women diet every Monday, eating very little all week, then overeat or even binge on the weekend. Others will attempt to eat only one meal per day — usually in the evening. However, once eating starts, it is difficult to stop. There is a feeling that "I've blown it — so I might as well keep eating!". The guilt that follows leads to more severe restriction on the next cycle, and the cycle intensifies. Some women will combine these two eating styles.

"Beyond Dieting" is offered in small groups (eight to ten women) for two hours a week over a twelve-week period. The program is advertised by media articles and appearances, public-service announcements, and posters. Women call and attend an information session to determine if they are willing to commit themselves to attending the program. The group is usually quite stable, with minimal dropout. Women are not willing to participate in the program unless they have experienced repeated weight loss with regain through a variety of programs. The women who do participate are more realistic about odds against a "magic cure," and are ready to listen to a nondieting "accept yourself" message.

Each weekly session is a combination of review, information sharing, experiential exercises, and the development and sharing of support within the group. Content themes are eating, self-esteem and body image, and the societal message of thinness as the only look for women. The program content can be summarized as:

- cultural imperative for thinness in women and the subsequent fear of fat, fat prejudice, and body/weight/shape preoccupation
- effect of dieting on eating, mood, behaviour, physical symptoms, and physical measurements

– effectiveness of reducing diets
– "set-point" and the metabolic adaptations the body makes in attempt to keep one's natural weight
– process and steps to normalize eating
– treating yourself like you are "worth it" — clothing, massage
– changing body image and self-esteem
– getting life off hold "until I lose weight"
– health risks of "overweight"
– the myth of the "overweight" personality
– the benefits of physical activity
– assertiveness
– strategies to reduce eating for emotional reasons
– dealing with the loss of the dream of being thin

Time in the group is primarily focused on the issue of eating. Years of dieting have led to a dulling of participants' perceptions of hunger and satiety. The process of "normalizing" eating is most successful when done as a progression of steps, firmly establishing one stage before beginning the next. We begin by addressing the pattern of eating the women have developed. We encourage them to eat three meals, initially to retrain them to recognize hunger and satiety. If meals are more than about four hours apart, a light snack between meals is helpful to keep from arriving at the next meal feeling famished — which often leads to rapid eating, ingestion of more food than would otherwise be eaten, and bingeing.

The next step is to focus on "forbidden foods." As do women with eating disorders, "yo-yo" dieters experience extremes of thinking in relation to food — there are diet foods for eating during the period of restriction and nondiet foods for binge times. The two types of food are rarely combined in one meal. Nondiet or "forbidden" foods are those most likely to induce a binge if restricted. The notion of never again eating chocolate sets up a feeling of deprivation, which may result in an eventual binge. All foods can be fattening, and all foods can be incorporated in a way which does not lead to weight gain. All foods can be eaten in moderation. In order to be able to eat previously forbidden foods without "overeating," it is helpful to eat these only after a meal; that is, one is more likely to eat several servings of a dessert if one is hungry and eats the dessert *instead* of a meal. Initially, feelings of guilt are associated with eating forbidden foods. However, eating some of these foods regularly will prevent bingeing and allow greater feeling of control over eating.

The third stage is to focus on the quantity of food intake. As previously stated, chronic dieters lose their ability to identify satiety. Participants are encouraged to experiment in finding a quantity of food which allows them to feel satisfied but not uncomfortably "stuffed." The end of a meal should be accompanied by feelings that they could fit more into their stomach, they are no longer hungry, and they have enjoyed the food. If one eats only food that is "good for you" but not enjoyable, one will want more food in order to feel satisfied. The emotional satisfaction of food must be acknowledged and accepted. Food is very pleasurable as well as biologically necessary for survival.

The last stage of retraining eating involves the quality of intake for health. Most chronic dieters know a great deal about nutrition, and may be eating in a very healthful style. Lowering fat intake and increasing complex carbohydrates and fibre intake are emphasized, with good health and energy, rather than weight loss, as the goal.

Different people take different lengths of time to get through this process. Some might successfully navigate all four stages in six weeks, while others may take twelve weeks or longer just to establish the pattern.

Attention to body image is a major content and experiential component of "Beyond Dieting." "Body image" refers to the mental picture we have of our bodies and the associated attitudes and feelings. Most women are dissatisfied with their body size, and view their bodies as larger than they are in reality. Several features of "Beyond Dieting" strive to reduce the body disparagement felt by participants. Some of the activities include exercises, such as drawing one's own silhouette and then having someone superimpose a tracing of one's actual body on the drawing. Participants are remarkably accurate about up-down proportions, such as where shoulders, hips, waist are, but most overestimate width. Another strategy is to make a list of how the body functions. Negative feelings about body size can be overshadowed by an appreciation of how well the body functions, and all of the pleasurable things it allows us to do.

Mild exercise (such as walking, dancing, or just movement to music for 15 to 20 minutes, three times per week) is encouraged. The participants need to get over the block of associating exercise with a diet program, and shift to focusing on exercise for positive body awareness, improved self-esteem, heightened mood, and the sense of "feeling good" that it brings.

Other strategies attempt to reduce the negative messages and increase the positive messages we give to our bodies. Giving up weigh scales and tape measures diminishes the external message of "not measuring up." Other means of pampering the body are encouraged, such as massage, stretching, and relaxation.

Self-esteem is another major content and experiential component. Cognitive-behavioural strategies and experiential exercises are used to help change the participants' underlying negative assumptions about themselves as lesser persons because they do not conform to cultural expectations. Group members explore their personal strengths in the areas of relationships, personality, and skills, and focus on these instead of repeating to themselves the negative messages about their bodies. The women come into the program minimizing and discounting their strengths "because I have fat thighs," as though size cancels out any positive characteristic. However, by the end of the program, they are more likely to describe their strengths and personalities, and not consider that their size affects those. Body size becomes more objective or neutral and less emotion laden.

Much discussion centres on dealing with the cultural norm for women to be thin, on building awareness of how far the prescribed ideal for thinness is from the reality of North American woman. How can one expect to look like the ideal when the average model is now 23 percent lighter than the average North American woman? Explanations for the endurance of this thin ideal are explored.

Information is shared regarding the medicalization of fat and the knowledge that the dangers of overweight are overstated. Several factors are more important than overall amount of fat or weight in determining health risks. For example, males have higher rates of illness and death than women, and this is particularly true for the "overweight" men: weight is more of a risk factor for stroke and heart disease in men than in women. In studies of families, and twins in particular, genetic inheritance has been shown to be as important as lifestyle in determining adult weight. Location of fat (in the abdominal region) is a greater risk factor for illness and death in adults than the overall amount of fat or weight.

Assertiveness techniques and other strategies are reviewed to help women deal with their own and others' fear of fat and weight prejudice. They role-play how to deal with uninformed family members who, through concern for health or through fat discrimination, are encouraging them to lose weight. In addition, they learn to deal with people who are rude to them (commenting on what they should be eating, how they should look), who, all too commonly, deny or delay service in consumer situations.

The process of changing one's identity from "dieter" to "nondieter" is not easy. It requires inner strength and support of others. It is not a continuous upward climb, but two steps forward, one step back. One very difficult part is dealing with grieving and loss — the loss of the dream to be thin — since so much of the participants' life energy has been spent on the goal of thinness. Anger erupts at society, for the pressure to look a certain way in order to be taken seriously, and at themselves for the delay in pursuing more meaningful goals. The group support is critical at this time.

The "Beyond Dieting" program has a significant effect on participants in increasing self-esteem and normalizing eating. Dieting is abandoned, and weight preoccupation reduced. If asked if they now like their bodies, participants still reply that they would like to be thinner, but are quick to add that it is no longer their goal in life. They now have energy to pursue more important issues of self-fulfilment through relationships, creative endeavour, education, and careers.

Publications about "Beyond Dieting" (see Ciliska 1990) have allowed other therapists to have detailed information about the content and process. Feedback has been received from around North America that the program is attended by women of all weights, as weight obsession is not the province solely of fat women. It has been adopted by public-health departments for community education for adults, and adapted for teens. There is recognition that even the teen years may be too late for preventing weight/shape and food preoccupation, and work is being done to further modify the program for preteens to build their resistance to the cultural message.

Recently, the ineffectiveness and dangers of dieting and the genetic basis of weight have received a lot of coverage in magazines and newspapers. One hopes this awareness will continue to grow until the cultural standards for women are more liberal and we are able to accept a wide range of body shapes and weights.

◆

FITNESS FOR LARGER WOMEN

Suzanne Bell

In a society obsessed with thinness, the needs of large women are seldom recognized and even less often addressed. A culture that has wholly embraced the media stereotype of the "beautiful body" sees the large women as having only one need: the need to get thin. Living a happy, successful life in a large body has not been considered a viable option; not by society and not by large women themselves. A fat woman aspiring to fitness would be generally regarded as a dreamer, indeed! Back in the early 1980s, "fat and fit" was a concept more likely to evoke ridicule than encouragement.

Coming to recognize fitness as a desirable and achievable goal for large women was not an overnight revelation. For me, it was a process that began more than a decade ago. Developing specialized fitness classes to further this goal, and working to combat the attitudes that inhibit its achievement, have been my focus for the past dozen years.

In 1981, I joined "Large As Life," a nonprofit organization whose motto was "Stop postponing your life until you lose weight and start living now!" At this stage in my career, it was a message I needed to hear. The founder and president of the group was Kate Partridge, a clinical psychologist who had developed the concept that large women needed to get on with their lives — to stop dieting and start exercising. The fitness program she envisioned for large women would include a safe, caring environment and, ideally, a qualified instructor. "Fat chance" was the general prognosis given such a proposal at the time.

As fate would have it, my "leadership potential" was spotted soon after I joined the organization. Before I knew what had hit me, I was being sent for training to become the first-ever fat fitness instructor! There I was, moving into the forefront as a fat woman — a prospect that scared me half to death. Imagine walking "large as life," into a YWCA class of 50 hardbodies and declaring your intention to train as a fitness leader. In 1981, when only the most perfectly endowed dared cross the threshold to teach, my audacity was, to say the least, unprecedented. Today, it is not uncommon to see fitness leaders of all shapes and sizes teaching specialized classes, but back in the dark ages, such diversity was unheard of. Well, not to be deterred by such minor considerations as abject terror, I proceeded with my leadership training at the "Y" in Vancouver. Fortune smiled on me, in the person of Debbie Harris, an enlightened instructor for her time. Luckily for me, and thousands of large women in years to come, she thought the concept was terrific. Her wholehearted support in that class was instrumental in my initial success.

During the forty-hour span of the training course, I learned several important lessons. First, I was much more fit than I would have given myself credit for. Second, I was able to bring more confidence and fun to my training role as an instructor than many of my superfit classmates. I also came to the realization that there needed to be much more information made available to women about living large in a thin society. By the time I finished the course, I felt the educational process had been somewhat reciprocal. Not only had I learned a lot, but I also felt I had caused some mainstream fitness types to see fat people in a new, more positive light. An outline of my future role (roles?) was beginning to form.

When I completed my training, passing with flying colours, two things happened. I started teaching immediately, and I was asked by Debbie Harris to return to the next training session to speak on the issue of fitness for large women. These two events shaped my career for many years to come.

I will never forget my first year of teaching. I was lucky to team up with Joan Del Santo, who had finished her training just as I did. Word traveled fast that two large women were teaching fitness at the community centre — and in hot pink tights, no less! Enrolment in the class trebled overnight.

There were no hard data available at this time to guide us in designing a fitness program specifically for large women. (Such data are still lacking — "fat and fit" does not seem to be a high-priority subject for study in the scientific community.) Going on gut instinct, personal experience, and common sense, Joan and I worked at adapting a program that was achievable and fun. As we saw it, the biggest obstacle to a large woman participating in fitness class was the looming spectre of failure. We worked hard that year to perfect a program that would meet all the needs of the large participant. We developed the idea and began team teaching in our class, long before it was used in the mainstream.

It is worth noting that the fitness industry was still in its infancy in 1981. It has gone through many changes since then, and continues to evolve to meet the changing demands of consumers and to reflect advances in knowledge about the body and how it works. Keeping current with new findings, and modifying our classes accordingly, remain an ongoing priorities for large-size fitness as well.

When we were starting out, a major concern was how the cardiovascular component of a fitness class would affect the large body. "Experts" has expressed concern that large women might collapse during a heavy cardio workout. We could see the validity of this concern if a large women (or anyone, for that matter) suddenly jumped up from a sedentary lifestyle and began working out at a maximum training rate. Common sense indicated that this hazard could be avoided by a careful and gradual approach to increased activity. Another safety feature we introduced was to teach participants to calculate and monitor their own heart rates. This allowed them not only to gauge the efficiency of their workout, but to take responsibility for their own safety as well.

In that first year, we worked on a warm-up concept that covered locomotion and stretching. One of our major objectives was to make our participants feel comfortable and safe right from the beginning. This goal was realized with humour and a lot of chatter, backed by upbeat, motivating music. The cardio portion of the class was, and still is, a no-bouncing, no-jumping, no-running workout with the heart-rate calculation used when applicable. (The standard we use is 200 minus your age maximum and 170 minus your age, as a minimum.) Besides its safety advantages, the beauty of this program is that it is immediately achievable for almost all participants. Teaching a participant to be responsible for her own safety is an important key. Education and communication can work wonders! Most adults respond positively when you explain that they are the only ones who can truly know if they are working too hard or not hard enough. This segment also included power walking, simple dance steps, knees up, and, of course, lots of combinations. In the beginning, cardio was 15 minutes long; today we are at 20–23 minutes. The type of cardio we teach allows participants to self-pace. Our team-teaching policy offers a comfort level and choices, as well as a non-competitive atmosphere. In our classes instructors say things like "Don't worry — this isn't a 'Get Fit In One Class' program" and "Is anyone watching what her neighbour is doing? No? Well, chances are she's not watching you either." Participants will look around and laugh, realize that no one is judging their performance, and relax into their own workout. A brief cool-down followed the cardio portion of a class. We took at least five minutes to strut around the room to funky music before we got a mat and took to the floor.

Over the years, the floor-work part of the session has undergone the most changes. The industry in general has moved towards a joint rotation practice that is ideal for large women. The basic concept is not to overwork any one joint or muscle at one time. For instance, you may do 20 pushups, then move to another muscle group before coming back to do more pushups. In the past, it was common to group all pushups together, resulting in joint overload, especially for large women. Futhering our concern for safety, our classes use peekups instead of sit-ups, and we avoid any unsupported forward flexion. Many exercises are modified to accomodate the large body, and we are particularly careful of any movement that could compromise the back.

Another concept we have stressed all along in our program, especially for beginners, is the importance of making a six-week commitment to get through the initial stages of becoming active. The first class feels great; the second seems harder; and so do the next few, as the muscles adjust. It seems that, with twice-weekly workouts, the six-week mark is the point where a beginner has worked past all the glitches and has a better chance of making a long-term commitment to fitness. Our participants do not usually have stiff muscles. Our long warmup to begin with, and the cooldown and stretching exercises to conclude, help to avoid this.

Hundreds of women over the years have come up at the end of a workout to tell us how relieved and grateful they were to be able to "do" the class. Many told of trying other classes, supposedly for beginners, where they could not keep up. It has also been my personal experience, that many so-called beginners' classes are sadly misnamed. The double whammy of failing at a beginners' class is that there is seemingly nowhere to go from there. It is still a pet peeve of mine that "beginners' classes" are too often inappropriately designed and paced, and are taught by instructors who have no concept of a beginner's needs or capabilities.

Though the number of women who were unable to "do" our class seemed small, over the years it became clear that we needed a very specialized class for women who were starting at the prebeginner level. We attracted women who had suffered previous injuries, those who felt they were hopelessly uncoordinated, and many who had been inactive for years and lacked confidence in their ability to participate in a fitness class. The great popularity of this class confirmed the need for it. It's a concept that could well serve to fill a gap in mainstream fitness as well.

I taught this class myself, and of all the thousands of classes I taught over the years, it was my favourite. There was a great sense of satisfaction in seeing so many women regain their confidence, as well as their fitness, and move on to our regular classes. For an instructor, it was a demanding assignment — lots of patience, kindness, and humour required — but very rewarding as the results were almost invariable positive. We laughed a lot in this class, and newcomers always seemed to feel welcome. We shared a lot of ourselves with each other, with everyone gaining in the exchange.

One other aspect of our program that has earned many expressions of appreciation from our participants is our concern for their safety. Many women have tried other classes where this did not seem to be a priority.

In the dozen years, since we started teaching fitness to large women, there have been many changes, both in our class structure and in our participants. The fact that literally thousands of large women have taken the plunge and started getting active has produced some very significant results. Having gained confidence in their physical abilities, many of these women ventured on to other activities they would never have dared to try before. Our alumni can be found in jazz dance, tennis, canoeing, cycling, and volleyball, to name just a few successful endeavours. One very large woman was even so bold as to take up riding white-water rapids. Many of our participants noticed positive effects on their health. Blood pressure was lower. Insulin users were decreasing their dosages. Resting heart rate slowed to healthier levels. Many women experienced an overall feeling of wellness. Many of our participants noticed positive changes in body shape. Some have gone on to mainstream classes where they have been able to modify the program to meet their comfort and safety needs.

One question I am asked every time I speak on this subject is "Do your participants lose weight?" My answer is that weight loss has never been the focus of our classes, nor our philosophy. We are not connected with, nor do we espouse, any weight-loss plan. Our purpose is to offer large women the opportunity and motivation to achieve fitness with the body they have. The reality is that most of our participants come to us initially at the same time they are starting a diet. Our biggest challenge is to keep them involved in fitness long after they fall off the diet. Some do lose weight, particularly if they are dieting, and often they drop out of fitness. But the unfortunate truth is that, in almost all cases, the weight comes back, especially if a fitness regimen is not maintained.

Convincing large women to make some form of regular physical activity a permanent addition to their lifestyle is not easy. But it is a challenge that can be met, particularly with specialized programming. The hundreds of women who started with us in the 1980s and have stayed active over the years are the best proof of this.

The impact of our fitness classes had also reached far beyond their effects on our participants. When we are working out in the community centres, we are a highly visible presence, and before long we are accepted as part of the community. People start referring relatives and friends to our classes. Seeing large women in such active physical roles has, in my opinion, had a subtle but positive effect on the collective consciousness, creating a tiny erosion of the "fat phobia" so ingrained in our culture. The exposure has resulted in media coverage of the "fat and fit" issue, leading to greater public awareness on the subject. Media attention has also stimulated interest across the country, inspiring other large women to start classes and programs in their own communities. For anyone who might be motivated in this direction here are a few points to consider: (a) use large instructors and limit participants to large-size women only; (b) take a leadership training program (YWCA or private); (c) check to see if there is a governing agency responsible for fitness certification in your province or state — you will want to be accredited; (d) A community centre — often they work on a contract — is a good place to start a class, but plan far in advance as they have early deadlines.

The fitness instructor herself is probably the single most important factor in the success of our classes. The job requires a high degree of physical ability coupled with exceptional interpersonal skills, exceeded only by a heroic dedication to the cause. It's a combination that is hard to find, and even harder to maintain. British Columbia has a provincial registration program for fitness instructors, with which we have always voluntarily complied. Also, we teach in some community centres that require provincial certification. This program includes a 40-hour training course, recognized by the governing BCRPA (British Columbia Recreation and Parks Association), as well as current CPR, a written examination, and teaching evaluation. Our instructors receive further specialized training after they have completed their BCRPA requirements. We find it takes a few months before they are ready to teach on their own.

Team teaching has served us well as an excellent vehicle to introduce a new instructor to a class. It is also an efficient method of addressing the problems of a multilevel fitness class. Whether or not a class is designated as such, it is crucial for an instructor to be aware that *all* classes are composed of individuals at varying levels of fitness and ability. A good leader will be tuned in to the fact that not all participants are created equal, and will be prepared to offer options to meet a range of needs. A major note of caution here — never, *never* make assumptions about fitness levels based on a person's appearance. Let me illustrate the importance of this.

The young woman who entered our fitness centre one day was very angry. She had, she told us with high indignation, just been insulted by a fitness instructor at another centre. This woman had been attending our classes regularly for about a year and had achieved a good fitness level.

That morning, a friend had invited her to come to her fitness class for a workout. She told us that, before the session started, the instructor had walked directly to her through the crowd and asked, without preamble, if she had checked with her doctor about the advisability of participating in the class. Embarrassed and humiliated, she had mumbled a reply that didn't satisfy, but at least got rid of, the offending instructor. She proceeded to do the class while fighting back the tears. This particular participant weighed about 200 pounds, and the leader in question had made a judgement about her which was not only inaccurate, but insulting and degrading.

What I really want to say about this incident (we've heard many variations on the theme) is that not all large participants are unfit — nor are they all fit. Like all fitness classes, ours are attended by people working out for the first time in years (or ever!) and by those, like the young woman above, who are advanced in their fitness level. We, as instructors, cannot assume people have, or have not, attained a certain level of fitness just by looking at them. So, how do we address the problem of teaching participants at diverse levels of fitness in the same one-hour class?

Two instructors working together can also avoid the problem of participants doing only what the instructor does, no matter what options he or she may offer verbally. Two instructors are right there, demonstrating different levels of movement, without ever having to say "this is the higher level" or "lower level" move. As a matter of fact, we try never to use such phrases; instead, we say things like "you can do this — or this."

We want our participants to take responsibility for themselves. After all, we don't know what their heart rates are, or how they feel. It is time we stopped being so maternal or paternalistic with fitness participants. While we must continue to maintain control of the class overall (much easier with two instructors), it is better, and even safer, for the individual participants to control their own workout.

Team teaching has other benefits, including some for the instructor. It raises the energy and interest level of the class, which can certainly make it more fun to teach. It helps reduce instructor "burnout syndrome," by giving the leader someone with whom to share the actual teaching responsibilities, and also someone with whom to compare notes. We have found our "teams" become just that — even instructors who have not had much in common before teaming up form a good bond.

The instructors who will not enjoy team teaching are those who are looking for centre stage. We all know them — the "performers," those whose egos require the fawning adoration of their participants. They will probably not be interested in sharing star billing with another instructor. Too bad. Teaming up adds a great new set of challenges and opportunities to the teaching experience.

What are those challenges? Well, you can't just get out there with a stranger and team teach. You have to do a little work together. You have to plan your class. I'm not saying you have to choreograph each step, but you must have an idea of the flow the class will take, and the confidence of having worked with your partner enough to have a general notion of where he or she is going next.

Team teaching works best in the cardio segment of the class. We often have only one instructor up front for warmup and the other acually in the class, maybe even at the back. During cardio, two instructors can have a lot of fun. With one at the front and one at the back, they can turn a class around and give a good sense of movement in what may be a small or crowded space. With both instructors side by side and up front, doing two levels of movement, we do what I mentioned earlier: give the participant a choice. If the instructors are actually demonstrating the movements, the participant is more likely to try them both and then choose the one best suited to his or her individual fitness level. During the floor work, we have one leader doing technique checking, something we all know is difficult for a single instructor to manage, and yet very, very important in a multilevel class.

I would just like to remind all instructors that, if you decide to introduce team teaching to your class, it shouldn't come as a surprise to your participants. Tell them, before the class, what you are going to do, how it works, and why you are doing it. Whether you are team teaching or not, it is always a good idea to arrive for your class a few minutes early. This gives your participants an opportunity to ask you questions or tell you of any concerns they may have. Best of all, it gives you an opportunity to confirm the theory that not all participants are created equal — thank goodness!

◆

"Getting Beyond Weight": Women's Health Clinic Weight Preoccupation Program

Catrina Brown and Robyn Zimberg

In 1985, the Women's Health Clinic in Winnipeg began an innovative program for women preoccupied with weight. Not only was this the first feminist program in Canada within a women's organization to deal with women's weight and shape issues from a woman-centred perspective, but it dealt with eating disorders as part of a continuum of weight preoccupation. It began to develop non-pathologizing ways of working with anorexia and bulimia. Central to this program was the fundamental belief that the "tyranny of slenderness" was oppressive to women. It was understood that women spend an inordinate amount of time, energy, and money in the pursuit of thinness, too often risking their health in the process. The program emphasized a nondieting, non–medical model approach, encouraging women to accept their bodies and themselves as they are.

We are writing about the program from our experiences as participants in the origin and development of the program. Catrina was the founder and initiator of the program. She coordinated the program for the first two years, doing work that included group facilitation, peer counseling, health education, outreach, and the development of a manual entitled *Getting Beyond Weight: Women*

Helping Women. Robyn has worked in many capacities in the program, including support group coordinator and facilitator, peer counselor, workshop facilitator, and community educator. She is currently the coordinator of the volunteer speakers program. Peer counseling and group practices are described in detail in the manual.

Perhaps what is unique about this program is the recognition that the proliferation of anorexia nervosa and bulimia among women could not be separated from the experiences most women have with their bodies in Western patriarchal society. Rather than understanding anorexia nervosa and bulimia as diseases, this program was based on the belief that these problems had to be understood in the context of a society obsessed with thinness, and on the philosophy that there is a continuum of weight preoccupation in which controlling weight is one way — albeit a precarious one — for women to feel more in control of their lives.

Recognizing that these problems exist on a continuum not only served to depathologize and demedicalize women's experiences with our bodies, but suggested that a feminist approach to therapy needed to be developed. It further meant that we needed to challenge the belief that women have to be thin to have social value. In addition to offering a feminist-therapy approach to working with women preoccupied with weight, this program was active in community education in an attempt to politicize these issues, to educate women about these issues, and to advocate a life free of weight preoccupation based on self-acceptance.

The Women's Health Clinic is an alternative health centre which offers nonjudgemental, women-centred health services. It emphasizes prevention, education, and informed choice. It is involved in public advocacy on health issues of concern to women, and health education to community and professional groups. The Women's Health Clinic also provides training for volunteers, and placements, training, and experience for students. Physicians, a nurse practitioner, a nutritionist, counselors, health educators, and client service workers comprise a multidimensional team who work together to provide woman-centred care to women. They offer a range of services, including individual care for pregnancy testing, unplanned pregnancy, birth control, post-partum stress, sexually transmitted diseases, AIDS testing and counseling, smoking-cessation groups, a teen clinic, and services for such health issues as PMS, menopause, and weight preoccupation.

The Women's Health Clinic has been involved in the "Getting Beyond Weight" program since 1983. Before the program formally began in 1985, significant work had already been done. Catrina approached the Women's Health Clinic in Winnipeg with a proposal to initiate and coordinate a woman-centred program for women preoccupied with weight. She subsequently worked alongside Marilyn Wolovick to develop a funding proposal for submission to the federal government's Health Promotions Directorate. [1]

In 1984, Catrina began co-facilitating support groups, and at the 1984 annual conference on women's health issues organized by the Women's Health Clinic, Catrina presented a talk entitled "The Tyranny of Slenderness." This event was extremely well attended, which provoked a great deal of interest in the program as well as considerable controversy. The then radical claims made by Catrina that the tyranny of slenderness is oppressive to women and that, instead of dieting, women should be encouraged to accept ourselves as we are, generated a significant amount of media attention. [2]

Through the process of writing and researching a Master's thesis in sociology on women's preoccupation with weight, Catrina became increasingly dissatisfied with traditional approaches to eating disorders and weight preoccupation, which pathologized and medicalized women's experiences. Clearly, women's experiences were not being heard. The accounts provided in the traditional literature and in mainstream therapy strategies focused on changing behaviour rather than on understanding the meaning and significance of behaviour. Medical-model literature and therapy addressed "obesity" as a disease, with an emphasis on weight loss, and the prevailing assumption was that fat was unhealthy. Underlying this work was the belief that fat women lacked will power, and were lazy and ugly, in addition to being unhealthy. These critiques resulted in Catrina's conceptualization of a woman-centred program for the continuum of weight preoccupation and eating issues experienced by women.

Popular weight-loss organizations and professionals working in the area of weight control not only perpetuated many myths about weight and eating but also promoted the idea that women must be thin in order to like themselves. In doing so, they reinforced the stigma associated with fatness and made women feel like failures. These "helpers," including dieticians, doctors, nurses, gym teachers, fitness instructors, and weight-loss counselors, appeared to be unable to examine critically the assumptions underlying their ideas about weight control, and even more unable to prevent their own "fat-phobia" and fat hatred from influencing the way they treated women who came to them for help. Women who already felt too fat, and were aware that society devalued them for being so, were chastized repeatedly by these so-called helpers. They were told in disapproving, moralistic, and often punitive tones that they would be happier thinner and that they should lose weight. Over and over again, the pain women felt being fat in our culture was only made worse by those trying to help: weight-preoccupied women seeking help were all too often revictimized.

The Women's Health Clinic sought to provide a service to women that challenged this approach, critically examining the underlying assumptions of weight control that have permeated our culture for so long. We asked, is it really true that fat is, in and of itself, unhealthy? We asked whether a truly feminist approach to women's well-being ought to encourage women to be preoccupied with weight and thereby sanction and reinforce society's obsession with slimness. The program chose to politicize the "tyranny of slenderness" and sought to provide the opportunity for women to empower themselves to be free from endless policing, self-denial, and constraint.

Women in the program were encouraged to explore the origins of their own weight preoccupation, and to discover whether they could learn to feel good about themselves, regardless of their body size. The program emphasized the importance of women learning to be in touch with their feelings and needs. We understood that it was critical that we not reinforce and perpetuate fat-phobic myths by assuming that women who are fat necessarily have a problem, eat "emotionally," eat more than a thin person, or want to lose weight. However, most women who chose to be a part of the program were able to begin to discover what was making them dissatisfied, what they needed in their lives, and to look at ways of empowering themselves to make changes they desired.

There were several features unique to this program. Of note was the way a group of women, including a nurse practitioner, medical practitioners, a dietician, community educators, peer counselors, and group facilitators, worked together to provide a comprehensive service for women within a feminist organization. Women were not weighed. They were never told what they should weigh, or to lose or gain weight. Instead, the staff at the Women's Health Clinic focused on what women themselves wanted and needed.

The program developed new ways of understanding and working with women who were anorexic or bulimic. Consistent with the clinic's overall woman-centred, non–disease model approach to women's health was the belief that forceful or coercive approaches to working with eating disorders were harmful. We did not believe that hospitalization was necessary for most women, and we believed that medical problems which resulted from an eating disorder could be dealt with more effectively most often on an "outpatient" basis. Because the Women's Health Clinic program had a team of helpers that included people with medical training, this approach worked effectively. In the time that we have worked at the clinic, not one woman has ever required hospitalization for her eating disorder. For more than six years in private practice, Catrina has also found this to be true.

The Women's Health Clinic program provided peer counseling, support groups, and nutritional and medical support where necessary. The focus was on helping women with eating disorders to figure out why they needed this "coping" strategy in their life, and to begin to develop self-esteem and to feel empowered enough to find alternative ways of coping. Not all women will decide to give up being weight preoccupied, and this is their choice. It was realized that women need to feel both safe and ready to let go of their anorexia, bulimia, or emotional eating. Moreover, the direction and timing of counseling must be determined by the woman. Women who were anorexic or bulimic were able to make changes around self-starvation, bingeing, and purging, by taking very slow, very tiny, baby steps, which felt safe. The program did not emphasize weight, or eating; instead, it focused on the meaning of the behaviour, body image, empowerment, and emotional needs.

The groups have included all women on the continuum of weight preoccupation, including anorexics and bulimics. These groups are now offered to approximately ten women, over a period of ten weeks, twice a year. They cover such issues as eating behaviour, body image, anger, self-esteem, control, relationships, communication, family of origin, abuse, sexuality, and psychoeducational material around dieting mythology. Methods of working include visualization, psychoeducation, journaling, small-group exercises, consciousness raising, roleplays, vignettes, and art work.

The philosophy of the program is based on an understanding of the social context of weight preoccupation, and, therefore, psychoeducation is often central in addressing issues, especially around dieting and weight control. Staff have been educated on the issues, and try to be consistent in putting forward an anti-dieting, body self-accepting message, and to address their own personal relationships to weight and shape issues and prejudices.

At this time, the the Women's Health Clinic continues to offer a variety of services to women, including group and individual counseling, nonjudgemental and respectful medical care, nutritional counseling, and community education. Originally the program was conceptualized as a grass-roots program where women used their own experiences and skills to support and assist other women through the healing process. This was done through a peer-counseling model which emphasized women taking control of their own healing and demedicalizing the treatment of eating disorders. Since 1991 the program has become more "professionalized" as the counseling services are being offered by more traditionally trained clinic staff.[3] As the clinic has employed therapists, the program has become less dependent upon trained peer counselors. The work that continues to be done on a peer level is community education. Over the past 2 years a considerable amount of energy has been invested in education within the school system, providing a crucial preventive service. Trained volunteer speakers facilitate discussions with young women from Grade 5 through Grade 12.

The program no longer has a program coordinator to organize and pull together a vision and direction for the program. However, the clinic remains committed to working with weight preoccupation as many of the clinic staff are involved in the weight-preoccupation program within the context of their own roles at the clinic.

Women's experiences are real and significant, regardless of where they appear on the weight-preoccupation continuum. Women who experience anorexia, bulimia, feelings of being trapped in a cycle of dieting, and the discrimination of living in a fat-phobic society often experience tremendous pain. While anorexia and bulimia are extensions of the common experience women have with their bodies and eating in a weight-obsessed society, they are not merely instances of dieting gone crazy. Women who adopt anorexic and bulimic behaviour are using their bodies and eating to work through a number of often complex emotional issues and needs. They are not self-centred, narcissistic, or irrational, as some would have it. Rather, they are speaking with and through their bodies about their pain and their needs. Feminist programs such as the weight-preoccupation program at the Women's Health Clinic provide an atmosphere of support and caring to women that facilitates a healing process which empowers women.

Like all new programs, especially those that challenge firmly embedded social values such as thinness, and traditional modes of therapy in which the therapist maintains most of the power and control, the Women's Health Clinic program was initially met with suspicion by some and welcomed by others. Some were unclear what a feminist perspective on these issues meant, and some were threatened by criticisms of traditional approaches. Not everyone was equally committed to an anti-dieting approach or to allowing anorexic and bulimic women the same opportunities for choice that women receiving counseling in other areas were given. But, today, almost ten years later, the clinic has disposed of all its weigh scales but one, which is used only when the client insists. Clients are not weighed in routine examinations. And the dietician does not give out "diets." These examples indicate the way the approach has permeated the entire clinic. Over the past decade, the Women's Health Clinic has provided necessary, important, and pioneering services to weight-preoccupied women. During these years, commitment to a feminist approach to working with weight preoccupation has grown alongside a feminist understanding of the issues.[4]

◆

NOTES

1. Marilyn Wolovick was central in getting this program off the ground and facilitated the first group with Catrina. As a staff person of the Women's Health Clinic, she served as an important liaison between Catrina and the clinic in the early stages, and strongly advocated the need for the program within the clinic. Margaret Clark, of the Health Promotions Directorate in Winnipeg, was also very supportive of the program and provided tremendous encouragement in securing funding. Additionally, the program was housed in the Women's Health Clinic, which provided it with significant credibility in the community.

2. Catrina was involved in outreach across Canada, producing materials such as pamphlets, and a manual entitled *Getting Beyond Weight: Women Helping Women* (1987), designed to help others interested in starting a woman-centred program for women preoccupied with weight.

3. This is simply an observation of some of the changes that have occurred as the program has evolved over time. It is interesting to note that this pattern of professionalizing women's organizations can be seen in many other agencies as well. One might question whether we have now created yet another elite group of experts who have harnassed control of knowledge and expertise. While we should examine this question, it is clear that feminist knowledge and skill differ from those of traditional experts. Feminist practitioners are conscious of the issues of power and control in a way that traditional practitioners often are not. Moreover, in feminist practice, clients are seen as their own best experts.

4. We would like to thank all women who have contributed to this program over the years, in particular the volunteers. It has taken a long time for these issues to be taken seriously as feminist concerns and we thank those who supported the need for this kind of work when most people did not, especially Lynn Crocker and Marilyn Wolovick. We learned the most from working with the women in the program and listening to the truth in our own personal experiences.

THE NATIONAL EATING DISORDER INFORMATION CENTRE: A PROFILE

Merryl Bear and Alisa Gayle

The National Eating Disorder Information Centre (NEDIC) was the first centre of its kind to be established in Canada. It continues to offer a unique service to people experiencing eating problems, family and significant others, educators, students, professionals, and laypeople. Recognizing the links between societal oppressions; women's life experiences; and food, weight, and shape issues has been integral in determining NEDIC's focus. With our description of the philosophy and practices of our Centre, we hope to provide an understanding of the nature of our work as a feminist agency. It is also our wish that these descriptions reflect the challenges we experience in working to dispel the pervasive myths and misperceptions about women's bodies which are embedded in our culture. This includes addressing the link not only between women's self-esteem and our physical being, but also between societal oppressions; women's life experiences; and food, weight, and shape issues. Understanding women's experiences within this cultural context has been an essential part of determining the focus of NEDIC. As we strive to deepen our analyses and improve our services, we recognize that this is the basis on which to begin to change both our experience and the perception of our bodies as the site of our resistance and our defence.

HISTORY AND SERVICES

The National Eating Disorder Information Centre (NEDIC) has been functioning as a community-based service since December 1985. As with most such service organizations, NEDIC has a history formed by the motivation and energy of a small group of advocates determined to raise the profile and meet the needs of people who are often casualties of a misinformed and unaware society.

A national needs assessment was undertaken in 1983 by the Health League of Canada. It resulted in a proposal to the Health Services and Promotional Branch of Health and Welfare Canada for initial funding of an eating-disorders information centre which would also focus on social and cultural factors that influence health-related behaviour of women. Funding for a two-year period began in October 1985. A telephone information and support line was established, while other activities included publication of informational materials, arranging public-speaking engagements, the establishment of a support group for people with anorexia or bulimia, compilation of an in-house national register of professionals and agencies serving people with eating problems, and sponsorship of the "Beyond Dieting" program.

On the collapse of the Health League, and with the exhaustion of funding from Health and Welfare, NEDIC was provided with sponsorship by Toronto General Hospital and moved onto their premises. The Centre sought and obtained provincial funding through the Community Mental Health Branch of the Ministry of Health. With a greater sense of the security of the agency, energy was channeled into a consolidation of the services provided by NEDIC.

In 1988, NEDIC made the first step towards concerted Canadian involvement in the international movement to increase awareness of eating disorders. Ongoing sponsorship and coordination of the Canadian Eating Disorder Awareness Week (EDAW) became another NEDIC function. Across the nation, with the assistance of NEDIC, events were hosted to provide up-to-date information and to garner public attention around the issues of eating disorders.

"Thinness isn't the answer ... It's what's inside that counts" and "Taking up space in a slender society: Celebrating our natural sizes" became slogans for Eating Disorders Awareness Week (EDAW). NEDIC's focus and intent around EDAW is to make connections between women's lived experiences and food, weight, and shape issues, across race, class, and other divisions.

From its inception, NEDIC has been devoted to contextualizing problematic eating behaviours. Over the years a number of innovative events have been organized under the auspices of EDAW. The links between rigid sex-role stereotypes, cultural constraints placed on women, and the narrow images of women portrayed in the media, and the continuum of problematic perceptions of food and weight were made increasingly explicit as the political consciousness of NEDIC staff members grew. NEDIC became increasingly responsive to the material conditions of women in the community, and began extensive networking with other organizations devoted to the eradication of the sociopolitical inequities experienced by women. At this time, close links were forged with the feminist community. Sharing of knowledge and ideas with these groups and organizations helped to inform NEDIC's understanding of the direct connection between eating disorders and women's experience of all forms of physical, psychological, and sexual violence. Simultaneously, NEDIC heightened awareness in the feminist community of the continuum of women's food, weight, and shape problems as a cultural and political oppression.

There has been increasing awareness of the interrelationship between diverse aspects of women's lives and the compulsion of the large majority of women to play out their emotional distress through both continued objectification of their bodies and chaotic eating patterns. This led to NEDIC staff members' increased incorporation of feminist philosophy and principles in our work, which is reflected in the direction and focus of NEDIC's public outreach events and materials, and our closer ties with other community agencies. It is particularly evident in the issues raised in the *NEDIC Bulletin*. These range from a challenge to diagnostic labeling, the concept that problematic eating behaviour is a response to a "food addiction," and an attempt to be as inclusionary as possible with regard to issues of sexual orientation, physical ability, race, class, and culture.

In 1991, increasing articulation of an holistic feminist perspective challenged the medical/psychiatric model with regard to such things as diagnostic labeling and "treatment." Subsequent to crises related to philosophical differences between NEDIC and some members of the hospital's staff — including concern that restructuring within the hospital would make NEDIC increasingly vulnerable to control by the Department of Psychiatry, and continued financial constraints — a new structure for the management of NEDIC was devised.

Procedures and processes were designed to ensure that NEDIC policy and functioning would be determined by the needs of the community it serves (a requirement of its funding body, the Community Mental Health branch of the Ontario Ministry of Health. Given its sponsorship by The Toronto Hospital, NEDIC remains fiscally responsible to a hospital-appointed administrative director. Autonomy of philosophy and day-to-day management of NEDIC was deemed to be protected by this structure. It is currently being tested to determine its efficacy.

As NEDIC began to address eating disorders as part of the "continuum" of women's food and weight problems, an understanding developed that body-image, food, and weight issues, including eating disorders as extremes, were situated within the context of women's oppression in a patriarchal and capitalist society. The prevention and promotion of awareness of eating disorders took on a different complexion and urgency. There was an increased drive to recognize and challenge the oppression of the beauty ideal, weight prejudice, and societal pressures to be "thin."

The recognition that these are deeply rooted in our Western, industrialized society, and that women's food, weight, and body-image pains are a direct consequence of a culture which objectifies and devalues women, has informed the development of the feminist principles by which NEDIC is guided. NEDIC's understanding is that food and weight problems are often a coping strategy: a means of survival for women who have diminished power, voice, and safety.

With this wider perspective, NEDIC not only became active in the war against society's unrealistic and dangerous standard of beauty, but also made the links between all forms of discrimination and its effect on our lives. NEDIC began to recognize and challenge the pervasiveness of all forms of oppression. We now attempt to ensure that these are an integral part of our analysis of issues related to our work.

NEDIC operates under a non–dieting, weight-acceptance philosophy. We do not refer clients to dieting centres, individuals, or services which advocate restrictive eating as a solution to food and weight or other problems. Dieting is intrinsically dangerous to women. It perpetuates women's feelings of low self-esteem, body-dissatisfaction, depression, food and weight preoccupation, and the painful pursuit of society's beauty ideal. Our belief is that dieting shrinks a woman's world, not her body.

NEDIC recognizes that many therapists and clients choose to view eating disorders and food and weight problems as addictions. Our work is based on a nonaddiction model. We oppose these models on the grounds that the "addictions" approach is a "disease" model that not only pathologizes, but also creates a permanence to women's food and weight problems. Thus women are made to feel that their particular struggle with food, weight, or body image is an eternal affliction and cannot be entirely overcome. They remain always "recovering anorexic/ bulimic/ diseased" women, and they are prevented from recognizing and fulfilling their own power and identity as women and as individuals.

NEDIC encourages clients both to articulate their subjective experiences and to seek support from professionals who understand and are willing to work with the complex issues raised by food and weight preoccupation.

FOCUS AND FUNCTION

While our ultimate goal is to work ourselves out of existence through the prevention and elimination of food and weight preoccupation, we recognize that this society has a long way to travel before we will be able to achieve that! In the interim, we have focused on smaller, more readily attainable goals on the long road to eradication of disturbed eating behaviours as a reflection of psychological pain.

Our primary links to the community are currently through public-speaking engagements and our telephone information, resource, and support line. During the past two years, we have received, on average forty telephone calls per day. Family members, friends, educators, students, health professionals, employers, and the media, in addition to women and men experiencing food and weight issues, call in. Despite the unique needs and circumstances of individuals, common themes reoccur. These themes, needs, and perspectives expressed by our clients play a central role in determining our direction and focus.

Having a client-centred philosophy recognizes the importance of continuously assessing our clients' needs. Given the temporal constraints of our telephone work, assessing client needs means that we need to rely on accurate records of our clientele base and the questions asked. Maintaining such records based on pertinent information is one way in which we attempt to ensure the provision of effective and appropriate services which are responsive to community needs. Through this and staff members' own accounts of contacts, we work to recognize who current clients are, who we are or are not reaching, and what gaps are occurring in the services we provide. We record who is making contact, based on several general categories (i.e., people experiencing food, weight, and shape issues; family/friends; health workers; non–health workers; educators; and students), what they need, from which province or area they are contacting us, and the amount of time we spend with them. Although our clientele may fluctuate, based on the demands of the school year, Eating Disorders Awareness Week, the holidays, etc., the majority of them consistently are women experiencing food, weight, and shape issues (98–99 percent are women; 1–2 percent are men).

Several needs are expressed by clients on a daily basis. The majority request printed materials and/or information on resources for food, weight, and shape difficulties in their area. Staffing our telephone line involves providing a medley of services, including referral, education, and support. NEDIC does not currently provide clinical services per se; however, our telephone work requires provision of support and counseling. Though we receive relatively few calls from women experiencing severe crises, many calls are from those who are extremely distressed and for whom calling our Centre has demanded a tremendous amount of courage. The age range of women for whom a call to our Centre is the first disclosure of their food and weight problems, and who are seeking support, guidance, and direction, is wide.

Many women are looking for local services: providing such resources is often a rather frustrating and complex task. Being client-centred, we believe in the importance of empowering our clients to explore these various options through increasing their knowledge base and encouraging critical enquiry. Yet, we simultaneously experience frustration around the fact that the vast majority of services fluctuate in availability, are unaffordable, or may not meet the clients' needs. This frustration is often shared by the client, and NEDIC staff are the recipients of much of this expressed dissatisfaction. As a way of diffusing our own sense of outrage, and as an act of political advocacy, dissatisfied clients are encouraged to write to the Minister of Health about concerns in respect to limited and inappropriate services. We often question our role as a *resource* agency based on feminist principles which can provide women with very few acceptable alternatives. In response to this, we make note of information we feel is important in accurately reflecting the needs and perspectives of our clients and the wider community.

Given that there are extremely few financially subsidized resources, we receive many calls from women seeking help who are unable to actually utilize them. Among these callers are women who do not have access in their area to subsidized services, including psychotherapy; who have chosen to explore hospital-based programs and must wait for three months to two years for a space; have chosen not to use psychiatric or government-funded services because they do not meet their needs; or are unable to pay for individual counseling. Also among them are clients who have not been helped, or have, in fact, been harmed by psychiatric practices, medical practitioners, and agency workers, and who recognize that these options do not meet their needs. We feel that it is important to document the number of clients who are unable to access services in order to have a firm basis for advocacy.

Our contact with clients is vital not only to our understanding of food, weight, and shape issues, but also to our ability to respond to the needs of our clients and the broader community. Clients' letters, telephone calls, and conversations are most effective in aiding and ensuring our understanding of women's experiences and needs, how we can reflect their experience through our services, and how we can most effectively respond to their needs.

Although, given our staff and funding constraints, we are not currently active in traditional "advocacy" work (i.e., for government funding for much-needed services for women experiencing food, weight, and shape issues), we believe that the work we do provides a voice and a space for the experiences of women. Our client's stories, needs, and perspectives determine our focus and direct our energies; for instance, they inform our topics for our newsletter, the *Bulletin*; themes for Eating Disorders Awareness Week forums and panels; and the information we disseminate. As well, our understanding of the dangers of diagnostic labeling stems from both our reading and our direct contact with clients. We regularly hear stories from women expressing distress, fear, and feelings of powerlessness around having been told by their doctor or psychiatrist, on the basis of their eating behaviours, that they have a psychiatric disorder. These women have then called us, looking for help for their "disease" or "personality disorder." While there continues to be controversy around the term "eating disorder" itself, we nonetheless strive to base our own understanding of the issues on our experience and analysis of clients' words and stories within their sociopolitical context.

As our mandate is to provide and disseminate "up-to-date" and accurate information on food, weight, and shape issues, we must make decisions about where we receive our information, our "facts" and "statistics." We are often asked to provide such statistics, studies, and references from the "traditional" literature. Given the nature and focus of this literature, we recognize that it is usually not an accurate reflection of all women's experience. People working within the dominant academic culture largely adopt a paradigm which asks particular questions within particular contexts and uses a particular methodology. The dominant paradigm excludes women of diverse backgrounds (including women in poverty, minority women, lesbians, etc.) from appropriate research on the assumption that food, weight, and shape issues, including anorexia, bulimia, yo-yo dieting, and body shame, are the "prerogative" experiences of females from specific profiles. These would include women in families where one or other parent is physically or psychologically absent, in middle to upper socio-economic status, in transition between class or culture, and generally of Western European descent. Feminist research, and our contact with a diverse range of women — callers, women who walk into our Centre, and those who attend workshops and meetings within the community — tells us that these issues cross all boundaries of race, class, age, sexual orientation physical ability, and culture. Therefore, we believe that we must include anecdotal and experiential evidence in our analysis and in our provision of "accurate" information.

As a form of primary and secondary prevention, NEDIC is mandated to raise awareness around the issues of food and weight preoccupation. Our focus has been to provide psychoeducational information and workshops to a wide range of audiences. These have included educators, health professionals, students, specific community groups, and the general population. Given the strong contention of workers in the area that sociocultural factors play a significant role in the precipitation/choice of and maintenance of problematic eating behaviour as a symptom of psychological dissonance, NEDIC has chosen to focus much of its intervention on raising consciousness about covert and overt societal expectations and norms that contribute to food, weight, and shape preoccupation.

The rationale for this approach is the belief that cultural imperatives are not immutable and are, in fact, open to amelioration, if not outright change. This is evident in behaviours that were previously socially unacceptable but are currently sanctioned (such as sexual behaviour). NEDIC thus chooses to be clear about situating body-image, food, and weight concerns firmly within a sociocultural context and targeting a diverse audience. A factor which feeds into the decision to use this prevention strategy is the notion that attitudinal and behavioural changes need to occur across generational and structural divisions to be effective and to offer support to individuals challenging entrenched mores. Although the efficacy of these interventions has not been objectively measured, anecdotal evidence is adequate to suggest that it is an example of work that can be done to shift cultural attitudes and to raise awareness of detrimental cultural stereotypes and practices.

To this end, the public-education work that NEDIC does focuses largely on providing current information and experiential exploration of the following issues:

a) sociocultural issues relating to food, weight, and shape preoccupation, including weight prejudice;

b) the psychological and physical dangers of restrictive and purgative eating behaviours;

c) early signs of food, weight, and shape preoccupation;
d) specific signs of eating problems; and
e) prevention and intervention strategies.

Staff at the Centre recognize the need to work with an appropriate developmental model of eating disorders in order to offer a coherent model of prevention. Current feminist understandings of the development of eating disorders are used as the basis for our own understanding thereof. The agency also attempts to make our work appropriate to the developmental phase of the audience and their "life tasks." Links are made between cultural prescriptions in respect of a narrow body ideal and how they feed into vulnerabilities and conflicts in completing perceived life-tasks, which in themselves are not culture or value free.

In addition to targeting children, parents, educators, and health workers, NEDIC sees great merit in challenging the media to become more responsible and aware of the messages that they disseminate with regard to the desirability and value of a thin body. With this in mind, NEDIC works cooperatively with such organizations as MediaWatch to create media-literacy and to debunk myths perpetuated by media-borne messages. NEDIC also works with the mass media with regard to disseminating information about eating disorders. At each opportunity, issues related to the media's role in perpetuating narrow images of women are raised. Since this stance is often conflictual with the revenue generated for the media by sponsorship and advertising by the beauty and diet industries, these comments are often excluded or softened by journatlists and editors. It is an economic reality that the enormous vested interests of these industries mitigate against primary preventative work being conducted through the mainstream media.

If we were asked to be concise in detailing our future focus (a difficult thing to be, in this job!), our priority would be to refine our preventative work. We strive to be as effective as possible given the parameters and resources of the agency. Our top priority would be to prevent problematic eating and the myriad of concomitant concerns, in addition to serving those who have developed these coping strategies. The continuation of our current services in a way in which access is assured for all is something towards which we continue to strive. The creation of a sustainable series of training workshops for people wanting to facilitate support groups is a project whose time has come. In accordance with our philosophy of inclusion, these will seek, through continued community liaison, to draw from and serve all sectors. As we build on previous staff's work, we continue to make the connections between all women's life experiences and food, weight, and shape issues. Thus, we recognize the increased pressures on women of particular class, race, ability, culture, and sexual orientation. These pressures are not only to deny our individual culture and conform to the white, middle-class "norm," but also to meet Western societies' beauty ideal — an injunction which is both oppressive and painful.

Finally, we would like to thank all previous staff members and volunteers for their contributions to the agency, and on whose work we continue to build.

◆

HERSIZE:
A WEIGHT-PREJUDICE
ACTION GROUP

Karin Jasper

In Toronto, during the summer of 1987, five women who identified themselves as having been affected by struggles with food, dieting, and weight got together to discuss the possibility of creating a
group to raise awareness of the factors contributing to widespread
body dissatisfaction among women. By the end of the summer, the
group had developed a mandate and plan of action. Some of the
women originally interested had left, and others had joined, resulting in a core group of four. They saw their immediate tasks as finding a name for the group; developing public-relations materials,
such as a brochure; and letting the media know of their existence.

Numerous brainstorming sessions led to establishing "Hersize"
as the name for the group. It was simple and snappy, and it connected the issues of being female with being concerned about size.
The group's desire to promote acceptance of a wide range of body
sizes was furthered by selecting a font with which to print "Hersize"
on the group's brochure and other materials in which each letter is
a different size and shape, making the medium the message.

Hersize group members developed a threefold purpose: to
increase public awareness of fat oppression (the group adopted a

radical fat-acceptance philosophy), to free women from overconcern with body size and shape, and to help prevent eating disorders. "A weight-prejudice action group" was chosen as a defining description, and the group's brochure outlined why. Weight prejudice, the habit of judging the personal and moral character of individuals by reference to their body size and shape — e.g., thin women are intelligent, sexy, and in control, while fat women are stupid, sexless, and weak-willed — was identified as critical to discrimination against fat people, a contributing factor in the increasing numbers of eating disorders, and a causal factor in yo-yo dieting. The brochure identified weight prejudice as a feminist issue because women learn to derive self-esteem from their appearance and because women are fatter by nature than men. Women are, therefore, disproportionately affected by weight prejudice. Hersize members chose to define themselves as an "action" group because they wanted to focus their efforts on speaking out to the largest audience possible, rather than providing, for example, support groups to small groups of women.

The group members began monitoring the media for inappropriate messages regarding women's weight and shape, and responding to those messages in writing. Letters were written to major newspapers, parents' magazines, women's magazines, and fashion magazines. A high proportion of letters written were either published or responded to directly. For example, published letters included those that were written to the *Toronto Star* in response to an article on Weight Watchers, to *Today's Parent* magazine regarding an article by a doctor urging parents to control the weights of their children from early ages, to *Now Magazine* for an ad it carried promoting a questionable weight-loss product, and to *Chatelaine* commenting on an article promoting stomach stapling. The Hersize group also complained to the *New York Times* about an ad it had carried for a book called *Responsible Bulimia*. The *Times* wrote back, acknowledging its error, and promised not to run further ads for the book. Even on occasions when letters were not published, the group members felt that, at least, consciousness was being raised and writers and publishers might be moved to think about future messages with greater care. Group members wrote articles for alternative publications such as *Rites Magazine, Healthsharing, Nurses for Social Responsibility Newsletter,* and the *Media Watch Bulletin,* as well as more mainstream publications.

Dissemination of the group's brochure as well as word-of-mouth resulted in some media coverage, which engendered more media coverage. Early on, a *Toronto Star* columnist visited the group during a meeting and wrote a very supportive column about its purpose and activities, and a CBC radio show, "Radio Noon," broadcast an interview with two of the group's members. Thereafter, Hersize members appeared on a variety of television and radio shows, as well as at public forums, passionately spreading the message that women should consider relaxing their concern about body size and shape and turn their attention to more substantive matters.

Energy was directed to finding more group members and developing an advisory board. The advisory board was intended to make professional expertise available in areas in which Hersize might require consultation, e.g., medicine, psychology, law, and feminism. Although consultation was not needed often, it was helpful for group members to be able to check controversial facts as well as to have input on written materials and strategies.

During the first winter of the group's existence, a set of slides (showing samples of weight-prejudiced advertising and giving information about weight control, fat prejudice, and eating disorders) was prepared for the group to use in making public presentations, and an annotated bibliography of resources for people who wanted to explore the issues related to women, weight, dieting, and eating disorders in greater depth was written. Considerable amounts of time, energy, and money were required for the diverse range of Hersize projects. Money came from the Hersize steering committee members themselves, as well as from the membership at large and from honoraria received for public speaking.

The fact that members of Hersize tended to identify themselves as having personally struggled with weight, shape, and eating issues made it possible for them to contribute uniquely when speaking in public. Most TV and radio shows or newspaper articles publicizing the issues draw their material from professionals, and from women in the throes of an eating disorder. Typically, the professional lays out the theories and facts as well as some statistics on prevalence and treatment, then the "victim" talks about the experience of being anorexic or bulimic, or fat. Anorexia, especially, has been "glamourized" as audiences (or readers) express shock but are *impressed* with the self-denial evident in the anorexic woman's behaviour. The ethics of this type of programming are highly questionable, since the predictable audience reaction constitutes a kind of reinforcement of anorexic self-denial. On TV or radio, or in front of an audience of students and teachers, Hersize speakers could provide a role model for women to challenge and resist the pressures to be thin and to encourage acceptance of a wide range of body sizes and shapes. These steps had been necessary for them as individuals resolving their own eating or weight issues. So they could talk about the experience, for instance, of having an eating disorder, contextualizing it appropriately, and thereby avoiding glamourization. From the position of having resolved their own issues about food, shape, and weight, they could invite women to join a counterculture in which they are encouraged to divest their energy from the obsession with weight and shape.

It is, however, of vital importance that women who do identify themselves as survivors of eating disorders exercise discretion when speaking publicly, especially when discussing details about self-harming behaviours that may have been part of their eating disorder. Some members of the audience will not be ready or willing to give up concern with body weight and shape and may instead use details to diversify the means by which they attempt to lose weight. It is also important that any information presented publicly as "fact" be backed up by research, otherwise the risk of having one's message being dismissed as the mere "rantings of an angry woman" are intensifed.

There are other risks connected with publicly acknowledging that one has struggled with an eating disorder. Some people respond differently once they have this knowledge. One can actually see their eyes change as it happens, searching for signs of remnants of the "disease." One has become "other." Not infrequently, one then hears the question: "Do people really ever completely recover from an eating disorder?" asked almost rhetorically. It gets worse as one senses the person shifting into a position of doubting what one has said — one has been transformed from a credible source of information into a person with a messianic mission. Over time, Hersize members became discriminating about when and to whom this personal information would be revealed.

Professionals often shake their heads over the fact that many women who have recovered or are trying to recover from an eating disorder want to help others with similar struggles. It is sometimes considered a kind of suspicious behaviour, indicating, perhaps, an unwillingness to give up the "illness." However, there is a simple explanation. It is natural for human beings who have suffered deeply to want to give meaning to that suffering and to desire that others not suffer similarly or needlessly. It is also natural, having been helped to recover, to want to pass that gift on to others. This is common to any area of human suffering.

Although it is not possible to prove the efficacy of activist groups in the overall prevention effort, members of Hersize report interesting anecdotal evidence that would support the belief that putting ones message in the public domain does make some difference. For instance, several reports of the following scenario have been made. In speaking casually to people about set-point theory and the disproportionate pressure on women to be thin, activists have found that people are often very sceptical. Once they see the activist on a television show or hear her on the radio, their willingness to believe her statements increases dramatically! TV and radio seem to bestow credibility that more mundane forms of communication do not.

In order to keep in touch with its membership-at-large as well as to spread the word, Hersize started a newsletter. The newsletter was intended to be a semiannual or quarterly publication, but in the end five issues were published over five years. Topics included fat phobia in the media, a critique of the "body mass index" for determining "healthy weights," body dissatisfaction, cosmetic and gastric surgery, and sexuality. Book and film reviews as well as updates on Hersize activities were also included in the newsletter. It was widely distributed at public-speaking events, during Eating Disorders Awareness Week, and at the International Women's Day Fair.

As the group became more widely known, it was sometimes asked to provide input to other group's projects. For instance, Hersize provided consultation to Katherine Gilday during the making of "The Famine Within" and participated in the development of a program called the "Bod Squad," a body-image workshop for Grades 9 and 10 students, created by the Nutrition Services Department of the Oxford County Board of Health in Ontario. Hersize and its members were also featured on major TV programs such as CBC's *The Journal* and CTV's *W5*, as well as the *Dini Petty Show* and *The Shirley Show*. An American newspaper, the *Chicago Tribune*, also featured an article about Hersize in the spring of 1990.

The *Tribune* article resulted in close to 100 letters from women in several American states, ranging from requests for information to requests for guidance in starting Hersize groups of their own. The Toronto group had assisted in setting up a Hersize branch in London, Ontario, and had learned that its already stretched members could not offer more than very limited support. Hence, American women who made this request were sent samples of Hersize materials, but were told that, being a volunteer organization, Hersize could offer no more than occasional telephone consultation. Whether any Hersize-type groups were generated in the

United States is unknown.

Two problems that plagued Hersize from the outset were finding new members for the steering committee and keeping up an activity level necessary for remaining in the public eye. Even impassioned volunteers have limits. Burnout became a reality, despite the arrival over a five-year period of many dedicated and energetic women.

Finding new members for the steering committee was challenging for a number of reasons. Women on the committee were expected to do writing, public speaking, and organizing. The issues related to weight prejudice are both politically and medically complex. The group needed to be sure that anyone who would be speaking or writing on behalf of the group would be able to answer a wide range of audience questions without losing credibility and without sacrificing the radical position on fat acceptance that Hersize espoused. Group members burned out one after the other.

Another problem related to diversity in the group. From the beginning, Hersize had committed itself to being a "model" group for women, that is, an organization (a) that was nonhierarchical in structure, (b) in which members were not competitive with regard to body size and shape, and (c) that was inclusive of a diverse range of women vis-à-vis ethnicity/race, economic background, and educational background. However, Hersize was nearly always made up of white, middle-class women. Efforts were made to diversify and enlarge the steering committee, including requests for participation from women of colour in the Hersize newsletter, a questionnaire circulated at a public meeting, sign-up sheets for various subcommittees at public events where Hersize speakers emphasized the desire to broaden the group's membership, and so on. These efforts bore little fruit.

How to interpret the meagre results became the focus of debate and argument within the group. Some committee members felt that Hersize was constitutionally unfriendly to women who were other than white, middle (or upper) class, and professional. They argued that the group needed to undergo antiracist training, a prospect they discovered would be very expensive and time-consuming, especially for a volunteer group, but which they considered essential. Other group members felt that the problems of weight prejudice, eating disorders, and body-image dissatisfaction were most intensely the problems of white middle-class women and were probably secondary problems for women dealing with racism. Therefore, they argued, women of colour were not likely to make it a priority to volunteer their time to fight weight prejudice. In response to this argument, a group member proposed changing the focus of Hersize from weight prejudice to "looksism," a more general issue that would encompass ageism, able-bodiedism, racism, and so on. These debates became the foundation for significant political disagreements and personal dissatisfactions, which finally rendered the group impotent. It had been difficult enough for the individuals participating to carry out the demanding Hersize agenda. With internal problems to deal with at every meeting, the Hersize output diminished considerably. During the early part of 1992, most Hersize members had either left the group or taken leaves of absence. A few members remained, mainly responding to mail and interview requests.

Five years of activist effort had, however, paid off. By 1992, general audiences were often already critical of media messages about the value of thinness; they were no longer in need of basic information about set-point theory, nor were their opinions about eating disorders and weight prejudice as naïve as they had been in 1987. Many women's groups were actively challenging their own beliefs about fat and the effort to be thin. While it would be untrue to suggest that the climate in which eating disorders easily develop had ceased to exist, certainly progress had been made. Hersize played a part in creating that change.

◆

REFERENCES

Abraham, S. and P. Beaumont. 1982. "Varieties of Psychosexual Experiences in Patients with Anorexia Nervosa." *International Journal of Eating Disorders* 1/3, 10-19.

Adisa, O. 1990. "Rocking in the Sunlight: Stress and Black Women." In *The Black Women's Health Book: Speaking for Ourselves*, ed. by E.White, 11-14. Seattle: Seal Press.

Allisen, S. 1992. "Lesbian Incest Survivors: A Particular Courage." *Lesbian Ethics*. Vol. 4/3.

American Psychiatric Association. 1980. *Diagnostic and Statistical Manual of Mental Disorders*, 3rd ed. (*DSM-III*). Washington, DC.

American Psychiatric Association. 1987. *Desk Reference to the Diagnostic Criteria from DSM-III-R*. Washington, DC.

Asian and Pacific Women's Resource Collection Network. 1989. *Asian and Pacific Women's Resource and Action Series — Health*. Kuala Lumpur: Asian and Pacific Development Centre.

Ault-Ritche, M. 1986. "A Feminist Critique of Five Schools of Family Therapy." In *The Family Therapy Collection: Women and Family Therapy*, ed. by J. Hansen and M. Ault-Ritche. Rockwell: Aspen Systems Corp.

Avis, J. 1988. "Deepening Awareness: A Private Study Guide to Feminism and Family Therapy." In *A Guide to Feminist Family Therapy*, ed. by L. Braverman. New York: Haworth Press.

Badgley R. et al. 1984. *Sexual Offences Against Children*. Vol. 1 and Vol. 2. Ottawa: Supply and Services Canada.

Bain, L., T. Wilson, and E. Chaikind. 1989. "Participant Perceptions of Exercise Programs for Overweight Women." *Research Quarterly* 60/2, 134-43.

Baines, C., P. Evans, and S. Neysmith, eds. 1991. *Women's Caring: Feminist Perspectives on Social Welfare*. Toronto: McClelland and Stewart.

Baker Miller, J. 1986. *Toward a New Psychology of Women*. Boston: Beacon Press.

Ballou, M. and N. Gabalac. 1985. *A Feminist Position on Mental Health.* Springfield, IL: Charles C. Thompson Press.

Banner, L. 1983. *American Beauty.* Chicago: University of Chicago Press.

Barrett, M. and R. Schwartz. 1987. "Couple Therapy for Bulimia." In *The Family Therapy Collection: Women and Family Therapy,* ed. by J. Hansen and M. Ault-Ritche. Rockwell: Aspen Systems Corp.

Bart, P. and P. O'Brien. 1985. *Stopping Rape: Successful Survival Strategies.* Elmsford, NY: Pergamon Press.

Bartky, S. 1990. *Femininity and Domination: Studies in the Phenomenology of Oppression.* New York and London: Routledge.

————. "Foucault, Feminity, and the Modernization of Patriarchal Power." In *Feminism and Foucault: Reflections on Resistance,* ed. by I. Diamond and L. Quinby. Boston: Northeastern University Press.

Bass, E. and L. Davis. 1988. *The Courage to Heal: A Guide for Women Survivors of Child Sexual Abuse.* New York: Harper and Row.

Beattie, M. 1987. *Codependent No More.* Center City, MI: Hazeldon.

Beckman, K. and G. Burns. 1990. "Relation of Sexual Abuse and Bulimia in College Women." *International Journal of Eating Disorders* 9/5, 487-92.

Beckman, L. 1978. "Sex Role Conflict in Alcoholic Women: Myth or Reality?" *Journal of Abnormal Psychology* 84, 408-17.

Belenky, M., B. Clinchy, N. Goldberger, and J. Tarule. 1986. *Women's Ways of Knowing.* New York: Basic Books.

Bell, R. 1985. *Holy Anorexia.* Chicago: University of Chicago Press.

Beller, A. 1977. *Fat and Thin: A Natural History of Obesity.* New York: Farrar, Straus and Giroux.

Bemis, K. 1987. "Current Approaches to the Etiology and Treatment of Anorexia Nervosa." *Psychological Bulletin* 85/3, 593-617.

Bennett, W. and J. Gurin. 1982. *The Dieters' Dilemma.* New York: Basic Books.

Benston, M. 1989. "Feminism and the Critique of the Scientific Method." In *Feminism from Pressure to Politics,* ed. by A. Miles and F. Finn, 57-76. Montreal: Black Rose Books.

Berg, F. 1992. "Who Is Dieting in the United States?" *Obesity and Health,* May/June, 48-49.

Berger, J. 1972. *Ways of Seeing.* London: BBC and Penguin Books.

Bernardez, T. 1987. "Gender-Based Countertransference of Female Therapists in the Psychotherapy of Women." *Women and Therapy* 6/1&2, 25-39.

Beumont, P., S. Abraham, and K. Simpson. 1981. "The Psychological Histories of Adolescent Girls and Young Women with Anorexia Nervosa." *Psychological Medicine* 11, 131-40.

Bion, W. 1963. *Elements of Psychoanalysis.* New York: Basic Books.

Bjorntorp, P. 1987. "Classification of Obese Patients and Complications Related to the Distribution of Surplus Fat." *American Journal of Clinical Nutrition* 45, 1120-25.

Bjorvell, H. and S. Rossner. 1990. "Long Term Treatment of Severe Obesity: Four Year Follow-Up of Combined Behavioural Modification Programme." *British Medical Journal* 291, 379-82.

Black, C., S. Bucky, and S. Wilder-Padilla. 1986. "The Interpersonal and Emotional Consequences of Being an Adult Child of an Alcoholic." *The International Journal of the Addictions* 21/2, 213-31.

Black, D. and M. Burckes-Miller. 1988. "Male and Female College Athletes: Use of Anorexia Nervosa and Bulimia Nervosa Weight Loss Methods." *Research Quarterly* 59/3, 252-56.

Blumenthal, J., L. O'Toole, and L. Chang. 1984. "Is Running an Analogue of Anorexia Nervosa?" *Journal of the American Medical Association* 252/4, 520-23.

Bograd, M. 1988. "Enmeshment, Fusion or Relatedness? A Conceptual Analysis." In *A Guide to Feminist Therapy,* ed. by L. Braverman. New York: Haworth Press.

Bollas, C. 1987. *The Shadow of the Object.* New York: Columbia University Press.

Bouchard, C., L. Perusse, and C. Leblanc. 1988. "Inheritance of the Amount and Distribution of Human Body Fat." *International Journal of Obesity* 12, 205.

Boskind-White, M. and W. White. 1983. *Bulimarexia: The Binge/Purge Cycle.* New York: W.W. Norton.

Bovey, S. 1989. *Being Fat Is Not a Sin.* London: Pandora.

Boyd, J. 1990. "Ethnic and Cultural Diversity in Feminist Therapy: Keys to Power." In *The Black Women's Health Book: Speaking for Ourselves,* ed. by E. White. Seattle: Seal Press.

Brand, D. and K. Sri Bhaggiyadatta. 1986. *Rivers Have Sources, Trees Have Roots: Speaking of Racism.* Toronto: Cross Cultural Communication Centre.

Brand, P., E. Rothblum, and L. Solomon. 1992. "A Comparison of Lesbians, Gay Men, and Heterosexuals on Weight and Restrained Eating." *International Journal of Eating Disorders* 11/3, 253-259.

Braverman, L. 1988. "Feminism and Family Therapy: Friends or Foes?" In *A Guide to Feminist Family Therapy*, ed. by L. Braverman. New York: Haworth Press.

Bray, G. and S. Inoue. 1992. "Pharmacological Treatment of Obesity." *American Journal of Clinical Nutrition* 55, S151-S319.

Bray, R. 1992. "Heavy Burden." *Essence* Vol. 22/9 (January), 52-54.

Brill, D. 1986. *Jump.* Vancouver: Douglas and McIntyre.

Brickman, J. 1984. "Feminist, Non-Sexist and Traditional Models of Therapy for Working with Incest." *Women and Therapy.* Vol.3/1, 49-61.

Brooks, C. 1991. Presentation at Women and Depression Forum. Toronto.

Brown, C. 1987a. "Feeding into Each Other: Weight Preoccupation and the Contradictory Expectations of Women." Master's Thesis, University of Manitoba, Department of Sociology, Winnipeg.

———. 1987b. *Getting Beyond Weight: Women Helping Women. A Self-Help Manual.* Winnipeg: Women's Health Clinic.

———. 1990a. "Contracting in Feminist Therapy for 'Eating Disorders'." Independent Enquiry Project, Carleton University, School of Social Work, Ottawa.

———. 1990b. "The 'Control Paradox': Understanding and Working with Anorexia and Bulimia." *National Eating Disorders Information Centre Bulletin,* (June, July) 1-3.

———. 1991. "The Meaning of Laxative Abuse." *National Eating Disorders Information Centre Bulletin,* (August), 1-2.

Brown, C. and D. Forgay. 1987. "An Uncertain Well-Being: Weight Control and Self Control." *Healthsharing,* (Winter), 11-15.

Brown, L. 1985. "Women, Weight, and Power: Feminist Theoretical and Therapeutic Issues." *Women and Therapy* 4, 61-71.

———. 1987. "Lesbians, Weight and Eating: New Analyses and Perspectives. In *Lesbian Psychologies: Explorations and Challenges*, ed by L. Brown, 294-309. Chicago: University of Illinois Press.

———. 1990. "What's Addiction Got to Do with It: A Feminist Critique of Codependence." *Psychology of Women* 17/1 (Winter),1-4.

Brown, L. and M. Root. 1990. *Diversity and Complexity in Feminist Therapy*. New York: Harrington Park Press.

Brown, L. and C. Gilligan. 1992. *Meeting at the Crossroads: Women's Psychology and Girls' Development*. Cambridge, MA: Harvard University Press.

Brown, S. 1987. *Treating Adult Children of Alcoholics*. New York: Wiley.

Brownell, K. and R. Jeffrey. 1987. "Improving Long-Term Weight Loss: Pushing the Limits of Treatment." *Behaviour Therapy* 18, 353-74.

Bruch, H. 1973. *Eating Disorders: Obesity, Anorexia Nervosa, and the Person Within*. New York: Basic Books.

————. 1978. *The Golden Cage*. Washington, DC: Howard University Press.

Brumberg, J. 1989. *Fasting Girls: The History of Anorexia Nervosa*. Markham, ON: Penguin Books.

Buchok, N. 1990. "Sexual Abuse and Eating Disorders: A Preliminary Study." Unpublished paper, York University, Toronto.

Buffalo, Y. 1990. "Seeds of Thought, Arrows of Change: Native Storytelling as Metaphor." In *Healing Voices: Feminist Approaches to Therapy with Women*, ed. by N. Laidlaw, C. Malmo, and Associates, 118-142. San Francisco: Jossey-Bass.

Bulik, C. 1987. "Drug and Alcohol Abuse by Bulimic Women and Their Families." *American Journal of Psychiatry* 144/12, 1604-6.

Burgess, A. and L. Holstrom. 1979. *Rape: Crisis and Recovery*. New York: Prentice-Hall.

Burstow, B. 1992. *Radical Feminist Therapy: Working in the Context of Violence*. London: Sage Publications.

Burstow, B. and D. Weitz, eds. 1988. *Shrink Resistant: The Struggle Against Psychiatry in Canada*. Vancouver: New Star Books.

Calam, R. and P. Slade. 1989. "Sexual Abuse and Eating Problems in Female Undergraduates." *International Journal of Eating Disorders* 8/4, 391-97.

Calles-Escandon, J. and E. Horton. 1992. "The Thermogenic Role of Exercise in the Treatment of Morbid Obesity: A Critical Evaluation." *American Journal of Clinical Nutrition* 55, S533-S537.

Campbell, J. 1985. "Anorexia Nervosa: Body Dissatisfaction in a High Risk Population." *CAHPER Journal* 52/4, 36-41.

Canada Fitness Survey. 1984. *Changing Times*. Ottawa.

Canadian Mental Health Association. Women and Mental Health Committee.

1987, April. *Women and Mental Health in Canada: Strategies for Change.* Toronto.

Canadian Native Women's Association. 1989. *Report on Childhood Sexual Abuse.*

Canning, H. and J. Muir. 1966. "Obesity — Its Possible Effects on College Acceptance." *New England Journal of Medicine* 275, 12-23.

Caplan, P. 1985. *The Myth of Women's Masochism.* New York: Dutton.

Caskey, N. 1986. "Interpreting Anorexia Nervosa." In *The Female Body in Western Culture,* ed. by S.R. Suleiman. Cambridge, MA: Harvard University Press.

Cauwells, J. 1983. *Bulimia. The Binge-Purge Compulsion.* New York: Doubleday.

Cermak, T. 1986a. *Diagnosing and Treating Co-Dependence: A Guide for Professionals Who Work with Chemical Dependents, Their Spouses, and Children.* Minneapolis: Johnson Institute.

———.1986b. "Diagnostic Criteria for Codependency." *Journal of Psychoactive Drugs* 18/1, 15-20.

Cermak, T. and S. Brown. 1982. "Interactional Group Therapy with Adult Children of Alcoholics." *International Journal of Group Psychotherapy* 32/3, 375-89.

Cermak, T. and A. Rosenfeld. 1987. *Therapeutic Considerations with Adult Children of Alcoholics.* New York: Haworth Press.

Chapkis, W. 1986. *Beauty Secrets: Women and the Politics of Appearance.* Boston: South End Press.

Chernin, K. 1981. *The Obsession: Reflections on the Tyranny of Slenderness.* New York: Harper and Row.

———. 1985. *The Hungry Self: Women, Eating, and Identity.* Toronto: Random House.

———. 1988. *Reinventing Eve.* New York: Harper and Row.

Chesler, P. 1972. *Women and Madness.* New York: Doubleday.

Chodorow, N. 1978. *The Reproduction of Mothering: Psychoanalysis and the Sociology of Gender.* Berkeley: University of California Press.

Chrisler, J. 1991. "Out of Control and Eating Disordered." In *Feminist Perspectives on Addictions,* ed. by N. Van Den Burgh. New York: Springer.

Ciliska, D. 1990. *Beyond Dieting: Psychoeducational Interventions for Chronically*

Obese Women. New York: Brunner/Mazel.

Ciliska, D. and C. Rice. 1989. "Body Image/Body Politics." *Healthsharing,* Summer, 13-17.

Clark, K. 1956. *The Nude: A Study in Ideal Form.* New Jersey: Princeton University Press.

Clarke, H. and W. Gwynne-Timothy. 1988. *Stroke.* Toronto: James Lorimer.

Claydon, P. 1987. "Self-Reported Alcohol, Drug, and Eating Problems among Male and Female Collegiate Adult Children of Alcoholics." *College Health* 36, 111-16.

Coalition for Feminist Mental Health Services. 1992, January. *Missing the Mark: Women's Services Examine Mental Health Programs for Women in Toronto.* Toronto.

Collins, P. 1990. *Black Feminist Thought: Knowledge, Consciousness and the Politics of Empowerment.* Boston: Unwin Hyman.

Cook, A. 1970. "Black Pride? Some Contradictions." In *The Black Woman: An Anthology,* ed. by Toni Cade, 149-161. New York: Penguin Books.

Criffin, S. 1979. *Rape: The Power of Consciousness.* San Francisco: Harper and Row Press.

Crisp, A. 1980. *Anorexia Nervosa: Let Me Be.* Linden: Academic Press.

Crosset, T. 1990. "The Abusive Coach." Unpublished paper, Brandeis University, Waltham, MA.

Dana, M. and M. Lawrence. 1989. *Women's Secret Disorder. A New Understanding of Bulimia.* London: Grafton Books.

Danica, E. 1990. *Don't: A Woman's Word.* Toronto: McClelland and Stewart

Davis, A.Y. 1983. *Women, Race and Class.* New York: Vintage Books.

Deutsche, H. 1926. "Occult Processes Occurring During Psychoanalysis." In *Psychoanalysis and the Occult,* ed. by G. Devereux, 133-46. New York: International Universities Press.

Diamond, N. 1985. "Thin Is a Feminist Issue." *Feminist Review* 1, 45-65.

Dolan, B. 1991. "Cross-Cultural Aspects of Anorexia Nervosa and Bulimia: A Review." *International Journal of Eating Disorders* 10/1, 67-78.

Donald, C. 1986. *The Fat Woman Measures Up.* Charlottetown, PEI: Ragweed Press.

Donnelly, P. 1986. "Youth Involvement in High Performance Sport." Paper presented at the 7th annual conference of the North American Society for the Sociology of Sport, Las Vegas, NV.

Doucette, J. 1986. *Violent Acts Against Disabled Women.* Toronto: DAWN.

Drinkwater, B. 1984. "Women and Exercise: Physiological Aspects." *Exercise and Sport Sciences Reviews* 12, 21-51.

Duke, L. 1988. "Worker Files Complaint with City over Cornrows." *The Washington Post,* January 6, B8.

Dunfee, S. 1982. "The Sin of Hiding: A Feminist Critique of Reinhold Niebuhr's Account of the Sin of Pride." *Soundings* 65/3 (Fall), 316-27.

Durrant, Michael. 1983. "Restructuring the Family's Reality—The Struggle of a Young Anorectic Woman and Her Family's Way of Viewing the World." Paper presented at the Fourth Australian Therapy Conference, Brisbane, September.

Dyrenforth, S., O. Wooley, and S. Wooley. 1980. "A Woman's Body in a Man's World: A Review of Findings on Body Image and Weight Control." In *A Woman's Conflict: The Special Relationship Between Women and Food,* ed. by R. Kaplan, 30-57. Englewood Cliffs, NJ: Prentice-Hall.

Eberts, M. and B. Kidd. 1985. *Athletes' Rights.* Toronto: Ministry of Tourism and Recreation.

Ehrenreich, B. and English, D. 1973. *Complaints and Disorders. The Sexual Politics of Sickness.* New York: The Feminist Press.

El-Guebaly, N. and D. Offord. 1977. "The Offspring of Alcoholics: A Critical Review." *American Journal of Psychiatry* 134, 357-65.

Epstein, B. 1983. "Family, Sexual Morality, and Popular Movement in Turn-of-the-Century America." In *Powers of Desire: The Politics of Sexuality,* ed. by A. Snitow, C. Stansell, and S. Thompson, 117-130. New York: Monthly Review Press.

Ernsberger, P. and P. Haskew. 1987. "Health Implications of Obesity: An Alternative View." *Journal of Obesity and Weight Regulation* 6/2, 58-137.

Ersek, R., J. Zambrono, G. Surak, and D. Denton. 1986. "Suction-Assisted Lipectomy for Correction of 202 Figure Flaws in 101 Patients: Indications, Limitations, and Applications." *Plastic and Reconstructive Surgery* 78, 615-26.

Ettorre, B. 1989. "Women and Substance Abuse: Towards a Feminist Perspective or How to Make Dust Fly." *Women's Studies International Forum* 12/6, 593-602.

Evans, P. 1991. "The Sexual Division of Poverty: The Consequences of

Gendered Caring." In *Women's Caring: Feminist Perspectives on Social Welfare,* ed. by C. Baines, P. Evans, and S. Neysmith. Toronto: McClelland and Stewart.

Ewen, S. and E. Ewen. 1982. *Channels of Desire: Mass Images and the Shaping of American Consciousness.* New York: McGraw-Hill.

Faludi, S. 1991. *Backlash: The Undeclared War Against American Women.* New York: Crown.

Feldman, W., E. Feldman, and J. Goodman. 1986. "Health Concerns and Health Related Behaviours of Adolescents." *Canadian Medical Association Journal* 134, 489-93.

Ferguson, M. 1983. *Forever Feminine: Women's Magazines and the Cult of Feminity.* London: Heinemann.

Firsten, T. 1991. "Violence in the Lives of Women on Psych Wards." *Canadian Women's Studies/ Les cahiers de la femme* Vol.11/4 (Summer), 45-48.

Fishman, H. 1979. "Family Considerations in Liaison Psychiatry: A Structural Approach to Anorexia Nervosa in Adults." *Psychiatric Clinics of North America* 2, 249-63.

Fleishmann, K. and A. Siegel. 1983. "For Debate: Are Some Compulsive Runners Really Closet Anorexics?" *Annals of Sports Medicine* 1/3, 98-99.

Folkins, C. and W. Sime. 1981. "Physical Fitness Training and Mental Health." *Archives of Physical Medicine and Rehabilitation* 36, 373-89.

Fossom, M. and M. Mason. 1989. *Facing Shame: Families in Recovery.* New York: Norton.

Foucault, M. 1979. *Discipline and Punish: The Birth of the Prison.* New York: Vintage Books.

———. 1982. *The History of Sexuality.* Vol. 1. Harmandsworth: Pelican Books.

———. 1988. *The History of Sexuality.* Vol. 3: *The Care of the Self.* New York: Vintage Books.

Freeman, B. 1989. "Twelve Steps Anonymous." *off our backs* (March) 20-21.

Freud, S. 1910. "The Future Prospects of Psycho-Analytic Therapy." *Standard Edition,* Vol. 11, 141-51.

———. 1915. "Observations on Transference-Love." *Standard Edition,* Vol. 12, 159-71.

Friedan, B. 1963. *The Feminine Mystique.* New York: Dell.

Friedman, M. 1985. "Bulimia." *Women and Therapy* 4/2 (Summer), 63-69.

Friedman, S. and D. Maranda. 1984. "The Tyranny of the Scale." *Heartwood*, 8, (Summer), 4-5.

Friel, J., R. Subby, and L. Friel. 1984. *Codependency and the Search for Identity.* Pompano Beach, FL: Health Communications.

Galanter, M. 1990. "Cults and Zealous Self-Help Movements: A Psychiatric Perspective." *American Journal of Psychiatry* 147/5 (May), 543-50.

Garfinkel, P. and D. Garner. 1982. *Anorexia Nervosa: A Multidimensional Perspective.* New York: Brunner/Mazel.

Garner, D. 1983. "The Sociocultural Epidemic of Eating Disorders." *Health News Digest* (March/April), 2-3.

Garner, D. and P. Garfinkel. 1980. "Cultural Expectations of Thinness in Women." *Psychological Reports* 47, 483-91.

———. 1985. *Handbook of Psychotherapy for Anorexia Nervosa and Bulimia.* New York: Guilford Press.

Garner, D., M. Olmstead, and P. Garfinkle. 1983. "Does Anorexia Nervosa Occur on a Continuum?" *International Journal of Eating Disorders* 2/4, 11-20.

Garner, D., M. Olmstead, J. Polivy, and P. Garfinkel. 1984. "Comparison Between Weight Preoccupied Women and Anorexia Nervosa." *Psychosomatic Medicine* 46/3 (May/June), 255-266.

Garner, D. and S. Wooley. 1991. "Confronting the Failure of Behavioral and Dietary Treatments for Obesity." *Clinical Psychology Review* 11, 729-80.

Gill, M. 1982. *Analysis of Transference.* Vol. 1: *Theory and Technique.* New York: International Universities Press.

Gilligan, C. 1982. *In a Different Voice.* Cambridge, MA: Harvard University Press.

Gilligan, C., N. Lyons, and T. Hanmer. 1990. *Making Connections.* Cambridge, MA: Harvard University Press.

Goffman, E. 1961. *Asylums. Essays on the Social Situation of Mental Patients and Other Inmates.* New York: Anchor Books.

Goldenberg, N. 1990. *Returning Words to Flesh: Feminism, Psychoanalysis, and the Resurrection of the Body.* Boston: Beacon Press.

Goldfarb, L. "Sexual Abuse Antecedent to Anorexia Nervosa, Bulimia, and Compulsive Overeating:Three Case Reports." *International Journal of Eating Disorders* 6/5, 675-80.

Gomberg, E. and J. Lisansky. 1984. "Antecedents of Alcohol Problems in Women." In *Alcohol Problems in Women*, ed. by S. Wilsnack and L. Beckman. New York: Guilford Press.

Goodrich, T., C. Rampage, B. Ellman, and K. Halstead. 1988. *Feminist Family Therapy: A Casebook.* New York: W.W. Norton.

Gorski, T. and M. Miller. 1984. "Relapse: The Family's Involvement." *Focus on the Family and Chemical Dependency* 7/1, 3-14.

Gray, James et al. 1987. "The Prevalence of Bulimia in a Black College Population." *International Journal of Eating Disorders* 6/6, 733-40.

Greaves. K. 1990. *Big and Beautiful.* London: Grafton Books.

Greenspan, M. 1983. *A New Approach to Women and Therapy.* New York: McGraw-Hill.

Gregory, D. 1992. "Hair-Raising Tales." *Essence* 22/9 (January), 56-57.

Greil, A. and D. Rudy. 1983. "Conversion to the World View of Alcoholics Anonymous: A Refinement of Conversion Theory." *Qualitative Sociology* 6/1 (Spring), 5-28.

Grinberg, L. 1979. "Countertransference and Projective Counteridentification." *Contemporary Psychoananlysis* 15, 226-47.

Haaken, J. 1990. "A Critical Analysis of the Co-dependence Construct." *Psychiatry* 53 (November), 396-406.

Haley, J. 1976. *Problem-Solving Therapy: New Strategies for Effective Family Therapy.* New York: Jossey-Bass.

Hall, R., L. Tice, T. Beresford, B. Wooley, and A. Klassen Hall. 1989. "Sexual Abuse in Patients with Anorexia Nervosa and Bulimia." *Psychosomatics* 30/1 (Winter), 73-79.

Halmi, K., J. Falk, and E. Schwartz. 1980. "Binge-Eating and Vomiting: A Survey of a College Population." *Psychological Medicine* 11, 697-706.

Hambidge, D. 1988. "Incest and Anorexia Nerovsa: What Is the Link?" *British Journal of Psychiatry* 152, 145-46.

Hamilton, J. 1989. "Emotional Consequences of Victimization and Discrimination in 'Special Populations' of Women." *The Psychiatric Clinics of North America.* Vol. 12/1, 35-51.

Hamilton, L., J. Brooks-Gunn, M. Warren, and W. Hamilton. 1988. "The Role of Selectivity in the Pathogenesis of Eating Problems in Ballet Dancers." *Medicine and Science in Sports and Exercise* 20/6, 560-65.

Hamilton, L., J. Brooks-Gunn, M. Warren, and W. Hamilton. 1986. "The Impact of Thinness and Dieting on the Professional Ballet Dancer." *CAH-PER Journal* 53/4, 30-35.

Hare-Mustin, R. 1978. "A Feminist Approach to Family Therapy." *Family Process* 17, 181-94.

Hargreaves, J. 1984. "Women and the Olympic Phenomenon." In *Five Ring Circus,* ed. by A. Tomlinson and G. Whannel, 53-70. London: Pluto.

Harper, J. and C. Capdevila. 1990. "Codependency: A Critique." *Journal of Psychoactive Drugs* 22/3 (July-September), 285-91.

Harris, M., R. Harris, and S. Bochner. 1982. "Fat, Four-Eyed and Female." *Journal of Applied Social Psychology* 6, 503-26.

Health and Welfare Canada. 1988a. *Promoting Healthy Weights: A Discussion Paper.* Ottawa.

———. 1988b. *Canadian Guidelines for Healthy Weights.* Report of an expert group convened by the Health Promotion Directorate. Ottawa.

———. 1989. *Nutrition Recommendations.* Report of the Scientific Review Committee. Ottawa.

———. 1991. *Report of the Task Force on Treatment of Obesity.* Ottawa.

Heilbrun, C. 1988. *Writing a Woman's Life.* New York: Ballantine Books.

Heinmann, P. 1950. "On Countertransference." *International Journal of Psychoanalysis* 31, 81-84.

Herman, E. 1988. "The Twelve-Step Program: Cure or Cover?" *Utne Reader,* (Nov/Dec), 52-63.

Herman, J. 1992. *Trauma and Recovery.* Cambridge, MA: Harvard University Press.

Herzog, D. 1982a. "Bulimia in the Adolescent." *American Journal of Disorders in Children* 136, 985-89.

———. 1982b. "Bulimia: The Secretive Syndrome." *Psychosomatics* 23, 481-84.

Heyward, C. 1989. *Touching Our Strength: The Erotic as Power and the Love of God.* San Francisco: Harper and Row.

Hollander, A. 1980. *Seeing Through Clothes.* New York: The Viking Press.

hooks, b. 1981. *Ain't I a Woman: Black Women and Feminism.* Boston: South End Press.

———. 1984. *Feminist Theory: From Margin to Center.* Boston: South End Press.

————. 1992. *Black Looks: Race and Representation.* Toronto: Between The Lines.

Hsu, L. 1987. "Are the Eating Disorders Becoming More Common in Blacks?" *International Journal of Eating Disorders* 6/1, 113-24.

Hudson, J., P. Laffer, and H. Pope. 1982. "Bulimia Related to Affective Disorders by Family History and Response to Dexamethasone Suppression Test." *American Journal of Psychiatry* 139, 685-87.

Hudson, J., H. Pope, and J. Jonas. 1983. "Hypothalamic-Pituitary-Adrenal-Axis Hyperactivity in Bulimia." *Psychiatry Research* 8, 111-17.

Hunter, A. 1992. "Numbering the Hairs of Our Heads: Male Social Control and the All-Seeing Male God." *Journal of Feminist Studies in Religion* 8/2, 7-26.

Hutchinson, M. 1985. *Transforming Body Image: Learning to Love the Body You Have.* New York: Crossing Press.

Hyde, N. and C. Watson. 1990. "Voices from the Silence: Use of Imagery with Incest Survivors." In *Healing Voices: Feminist Approaches to Therapy with Women,* ed. by T. Laidlaw, C. Malmo, and Associates. San Francisco: Jossey-Bass.

Inches, P. 1985. "Anorexia Nervosa." *Maritime Medical News* (April) 7/4, 73-75.

Issajenko, A. 1990. *Running Risks.* Toronto: Macmillan.

Illich, I. 1981. "Medical Nemesis." In *The Sociology of Health and Illness: A Critical Perspective,* ed. by P. Conrad and R. Kern, 426-433. New York: St. Martin's Press.

Jack, D. 1991. *Silencing the Self.* Cambridge, MA.: Harvard University Press.

Jaffee, L., J. Lutter, and N. Straiton. 1990. "Larger Women in a Society Over-occupied with Thinness." *Melpomene Journal* 9/2, 18-25.

James, C. 1990. *Making It: Black Youth, Racism and Career Aspirations in a Big City.* Oakville, ON: Mosaic Press.

James, K. and D. McIntyre. 1983. "The Reproduction of Families: The Social Role of Family Therapy." *Journal of Marital and Family Therapy* 9, 119-29.

Jasper, K. and S. Maddocks. 1992. "Body Image Groups." In *Psychotherapy for Eating Disorders,* ed. by H. Harper-Giuffre and K. MacKenzie. Washington, DC: American Psychiatric Press.

Jordan, J., A. Kaplan, J. Miller, I. Stiver, and J. Surrey. 1991. *Women's Growth in Connection: Writings from the Stone Center.* New York: Guilford Press.

Jordon, J. 1980. *Passion: New Poems, 1978-1980*. Boston: Beacon Press.

Kano, S. 1985. *Making Peace with Food: A Step-by-Step Guide to Freedom from Diet/Weight Conflict*. New York: Harper and Row.

Kaplan, A. and D. Woodside. 1987. "Biologic Aspects of Anorexia Nervosa and Bulimia." *Journal of Clinical and Consulting Psychology* 55, 645-53.

Kasperowski, U. 1991. "The Body Speaks: Eating Disorders and Sexual Abuse." Thesis, Ontario Institute for Studies in Education, Toronto.

Kaufman, G. 1989. *The Psychology of Shame: Theory and Treatment of Shame-Based Syndromes*. New York: Springer.

Kearney-Cooke, A. 1988. "Group Therapy of Sexual Abuse Among Women with Eating Disorders." *Women and Therapy* 7/1, 5-21.

Keller, C. 1986. *From a Broken Web: Separation, Sexism, and Self*. Boston: Beacon Press.

Kelly. 1983. "Medical Crimes." In *Shadow on a Tightrope: Writings by Women on Fat Oppression*, ed. by L. Schoenfielder and B. Wieser, 185-186. San Francisco: Spinsters/Aunt Lute Press.

Keyes, A., J. Brozek, A. Henschel, O. Mickelson, and H. Taylor. 1950. *The Biology of Human Starvation*, Vol. 1. Minneapolis: University of Minnesota Press.

Kiceluk, S. 1991. "Made in His Image: Frankenstein's Daughters." In *The Female Body: Figures, Styles, Speculations*, ed. by L. Goldstein. Ann Arbor: University of Michigan Press.

Kissebah, A., D. Freedman, and A. Peris. 1989. "Health Risks of Obesity." *Medical Clinics of North America* 731/1, 111.

Klein, M. 1946. "Notes on Some Schizoid Mechanisms." *International Journal of Psychoanalysis* 31, 81-84.

Kloss, S. 1989. "A Coach's Guide to Eating Disorders." *NSCA Journal* 11/6, 68-72.

Kramer, F., R. Jeffery, J. Forster, and M. Snell. 1989. "Long-Term Follow-Up of Behavioral Treatment for Obesity: Patterns of Weight Regain among Women and Men." *International Journal of Obesity* 13, 123-26.

Krestan, J. 1991. "The Baby and the Bathwater." *Journal of Feminist Family Therapy* 3/ 1&2 (June), 216-32.

Krestan, J. and C. Bepko. 1990. "Codependency: The Social Reconstruction of Female Experience." *Smith College Studies in Social Work* 60/3 (June), 216-32.

Kristeva, J. 1980. *Desire in Language: A Semiotic Approach to Literature and Art*, ed. by Leon S. Roudiez. New York: Columbia University Press.

Kurtz, E. 1983. "Why AA Works: The Intellectual Significance of Alcoholics Anonymous, Part Two." *Digest of Alcoholism Theory and Application* 2/2 (January), 57-70.

Lackey, D. 1990. "Sexual Harassment in Sports." *Physical Educator* 47/2, 22-26.

Lagones, M. 1990. "Playfulness, World-Travelling and Loving Perception." In *Making Face, Making Soul — Haciendo Cara: Creative and Critical Perspectives by Women of Colour*, ed. by E. Anzaldua. San Francisco: Aunt Lute Books.

Laidlaw, T., C. Malmo, and Associates. 1990. *Healing Voices: Feminist Approaches to Therapy with Women*. San Francisco: Jossey-Bass.

Lawrence, M. 1979. "Anorexia Nervosa: The Control Paradox." *Women's Studies International* 2, 93-101.

———. 1984. *The Anorexic Experience*. London: The Women's Press.

Lawrence, M. and M. Dana. 1990. *Fighting Food. Coping with Eating Disorders*. London: Penguin Books.

Lawrence, M. and C. Lowenstein. 1979. "Self Starvation." *Spare-rib* 83 (June), 41-43.

Lenskyj, H. 1986. *Out of Bounds: Women, Sport and Sexuality*. Toronto: Women's Press.

———. 1993 (forthcoming). "Playing a Different Game: Sex-Related Trends in Sport Socialization." In *Psychology and Sociology of Sport: Current Selected Research III*, ed. by L. Vander Velden. New York: AMS Press.

Leon, G. 1984. "Anorexia Nervosa and Sport Activities." *Behavior Therapist* 7, 9-10.

Leon, G., K. Carroll, B. Chernyk, and S. Finn. 1985. "Binge Eating and Associated Patterns within College Student and Identified Bulimic Populations." *International Journal of Eating Disorders* 4/1, 43-57.

Lerman, H. and N. Porter, eds. 1990. *Feminist Ethics in Psychotherapy*. New York: Springer.

Lerner, H. 1988. "Is Family Systems Theory Really Systemic? A Feminist Communication." In *A Guide to Feminist Family Therapy*, ed. by L. Braverman. New York: Haworth Press.

———. 1989. *Women in Therapy*. New York: Harper and Row.

———. 1991. "12 Stepping It: Women's Roads to Recovery. A Psychologist Tells WHY." *Lilith*, Spring, 15-16.

Levenkron, S. 1982. *Treating and Overcoming Anorexia Nervosa*. New York: Warner Books.

Levine, H. 1981. "Feminist Counselling: Approach or Technique?" In *Perspectives of Women in the 80s*. ed. by J. Turner and L. Emery, 74-87. Winnipeg: University of Manitoba Press.

Levine, H. 1982. "The Personal Is Political: Feminism and the Helping Professions." In *Feminism in Canada: From Pressure to Politics*, ed. by A. Miles and G. Finn. Montreal: Black Rose Books.

Libow, J., P. Raskin, and B. Caust. 1982. "Feminist and Family Systems Therapy: Are They Irreconcilable?" *Journal of Family Therapy* 10, 3-12.

Lissner, L. and K. Brownell. 1992. "Weight Cycling, Mortality, and Cardiovascular Disease: A Review of Epidemiologic Findings." In *Obesity*, ed. by P. Bjorntorp and B. Brodoff, 653-61. New York: Lippincott.

Little, M. 1951. "Countertransference and the Patient's Response to It." *International Journal of Psychoanalysis* 33, 32-40.

Lorde, A. 1984. *Sister Outsider*. Freedom, CA: Crossing Press.

Lucie-Smith, E. 1981. *Images of the Nude*. London: Thames and Hudson.

Lupis, E. 1989. "Male Violence in the Home." In *Canadian Social Trends*.

Lurie, A. 1981. *The Language of Clothes*. New York: Vintage Books.

Lyons, P. 1989. "Fitness, Feminism and the Health of Fat Women." *Women and Health* 8/3, 65-77.

McCann, L. and D. Holmes. 1984. "Influence of Aerobic Exercise on Depression." *Journal of Personality and Social Psychology* 46/5, 1142-47.

Madanes, C. 1981. *Strategic Family Therapy*. San Francisco: Jossey-Bass.

Mallick, M., T. Whipple, and E. Huerta. 1987. "Behavioral and Psychological Traits of Weight-Conscious Teenagers." *Adolesence* 22/85, 157-66.

Maltz, W. 1991. *The Sexual Healing Journey: A Guide for Survivors of Sexual Abuse*. New York: HarperCollins.

Mayer, V. 1983a. "The Fat Illusion." In *Shadow on a Tightrope: Writings by Women on Fat Oppression*, ed. by L. Schoenfielder and B. Wieser, 3-14. San Francisco: Spinsters/Aunt Lute Press.

———. 1983b. "The Questions People Ask." In *Shadow on a Tightrope: Writings by Women on Fat Oppression*, ed. by L. Schoenfielder and B.

Wieser, 23-36. San Francisco: Spinsters/Aunt Lute Press.

Meador, B. 1990. "Thesmorphia: A Woman's Fertility Ritual." In *To Be a Woman*, ed. by C. Zweig. New York: St. Martin's Press.

Millar, W. 1991. "A Trend to a Healthier Lifestyle." *Health Reports* 3/4, 363-70.

Miller, D. 1987. *Children of Alcoholics: A Twenty-Year Longitudinal Study.* San Francisco: Institute for Scientific Analysis.

Miller, K. 1990. "Childhood Sexual Abuse as a Factor in Eating Disorders in Women: Prevalence and Symptom Severity." Paper presented at the 4th International Eating Disorders Conference, New York.

Millman, M. 1980. *Such a Pretty Face: Being Fat in America.* New York: W.W. Norton.

Minister, K. 1991. "A Feminist Frame for the Oral History Interview." In *Women's Words: A Feminist Practice of Oral History*, ed. by S. Gluck and D. Patai. New York: Routledge.

Minuchin, S. 1974. *Families and Family Therapy.* San Francisco: Jossey-Bass.

Minuchin, S., B. Rosman, and L. Baker. 1978. *Psychosomatic Families: Anorexia Nervosa in Context.* Cambridge, MA: Harvard University Press.

Morega, C. 1983. *Loving in the War Years.* Boston: South End Press.

Morgan, E. 1985. *Descent of Woman.* London: Souvenir Press.

Moriarty, D. and M. Moriarty. 1986. "Sport/Fitness Programs and Sociocultural Influences in Eating Disorders." *CAHPER Journal* 53/4, 4-9.

Morrison, T. 1992. *Jazz.* Toronto: Alfred A. Knopf Canada.

Mueller, W., R. Shoup, and R. Malina. 1982. "Fat Patterns in Athletes in Relation to Ethnic Origin and Sport." *Annals of Human Biology* 9/4, 371-76.

National Institutes of Health. 1991. "Gastrointestinal Surgery for Severe Obesity." *National Institutes of Health Consensus Development Statement,* (March), 25-27.

Ngcobo, L., ed. 1987. *Let It Be Told: Essays by Black Women in Britain.* London: Virago.

Nopper, S., and J. Harley. 1986. "How Society's Obsession with Thinness Is Consuming Women." *Herizons* 4/7, 25-29.

Norwood, R. 1985. *Women Who Love Too Much.* New York: Pocket Books.

O'Neill, J. 1985. *Five Bodies: The Human Shape of Modern Society.* Ithaca, NY: Cornell University Press.

Oppenheimer, R., K. Howells, R. Palmer, and D. Chaloner. 1985. "Adverse Sexual Experiences in Childhood and Clinical Eating Disorders: A Preliminary Description." *Journal of Psychiatric Research* 19/ 2&3, 357-61.

Orbach, S. 1978. *Fat Is a Feminist Issue.* New York: Paddington Books.

———. 1982. *Fat is a Feminist Issue II.* New York: Berkeley Books.

———. 1985. "Accepting the Symptoms: A Feminist Psychoanalytic Treatment of Anorexia Nervosa." In *Handbook of Psychotherapy for Anorexia Nervosa and Bulimia*, ed. by D. Garner and P. Garfinkel. New York: Guilford Press.

———. 1986. *Hunger Strike: The Anorectic Struggle as a Metaphor for Our Age.* New York: W.W. Norton

———. 1992. Cited in *Caversham Newsletter* 5, 1-2.

Paglia, C. 1991. *Sexual Personae: Art and Decadence from Nefertiti to Emily Dickinson.* New York: Vintage.

Palmer, R. 1980. *Anorexia Nervosa.* Markham, ON: Penguin Books.

Palmer, R., R. Oppenheimer, A. Dignon, A. Chaloner, and K. Howells. 1990. "Childhood Sexual Experiences with Adults Reported by Women with Eating Disorders: An Extended Series." *British Journal of Psychiatry* 156, 699-703.

Parades, M. 1992. *Report for Education on Sexual Assault.* Toronto.

Penfold, P. and G.Walker. 1983. *Women and the Psychiatric Paradox.* Montreal: Eden Press.

Picker, R. 1978. "On the Path: A Moving Experience." In The *Holistic Health Handbook*, ed. by E. Bauman, A. Brent, L. Piper, and P. Wright. Berkeley, CA: And/Or Press.

Philip, M. 1989. *She Tries Her Tongue: her silence softly breaks.* Charlottetown, PEI: Ragweed Press.

Plummer, K. 1975. *Sexual Stigma: An Interactionist Account.* London: Routledge and Kegan Paul.

Polhemus, T., ed. 1978. *Social Aspects of the Human Body.* New York: W.W. Norton.

Prior, J. and Y. Vigna. 1987. "Conditioning Exercise and Premenstrual Symptoms." *Journal of Reproductive Medicine* 32/6, 423-28.

Probyn, E. 1987. "The Anorexic Body." *Canadian Journal of Political and Social Theory* 1-2, 111-19.

Pyle, R., J. Mitchell, and E. Eckert. 1981. "Bulimia: A Report of 34 Cases." *Journal of Clinical Psychiatry* 42, 60-64.

Racker, H. 1957. "The Meanings and Uses of Countertransference." *Psychoanalytic Quarterly* 26, 303-57.

———. 1968. *Transference and Countertransference.* New York: International Universities Press.

Rand, C., and J. Kuldau. 1992. "Epidemiology of Bulimia and Symptoms in a General Population: Sex, Age, Race and Socioeconomic Status." *International Journal of Eating Disorders* 11/1, 37-44.

Rice, C. 1988. "Society's Obsession with Thinness." *National Eating Disorders Information Centre Bulletin.* (February), 1-3.

Roberto, L. 1987. "Bulimia: Transgenerational Family Therapy." *The Family Therapy Collections* 20, 1-11.

———. 1991. "Impasses in the Family Treatment of Bulimia." In *Family Approaches in Treatment of Eating Disorders,* ed. by D. Woodside and L. Shekter-Wolfson. Washington, DC: American Psychiatric Press.

Robbins, J., and R. Siegel. 1985. *Women Changing Therapy. New Assessments, Values and Strategies in Feminist Therapy.* New York: Harrington Park Press.

Robinson, B. 1985. "The Stigma of Obesity: Fat Fallacies Debunked." *Melpomene Report* 4/1, 9-11, 13.

Romeo, F. 1984. "The Physical Educator and Anorexia Nervosa." *The Physical Educator* 41/1, 2-5.

Root, M. 1989. "Treatment Failures: The Role of Sexual Victimization in Women's Addictive Behaviour." *American Journal of Orthopsychiatry* 59/4 (October), 542-49.

Root, M., and P. Fallon. 1988. "The Incidence of Victimization Experiences in a Bulimic Sample." *Journal of Interpersonal Violence* 3/2 (June), 161-73.

———. 1989. "Treating the Victimized Bulimic: The Functions of Binge-Purge." *Journal of Interpersonal Violence* 4/1 (March), 90-100.

Root, M., P. Fallon, and W. Friedrick. 1986. *Bulimia: A Systems Approach to Treatment.* New York: W.W. Norton.

Rosen, L., C. Shafer, G. Dummer, Cross, G. Deuman, and S. Malmberg. 1988. "Prevalence of Pathogenic Weight-Control Behaviours among Native American Women and Girls." *International Journal of Eating Disorders* 7/6, 807-811.

Rosen, L. and D. Hough. 1988. "Pathogenic Weight-Control Behaviors of

Female College Gymnasts." *Physician and Sportsmedicine* 16/9, 140-46.

Rosenhan, D. 1973. "On Being Sane in Insane Places." *Science*, 179 (January), 250-258.

Roth, G. 1989. *Why Weight? A Guide to Ending Compulsive Eating.* New York: Plum.

Rule, S. 1992. "Director Defies Odds with First Feature, 'Daughters of the Dust.' "*The New York Times,* February 12, C15.

Runtz, M., and J. Briere. 1986. "Adolescent 'Acting-Out' and Childhood History of Sexual Abuse." *Journal of Interpersonal Violence* 1/3 (September), 326-34.

Russell, D. 1982. *Rape in Marriage.* New York: Collier-MacMillan.

———. 1984. *Sexual Exploitaion: Rape, Child Sexual Abuse and Workplace Harrassment.* Newbury Park, CA: Sage.

Ryan, W. 1971. *Blaming the Victim.* New York: Vintage Books.

Sanchez, R. 1988. "Cornrows Win Brush with Controversy." *The Washington Post,* May 9, D4.

Sady, S. and P. Freedman. 1984. "Body Composition and Structural Comparisons of Female and Male Athletes." *Clinics in Sports Medicine* 3/4, 140-46.

Saiving, V. 1979. "The Human Situation: A Feminine View." In *Womanspirit Rising: A Feminist Reader in Religion,* ed. by C. Christ and J. Plaskow. San Francisco: Harper and Row.

Sandler, J. 1976. "Countertransference and Role Responsiveness." *International Review of Psychoanalysis* 3, 43-47.

Sargent, J., R. Liebman, and M. Silver. 1985. "Family Therapy for Anorexia Nervosa." In *Handbook of Psychotherapy for Anorexia Nervosa and Bulimia,* ed. by D. Garner and P. Garfinkel. New York: Guilford Press.

Schaef, A. 1986. *Co-Dependence: Misunderstood-Mistreated.* San Francisco: Harper and Row.

Scheff, T. 1968. "The Societal Reaction to Deviance: Ascriptive Elements in the Psychiatric Screening of Mental Patients in a Midwestern State." In *The Mental Patient: Studies in the Sociology of Deviance,* ed. by S. Spitzer and N. Denzin, 276-293. New York: McGraw-Hill.

Schechter, J., M. Schwartz, and D. Greenfeld. 1987. "Sexual Assault and Anorexia Nervosa." *International Journal of Eating Disorders* 6/2, 313-16.

Schwartz, D., M. Thompson, and C. Johnson. 1985. "Anorexia Nervosa and Bulimia: The Socio-Cultural Context." *International Journal of Eating Disorders* 1/3, 20-36.

Schwartz, R. and M. Barrett. 1988. "Women and Eating Disorders." In *A Guide to Feminist Family Therapy*, ed. by L. Braverman. New York: Haworth Press.

Schwartz, R., M. Barrett, and G. Saba. 1985. "Family Therapy for Bulimia. "In *Handbook of Psychotherapy for Anorexia Nervosa and Bulimia*, ed. by M. Garner and E. Garfinkel. New York: Guilford Press.

Segal, H. 1975. "Countertransference." Paper presented at Symposium on Countertransference, London, England.

Seid, R.P. 1989. *Never Too Thin: Why Women Are at War with Their Bodies*. Scarborough, ON: Prentice-Hall.

Selvini Palazzoli, M. 1974. *Self-Starvation: From Individual to Family Therapy in the Treatment of Anorexia Nervosa*. New York: Jason Aronson.

Selvini Palazzoli, M., L. Boscolo, G. Cecchin, and G. Prata. 1978. *Paradox and Counterparadox*. New York: Jason Aronson.

Sheinin, R. 1990. "Body Shame." *National Eating Disorder Information Centre Bulletin* 5/5, 1.

Sheppard, K. 1989. *Food Addiction: The Body Knows*. Deerfield, FL: Health Communications Inc.

Showalter, E. 1985. *The Female Malady: Women, Madness and English Culture, 1830-1980*. London: Virago.

Siegel, A., E. Stewart, and B. Barone. 1990. "Body Image Assessment and Eating Attitudes in Marathon Runners." *Annals of Sports Medicine* 5, 67-70.

Silvera, M. 1988. *Silenced*. Toronto: Sister Vision Press.

Sloan, G. and P. Leichner. 1986. "Is There a Relationship between Sexual Abuse or Incest and Eating Disorders?" *Canadian Journal of Psychiatry* 31/7 (October), 656-60.

Smith, D. and S. David, eds. 1975. *I'm Not Mad, I'm Angry*. Vancouver: Press Gang.

Smith, N. 1980. "Excessive Weight Loss and Food Aversion in Athletes Simulating Anorexia Nervosa." *Pediatrics* 66/1, 139-42.

Smolak, L., M. Levine, and E. Sullins. 1990. "Are Child Sexual Experiences Related to Eating-Disordered Attitudes and Behaviours in a College Sample?" *International Journal of Eating Disorders* 9/2, 167-78.

Sobal, J. and A. Stunkard. 1989. "Socioeconomic Status and Obesity." *Psychological Bulletin* 2, 260-75.

Spender, D. 1982. *Invisible Women: The Schooling Scandal.* London: Writers and Readers Publishing Cooperative.

———. 1985. *Man Made Language,* 2nd ed. London: Routledge and Kegan Paul.

———. 1990. *Woman of Ideas.* London: Pandora Press.

Squire, S. 1984. *The Slender Balance.* New York: Pinnacle Books.

Staffieri, J. 1967. "A Study of Social Stereotype of Body Image in Children." *Journal of Personality and Social Psychology* 1, 101-4.

Steiner-Adair, C. 1986. "The Body Politic: Normal Female Adolescent Development and the Development of Eating Disorders." *Journal of the American Academy of Psychoanalysis* 14, 95-114.

———. 1989. "Developing One Voice of One Wise Woman: College Students and Bulimia." In *The Bulimic College Student. Evaluation Treatment and Prevention,* ed. by L. Whitaker and W. Davis. New York: The Haworth Press.

———. 1989. "The Politics of Prevention: Weight Preoccupation, Weight Prejudice and Eating Disorders." Paper presented at the public forum during the Nurturing the Hungry Self Conference, Toronto, October.

———. 1990. Paper presented on a panel called "The Psychology of Women and the Treatment of Eating Disorders." At the International Conference on Eating Disorders, New York.

Stephenson, J. 1991. "Medical Consequences and Complications of Anorexia Nervosa and Bulimia Nervosa in Female Athletes." *Athletic Training* 26/2, 130-35.

Sternhell, C. 1985. "We'll Always Be Fat But Fat Can Be Fit." *Ms.,* (May), 66, 68, 142-44, 146, 154.

Striegel-Moore, R., L. Silberstein, and J. Rodin. 1986. "Toward an Understanding of Risk Factors for Bulimia." *American Psychologist* 41/3, 246-63.

Strupp, H. and J. Binder. 1984. *Psychotherapy in a New Key: A Guide to Time-Limited Dynamic Psychotherapy.* New York: Basic Books.

Stunkard, A., M. Coll, L. Lindquist, and A. Meyers. 1980. "Obesity and Eating Style." *Archives of General Psychiatry* 37, 1127-29.

Stunkard, A., T. Sorenson, C. Hanis, T. Teasdale, R. Chakraborty, W. Schull, and F. Schulsinger. 1986. "An Adoption Study of Human Obesity." *New England Journal of Medicine* 314, 193-98.

Stunkard, A., T. Foch, and Z. Hrubec. 1986. "A Twin Study of Human Obesity." *Journal of the American Medical Association* 256, 51-54.

Surrey, J. 1991. "Eating Patterns as a Reflection of Women's Development." In *Women's Growth in Connection: Writings from the Stone Center*. New York: Guilford Press.

Surrey, J. and J. Kilbourne. 1986-91. "Women, Addiction, and Co-dependecy." *Work in Progress*, Tape A1. Wellesley: The Stone Center for Developmental Services and Studies.

Szasz, T. 1968. "The Myth of Mental Illness." In *The Mental Patient: Studies in the Sociology of Deviance*, ed. by S. Spitzer and N. Denzin, 22-30. New York: McGraw-Hill.

———. 1970. *Ideology and Insanity. Essays on the Psychiatric Dehumanization of Man*. New York: Doubleday.

———. 1971. *The Manufacture of Madness: A Comparative Study of the Inquisition and the Mental Health Movement*. New York: Dell Books.

———. 1974. *The Myth of Mental Illness: Foundations of a Theory of Personal Conduct*. New York: Harper and Row.

Székely , É 1987. "Society, Ideology, and the Relentless Pursuit of Thinness." *Practice* 3, 34-49.

———. 1988a. *Never Too Thin*. Toronto: Women's Press.

———. 1988b. "Reflections on the Body in the 'Anorexia' Discourse." *Resources for Feminist Research/Documentation sur la recherche feministe* 4, 8-11.

———1989. "From Eating Disorders to Women's Situations." *Counselling Psychology Quarterly* 2, 167-84.

Taggart, M. 1985. "The Feminist Critique in Epistemological Perspective: Questions of Context in Family Therapy." *Journal of Marital and Family Therapy* 11, 113-26.

Tallen, B. 1990. "Twelve Step Programs: A Lesbian Feminist Critique." *NWSA Journal* 2/3 (Summer), 390-407.

Tannen, D. 1990. *You Just Don't Understand: Women and Men in Conversation*. New York: Ballantyne Books.

Tenzer, S. 1989. "Fat Acceptance Therapy." In *Overcoming Fear of Fat*, ed. by L. Brown and E. Rothblum, 39-48. New York: Harrington Park.

"The 10 Percent Dilemma." 1987. *Women's Sports and Fitness* 9/12, 72.

Teskey, S. 1986. "Hooked on Perfection." *Verve*, (Aug./Sept.), 40-46.

Theroux, P. 1982. "The Size 7 Soul." *American Health*, (May), 46.

Thompson, R. 1987. "Management of the Athlete with an Eating Disorder." *The Sport Psychologist* 1, 114-26.

Tomkins, S. 1987. "Shame." In *The Many Faces of Shame*, ed. by Donald Nathanson. New York: Guilford Press.

Tomm, K. 1984a. "One Perspective on the Milan Systemic Approach. Part I: Overview of Development, Theory and Practice." *Journal of Marital and Family Therapy* 10, 113-26.

———. 1984b. "One Perspective on the Milan Systemic Approach. Part II: Description of Session Format, Interviewing Style and Intervention." *Journal of Marital and Family Therapy* 10, 253-72.

Tower, L. 1956. "Countertransference." *Journal of the American Psychoanalytic Association* 4, 224-25.

Vancouver Women's Research Collective. 1989. *Recollecting Our Lives: Women's Experiences of Childhood Sexual Abuses.*

Van Den Bergh, N., ed. 1991. *Feminist Perspectives on Addictions.* New York: Springer.

Vandereycken, W., E. Kog, and J. Vanderlinder. 1989. *The Family Approach to Eating Disorders.* New York: PMA Publishing Corp.

Waller, G. 1991. "Sexual Abuse as a Factor in Eating Disorders." *British Journal of Psychiatry* 159, 664-71.

The Washington Post. 1988. "Md. ACLU to Assist in Cornrow Case." April 19, D7.

Wegscheider, S. 1981a. *Another Chance: Hope and Healing for the Alcoholic Family.* Palo Alto, CA: Science and Behavior Books.

———. 1981b. "From the Family Trap to Family Freedom." *Alcoholism*, Jan.-Feb., 36-39.

———. 1985. *Choice-Making: For Codependents, Adult Children and Spirituality Seekers.* Deerfield Beach, FL: Health Communications.

Weight, L. and T. Noakes. 1987. "Is Running an Analog of Anorexia?" *Medicine and Science in Sports and Exercise* 19/3, 213-17.

Westerlund, E. 1992. *Women's Sexuality after Childhood Incest.* New York: W.W. Norton.

Wheeler, L. 1988. "Hotel Worker Fights to Keep Cornrows." *The Washington Post,* January 5, D3.

White, E. 1991. "Unhealthy Appetites." *Essence,* 22/5 (September), 28-30.

White, M. 1983. "Anorexia Nervosa: A Transgenerational System Perspective." *Family Process* 22, 255-73.

———. 1987. "Anorexia Nervosa: A Cybernetic Perspective." In *The Family Therapy Collection,* ed. by J.C. Hansen and J.E. Harkaway. Rockwell: Aspen Publishing Inc.

Whitfield, C. 1984. "Co-alcoholism: Recognizing a Treatable Illness." *Family and Community Health* 7, 16-25.

———. 1987. *Healing the Child Within.* Pompano Beach, FL: Health Communications Inc.

———. 1989. "Co-dependence: Our Most Common Addiction — Some Physical, Mental, Emotions, and Spiritual Perspectives." *Alcoholism Treatment Quarterly* 6/1, 19-36.

Wilson, E. 1985. *Adorned in Dreams: Fashion and Modernity.* London: Virage.

Wilson, C. and J. Orford. 1978. "Children of Alcoholics: Report of the Preliminary Study and Comments on the Literature." *Journal of Studies on Alcohol* 39, 121-42.

Woititz, J. 1983. *Adult Children of Alcoholics.* Hollywood, CA: Health Communications Inc.

Wolf, N. 1990. *The Beauty Myth.* Toronto: Vintage Books.

Wolfe, L. 1983. "Weight Loss Surgery." In *Shadow on a Tightrope: Writings by Women on Fat Oppression,* ed. by L. Schoenfielder and B. Wieser, 162-166. San Francisco: Spinsters/Aunt Lute Press.

Woodman, M. 1985. *The Pregnant Virgin.* Toronto: Inner City Books.

Woodside, D. and L. Shekter-Wolfson. 1991. *Family Approaches in Treatment of Eating Disorders.* Washington, DC: American Psychiatric Press.

Wooley, S. 1987. "A Woman's Body in a Man's World." *Shape,* (October) 7/2, 70-71.

Wooley, S. and A. Kearney-Cooke. 1986. "Intensive Treatment of Bulimia and Body Image Disturbance." In *Handbook of Eating Disorders: Physiology, Psychology and Treatment of Obesity, Anorexia and Bulimia,* ed. by K. Brownell and J. Foreyt. New York: Basic Books.

Wooley, S. and O. Wooley. 1980. "Eating Disorders: Obesity and Anorexia. In

Women and Psychotherapy: An Assessment of Research and Practice, ed. by A. Brodsky and R. Hare-Mustin, 135-158. New York: Guilford Press.

Wooley, S., and O. Wooley. 1979. "Obesity and Women: A Closer Look at the Facts." *Women's Studies International Quarterly* 2, 69-79.

———. 1984. "Should Obesity Be Treated at All?" In *Eating and Its Disorders*, ed. by A. Stunkard and E. Stellar. New York: Raven Press.

———. 1985. "Women and Weight: Obsession Toward a Redefinition of the Underlying Problem." In *For Alma Mater*, ed. by T. Reichler, C. Kramerae and B. Stafford, 350-372. Chicago: University of Illinois Press.

———.1986. "Editorial: The Beverly Hills Eating Disorder: The Mass Marketing of Anorexia Nervosa." *International Journal of Eating Disorders* 1/3, 57-69.

Wooley, S., O. Wooley, and S. Dyrenforth. 1979. "Theoretical, Practical, and Social Issues in Behavioral Treatments of Obesity." *Journal of Applied Behavioral Analysis* Vol. 12, 3-15.

Worchester, N. and M. Whatley. 1985. *Women's Health: Readings on Social, Economic and Political Issues.* Dubuque, IA: Kendall House.

Yates, A., K. Leehey, and C. Shisslak. 1983. "Running: An Analogue of Anorexia Nervosa?" *New England Journal of Medicine* 308 (Feb. 3), 251-55.

Young-Eisendrath, P. and F. Wiedemann. 1987. *Female Authority.* New York: Guilford Press.

Zellner, D., D. Harner, and R. Adler. 1989. "Effects of Eating Abnormalities and Gender on Perceptions of Desirable Body Shape." *Journal of Abnormal Psychology* Vol. 98/1, 93-96.

Zillman, D. and J. Bryant. 1982. "Effects of Exposure to Pornography" In *Pornography and Sexual Aggression.* ed by N. Malamuth and E. Donnerstein. New York: Academic Press.

Zola, K. 1981. "Medicine as an Institution of Social Control." In *The Sociology of Health and Illness. A Critical Perspective*, ed. by P. Conrad and B. Kern, 511-526. New York: St. Martin's Press.

◆

NOTES ON CONTRIBUTORS

MAXENE ADLER is a writer residing in Winnipeg. She holds a M.S.W. from the University of Toronto with a specialty in clinical social work. Most of Maxene's career has focused on creating policy changes in health care for women. She has devoted a great deal of time to the creation and support of grassroots women's organization and maintains a special interest in the area of family violence.

MERRYL BEAR, M. Ed. (Psych), is the current program coordinator for NEDIC (National Eating Disorder Information Centre). She has a background in psychology and education, having taught and counseled at both secondary and tertiary levels. She has worked as a school psychologist in primary and secondary schools. Merryl worked as a rape crisis counselor, educator, and consultant for several years.

SUZANNE BELL has devoted over a decade of her life to fighting "fat phobia," as a pioneer in the development of fitness programs for large women, as an innovator in creating and marketing large and supersize fashions in exciting syles and fabrics, and as an outspoken champion of many "fat issues." From her base in Vancouver, B.C., she acts as an unofficial spokesperson for the empowerment of fat women in their uphill battle against the prejudice, abuse, and neglect of our thin-fixated society. Suzanne has spoken to hundreds of groups on issues of self-esteem and fat acceptance, participated in documentary film projects, and appeared on dozens of local and national radio and television shows in her determination to spread her message.

Catrina Brown, M.A., M.S.W., is a feminist psychotherapist and community educator in private practice in Toronto. She is the founder of the "Getting Beyond Weight" program at the Women's Health Clinic in Winnipeg and author of *Getting Beyond Weight: Women Helping Women*. She is currently completing her doctoral studies in social work at the University of Toronto, researching the relationship between eating disorders and sexual violence.

Kim Shayo Buchanan did her undergraduate degree in sociology at Queen's University, focusing primarily on race, gender, and representation. She is now studying law at the University of Toronto, where she is continuing her work in Black and anti-racist advocacy; she is also involved in legal aid clinic work.

Donna Ciliska, R.N., Ph.D. is an associate professor of Health Sciences at McMaster University, a clinical nurse consultant at the Hamilton-Wentworth Region Department of Public Health Services, a research associate at Toronto General Division of The Toronto Hospital, and a career scientist supported by the Ontario Ministry of Health. She is author of *Beyond Dieting*, which details a psychoeducational intervention and its evaluation for large women, aimed at improving their self-esteem, "normalizing" eating patterns, and stopping dieting.

Connie Coniglio is a counselor/therapist with the Counseling and Career Development Services at the University of Western Ontario. Connie has extensive experience working both with individuals and in groups with women from "unhealthy homes": adult children of alcoholics and survivors of sexual, emotional and physical abuse. Connie is currently completing her doctorate in Education, Applied Psychology, and Counseling at the Ontario Institute for Studies in Education. Connie's dissertation project, entitled "Making Connections," is an exploration of the connections between experiences of childhood trauma and the development of eating problems among adult women.

PATRICIA DEFAZIO received her B.A. in psychology from McMaster University. She is currently working part-time as a counselor in residential treatment centres.

ELLEN DRISCOLL is a psychotherapist specializing in women's issues, particularly substance abuse, body-image and eating-disordered patterns, and spirituality. She is a Ph.D. candidate at the University of Ottawa where she is pursuing research in the psychology of women and feminist studies in religion. She teaches courses on these topics at the University of Prince Edward Island.

SANDY FRIEDMAN, B.S.W., M.A., is a counselor, educator, and program developer who has worked with women with eating disorders and weight preoccupation since 1980. She is currently the Eating Disorder Consultant for Boundary Health Unit where she is working with public health nurses in Surrey, Delta, and White Rock, B.C., to develop prevention programs for preadolescent and adolescent girls. She is also in private practice in Vancouver.

ALISA GAYLE is currently assistant program coordinator of the National Eating Disorder Information Centre. She has a wide experience in working with food, weight, and shape preoccupation and runs a support group for women. Alisa is also engaged in social activism against oppression.

KARIN JASPER, Ph.D., M.Ed., is in private practice at the College Street Women's Centre for Health Education and Counselling, specializing in the area of weight preoccupation and eating disorders. A co-founder of the activist group Hersize, Karin is also author of a children's book *Are You Too Fat, Ginny?* (Is Five Press 1988). She is assistant professor in the Department of Psychiatry at the University of Toronto, where she teaches feminist principles in psychotherapy.

JAN LACKSTROM, a social worker, is the coordinator of Family Therapy in the Eating Disorder Day Hospital at The Toronto Hospital. Jan is also an adjunct field practice professor at the University of Toronto, Faculty of Social Work, and a sessional instructor at the School of Social Work, York University. She is a co-author of a book on marriage and eating disorders.

HELEN JEFFERSON LENSKYJ teaches feminist studies at the Ontario Institute for Studies in Education (OISE). She has published two books: *Out of Bounds: Women, Sport and Sexuality* (Women's Press, 1986) and *Women, Sport and Physical Activity: Research and Bibliography* (Fitness and Amateur Sport, 1991).

PATTI MCGILLICUDDY works as a counselor, teacher, and anti-oppression activist in the Toronto area.

BETH MACINNIS describes herself as a fat, radical feminist who has recently come to realize that taking up space in a slender society is a daily act of resistance. She works as a women's advocate in a shelter for abused women, and is completing her doctorate at OISE.

SASHA MAZE works as a performing artist and anti-oppression activist in the Toronto area.

NIVA PIRAN, Ph.D., C.Psych., is assistant professor in the Department of Applied Psychology at OISE. She is author of many articles on group approaches to eating disorders.

FARAH M. SHROFF is a community health worker with experience in many parts of the world. She teaches at Ryerson Polytechnic University in the first university program in midwifery in Canada. Her current research focuses on holistic medicine, health promotion, and health policy. For the last fifteen years, she has been active in community-based movements for social justice.

ANDRIA SIEGLER, B.SC.S.W., C.S.W., is a social worker in private practice in Toronto. She specializes in the area of food, weight, and shape preoccupation issues. She counsels women in individual therapy and in the "Beyond Dieting" program to give up weight cycling, improve self-esteem and body-image, and "normalize" eating. She also works in the area of childbearing issues such as postpartum adjustment, infertility, and reproductive loss.

Éva A. Székely is a psychologist at Centenary Health Centre and associate member of the Graduate Faculty at OISE (University of Toronto). She is author of a *Never Too Thin* (Women's Press 1988) and of several articles on the relentless pursuit of thinness among women.

ROBYN ZIMBERG, B.A. Honors, B.S.W., is a feminist social worker who is committed to working in the area of women and weight preoccupation. For the past seven years, Robyn's work has included individual and group counseling, facilitating workshops, and community education. She is currently the coordinator of the Volunteer Speaker's Program at the Women's Health Clinic in Winnipeg, Manitoba, and is a member of the Eating Disorders-Weight Preoccupation Network of Manitoba.

◆